Disability

Also Available from Lyceum Books, Inc.

Advisory Editor: Thomas M. Meenaghan, *New York University*

EMPOWERING VULNERABLE POPULATIONS
Mary Keegan Eamon

CASE MANAGEMENT: AN INTRODUCTION TO CONCEPTS AND SKILLS,
2ND EDITION
Arthur J. Frankel and Sheldon R. Gelman

STRAIGHT TALK ABOUT PROFESSIONAL ETHICS
Kim Strom-Gottfried

ENDINGS IN CLINICAL PRACTICE: EFFECTIVE CLOSURE IN DIVERSE SETTINGS
Joseph Walsh

SHORT-TERM EXISTENTIAL INTERVENTION IN CLINICAL PRACTICE
Joseph Walsh and Jim Lantz

SOCIAL WORK EVALUATION: ENHANCING WHAT WE DO
James R. Dudley

ESSENTIAL SKILLS OF SOCIAL WORK PRACTICE: ASSESSMENT, INTERVENTION,
EVALUATION
Thomas O'Hare

CONTEMPORARY PSYCHODYNAMIC THEORY AND PRACTICE
William Borden

DIVERSITY, OPPRESSION, AND CHANGE
Flavio Francisco Marsiglia and Stephen Kulis

CRITICAL MULTICULTURAL SOCIAL WORK
Jose Sisneros, Catherine Stakeman, Mildred C. Joyner, and Cathryne L. Schmitz

Disability

A Diversity Model Approach in Human Service Practice

SECOND EDITION

Romel W. Mackelprang
Eastern Washington University

and

Richard O. Salsgiver
California State University, Fresno

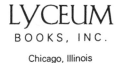

LYCEUM
BOOKS, INC.

Chicago, Illinois

Published by LYCEUM BOOKS, INC.
5758 S. Blackstone Ave.
Chicago, Illinois 60637
773 + 643-1903 (Fax)
773 + 643-1902 (Phone)
lyceum@lyceumbooks.com
http://www.lyceumbooks.com

6 5 4 3 2 1   09 10 11 12

ISBN 978-1-933478-59-3

Library of Congress Cataloging-in-Publication Data

Mackelprang, Romel W., 1955–
    Disability : a diversity model approach in human service practice / Romel W. Mackelprang
and Richard Salsgiver.—2nd ed.
        p.   cm.
    ISBN 978-1-933478-59-3
    1. People with disabilities—Care—United States.   2. People with disabilities—Services
for—United States.   I. Salsgiver, Richard O., 1946–   II. Title.
HV1553.M33   2009
362.4'0480973—dc22

                                                                        2008043801

Manufactured in Canada

To Susan, my wife and favorite person in the world. And to our children and their families, who teach and inspire us. Thanks also to Dad and Mom. Finally, my gratitude goes to my disabled brothers and sisters who have struggled for human rights and who are role models for generations to come.

—Romel Mackelprang

To all those people with disabilities throughout the world who have struggled and continue to struggle to be a part of the mainstream of society. I know and have known many of you, and it has been a privilege.

—Richard Salsgiver

Contents

Figures, Tables, and Boxes

About the Authors

Romel W. Mackelprang (MSW, DSW, University of Utah) is professor of social work and the director of the Center for Disability Studies and Universal Access at Eastern Washington University. He has been involved in the disability rights and independent living movements since 1980. He has worked as a hospital-based rehabilitation social worker for people with spinal cord injury, brain injury, and other neurological disabilities. He was a founder and chair of the Council on Social Work Education task force on disability and has been involved in the Council on Social Work Education and the National Association of Social Workers in promoting disability as a form of diversity. In recent years, his activities have expanded to Canada, Europe, Africa, and Australia. He is currently involved in promoting diversity through the application of universal access.

Richard O. Salsgiver (MSW, University of Pittsburgh; DA, Carnegie Mellon University) is professor of social work education at California State University, Fresno. Professor Salsgiver is a person with disability, having cerebral palsy since birth. He has taught at both the high school and college levels. In addition, he has served in various practice and administrative positions in social welfare and higher education, including as executive director of the California Association of the Physically Handicapped Independent Living Center in Fresno, California, and as director of diversity programs in the California State University Office of the Chancellor. He is active in various disability issues in both the community and university.

Preface

Disability: A Diversity Model Approach in Human Service Practice was first published in 1999. It was written primarily to prepare students for human service careers that are directly related to working with persons with disabilities. Human service careers can include social work, psychology, rehabilitation counseling, family counseling, and school and university counseling. This primary educational objective remains in the second edition, which now includes international information and perspectives.

As in the first edition, the language of the work reflects the overriding concept that disability needs to be understood from a perspective of diversity and of oppression rather than as a condition of psychological or physical dysfunction. This concept incorporates the need to understand the limitations presented by psychological and physical conditions but reinforces the need to place these limitations within a diversity/oppression framework. It advocates universal access to society's resources for people with disabilities as well as all groups. The voice of our work centers on the theme that the origin of the vast majority of problems of persons with disabilities does not reside in "distorted ego function" or "crooked limbs," but in the way society views disability, and how it reacts to and treats persons with disabilities in light of its limited vision. We acknowledge the existence of a Disability culture and a disability history. We assert that persons with disabilities as a group have more commonalities than dissimilarities. We propose that the answers to the "disability problem" lie in interventions not only with individuals but with the society in general. It is a language that promotes the empowerment of persons with disabilities in the economic and political arenas. It is a language that celebrates disability as an important piece of the great mosaic of diversity that makes up our society. The language of our work calls upon human service professionals to challenge old models of conceptualizing disability and to embrace a model of difference rather than dysfunction.

Much like in our first edition, the second edition of our textbook invites controversy and discussion. We seek to probe old ideas and ways of looking at both human service practice and persons with disabilities. We ask students to grab hold of the lion's tail and get ready for a wild and different ride. We urge students to reach deep within and examine their beliefs and attitudes about disabilities. We encourage students to examine old ways of categorizing disabilities and persons with disabilities. We challenge students to view persons with disabilities in terms of their strengths rather than their "dysfunctions." And we call upon students to become politically involved in the struggle. Politics is the biggest game in town!

We also wish to challenge instructors and other professionals. Many of the concepts presented in this book are controversial at best, and downright heresy at worst. Some professionals may have trouble seeing disability as a social construct rather than primarily as a function of people's biological and psychological problems. Some may find it difficult to accept our focus on disabled people's commonalities rather than on classifications of disabilities. Some may continue to see proponents of the independent living movement as paraprofessionals. And some may continue to believe that those with disabilities need to be taken care of by professionals. However, the text truly reflects the winds of change, as demonstrated by visionaries in human services and as reflected in the changing ethical standards of many professions. We also challenge professionals to look beyond the boundaries of the United States to the rest of the world, throughout which the seeds of change first planted in America have spread.

The textbook is divided into three sections. The first section establishes a nontraditional view of disability. We invite readers to move away from the perspective that persons with disabilities are sick, passive, and deviant. We create a context that acknowledges the devaluation and oppression of persons with disabilities, that recognizes the development of a culture built upon the experience of oppression, and that suggests the need for an aggressive political struggle to end that oppression. It advocates the universal access made possible by a society constructed for the broad range of diverse people rather than one built for the mainstream that then accommodates those who are atypical.

The second section looks at groupings of disabilities placed within the context of the social definition of disability. Each chapter discusses the implications of various disabilities on people's lives. Each also contains a personal account of someone living with these disabilities. Readers will find many common themes in the lives of people with different disabilities.

The third section discusses human service practice with persons with disabilities, using the frames of reference presented in the first and second sections. Chapter 13 addresses issues in assessing people with disabilities. Chapter 14 presents various models of intervention. The final chapter presents guiding principles of practice that we believe practitioners should use when working with people with disabilities. They represent our guiding principles in the textbook as a whole and in our professional lives. We introduce them here.

1. People with disabilities are capable, have potential, and are important members of society.

2. Devaluation and a lack of resources, not individual pathology, are the primary obstacles facing persons with disabilities.
3. Disability, like race and gender, is a social construct, and intervention with people with disabilities must be political in nature.
4. There is a Disability culture and history that professionals should be aware of in order to facilitate the empowerment of persons with disabilities.
5. There is a joy and vitality to be found in disability.
6. Persons with disabilities have the right to self-determination and the right to guide professionals' involvement in their lives.

Acknowledgments

So many people deserve to be recognized in our endeavor of writing this book. There are the many theorists and writers from whom we have borrowed. All the people who shared their personal narratives deserve special recognition. Their stories remind us of people's value and potential. Their insights are invaluable. We would like to thank the many colleagues who reviewed the book at various stages.

We acknowledge those who have developed and nurtured Disability culture. These include the individuals who have, through their strength and commitment, initiated the process of changing the way society views and deals with disability. These individuals are the primary players in disability history and provide the foundation for Disability culture. Some of them are found in our book. Others are not. All of you, alive and dead, are the pioneers and the role models who have made and will continue to make a better place for those who follow.

Part I

Context for Practice

One of the most important tools for effective human service practitioners is an understanding of our personal values. This particularly holds true for those who work with persons with disabilities. Our internalized values and beliefs come from a variety of sources, including the aggregate culture, various subcultures, family teaching, life journeys, and educational experiences. Values and beliefs concerning disability affect the work that you will be doing with one of the largest minority groups in the world—persons with disabilities.

To understand personal views regarding persons with disabilities, it is necessary to explore the various ways societies and cultures perceive persons with disabilities. This understanding is also extremely important in determining intervention approaches and activities that facilitate or support the development of enfranchised, empowered, and independent human beings.

How does the society in which you live view disability and where do these perceptions come from? What are your views of disability, and how are they connected to history, culture, and society? A current cultural perspective on disability involves the idea that persons with disabilities are objects of pity who exist to be taken care of. Some fear persons with disabilities either because they feel they may tear the very fabric of society or because they remind nondisabled folks of their own vulnerability and mortality. Others see disabled persons as sick. Some see them as perpetual children, sexless and in need of care. Still others see persons with disabilities as incompetent. Some see them as freaks. Others see them as either a gift or curse from God. And some see persons with disabilities merely as people who are, in superficial ways, different from people without disabilities. They recognize that persons with disabilities are, like everyone else, striving to get by, to live, to have good jobs, to have nice homes, to have fun, to lead fulfilling lives.

The etiology of these various beliefs and viewpoints can be traced to a myriad of sources. They stem from various religious beliefs and ideologies.

They stem from the idea that humans should be, and are capable of being, perfect. And they can stem from creative thinking, research, and political action.

The origins of beliefs about disability, their impact on society, and their impact on the human service professions influence each of us as professionals. How we choose to approach persons with disabilities depends on how we view disability and being disabled. If we see disability as a curse from God, our assessment will look for unchangeable deficiency or immorality. If we see persons with disabilities as incompetent or as perpetual children, we will expect them to be helpless. If we perceive persons with disabilities as competent and having potential for success, we will recognize the strengths they possess and that they can use to empower themselves.

Our values and beliefs about disability also guide our work with persons with disabilities. If we see persons with disabilities as sick or incapable, we will take care of them. If we see them as a menace, we will segregate them by locking them away in institutions or hiding them in their homes. If we see them as a minority group that has been stereotyped and subjected to discrimination, we will advocate social justice and seek the changes in society, economics, and politics that will empower them.

The first five chapters of this text provide a context for human service practice with persons with disabilities. We explore historical and current societal values and beliefs about disability. We examine the effects of these beliefs in the lives of disabled folks. We also explore how societal values influence human service practice.

Chapter 1 reviews the history of disability, including the origins and impacts of models used to define disability. Chapter 2 explores theories of human behavior and disability and these theories' implications for practice with persons with disabilities. It reviews multiple perspectives including psychosocial development, social, and economic theories and discusses their limitations as they apply to disability. Chapter 3 examines, in depth, the various stereotypes applied to persons with disabilities and how these stereotypes emerge from social constructions of disability. It addresses the influences of various professions on how practitioners approach practice with persons with disabilities. It also offers ways you can begin to examine your own values and beliefs about disability. Chapter 4 introduces the unique view that, out of their minority status, persons with disabilities have created a culture of Disability with a characteristic history, language, and values. Chapter 5 presents readers with an overview of the evolution of perspectives on disability around the world and provides readers with samples of important American and international social policies and legislative milestones.

1

The Meanings and History of Disability in Society

STUDENT LEARNING OBJECTIVES

1. To understand the complex history of persons with disabilities and how it affects current human service practice methodology toward disabled people
2. To understand the impact of disability history on the identity development of people with disabilities
3. To understand the ever-developing language used to describe disability

DISABILITY IN HISTORY

Throughout history, societies have attempted to explain the place of disability in the social order. Neolithic tribes believed disabilities were caused by spirits (Albrecht, 1992), and skull surgeries were performed to release evil spirits. The Spartans, with their rugged individualism, left persons with disabilities, both young and old, to die in the countryside. Ancient Greeks believed disabled persons were not human and that they should be abandoned to die (DePoy & Gilson, 2004; Plato, 1991). Plato, to whom we owe much of our ethical framework, saw persons with disabilities as standing in the way of a perfect world. He wrote in Book 5 of *The Republic* that "the offspring of the inferior, or of the better when they chance to be deformed, will be put away in some mysterious, unknown place, as they should be" (Plato, 1991, p. 183).

The Romans, who borrowed the concept of reciprocity from the Greeks, gave assistance to adult persons with disabilities with the expectation they would express their appreciation through complacency (Morris, 1986). But like the Greeks, they also at times abandoned disabled and deformed infants to die, justifying their actions by defining those children as not fully human. However, the Romans did not perceive all disabilities as problematic, particularly those disabilities that did not manifest in physical differences. For example, Julius Caesar had epilepsy, known as falling sickness, and claimed that he had visions during his seizures.

In ancient Asia, disability was viewed similarly to the way it was viewed in Western culture. Life with disability was viewed as substandard, and people with disabilities were often forced to beg for sustenance. However, because religious vows of poverty were common in some parts of Asia, the act of begging may not have been viewed as negatively as in Western culture. Both heroic and malevolent disabled characters are featured in ancient Asian history. Yet ancient Zoroastrian scripture dating back 2,500 years in Persia envisioned a perfect world without disabilities (Miles, 2002).

Judeo-Christian thought, upon which much of Western culture is based, teaches that humans are made in God's image and are different from and superior to the rest of the animal kingdom. Livneh (1980) contends that persons with disabilities remind those without disabilities of humankind's link with the rest of the animal kingdom and bring to consciousness their fallibility. Thus, disabilities remind people of humankind's imperfections and dissimilarities to God while illuminating humankind's relationship to the imperfect animal kingdom.

Judeo-Christian and Muslim scripture portray disability negatively. The Bible and Koran are full of references linking disability to sin and evil. The Koran depicted the deaf, blind, and "dumb" as being without understanding. Disability signified sinners to the ancient Hebrews, and people with disabilities were thought to be possessed by demons. The Old Testament prohibited people who were deformed, crippled, or of short stature from officiating in priesthood rites. The Old Testament forbade the blind or lame from entering the houses of believers (Wright, 1983). However, disability was not universally condemned. For example, according to the texts of both the Koran and the Torah, although Moses lived with a significant speech impairment, it did not disqualify him from leading the Israelites out of Egypt.

The New Testament portrayed disability as arising from sin and spiritual deficiency. Blindness and other disabilities were believed to be caused by the sins of disabled people or their parents. Those with disabilities that are characterized today as "mental illness" were thought to be possessed by demons. However, Jesus also displayed compassion for disabled persons, setting a model for subsequent charitable efforts in Western culture.

Judeo-Christian tradition was prevalent among Europeans during the Middle Ages and beyond; during this time, persons with disabilities were thought to be expressions of God's displeasure (Livneh, 1982). Although Judeo-Christian philosophy did not advocate their killing, people with disabilities were ostracized and stereotyped.

In the Middle Ages, disability continued to be explained in moral and spiritual terms. People with disabilities were perceived as being out of harmony with God or the natural order of the universe. When disabilities were believed to arise from demonic or other evil influences, people with disabilities were rejected by society. Some were even burned at the stake. On the other hand, churches sometimes articulated the belief that the presence of disabled folks created the opportunity for the nondisabled to practice charity. People with leprosy were segregated to protect society physically and spiritually; however, some believed lepers' infirmities helped them achieve salvation faster than others. Thus, while moral explanations prevailed during the Middle Ages, explanations for the meaning of disability for individuals varied widely (Metzler, 2006).

The Enlightenment brought a new emphasis on rational inquiry that competed with traditional religious and spiritual explanations of disability. As early as 1600, Francis Bacon refuted the idea that "madness" was a form of moral punishment. Disability from birth was considered a monstrosity, while acquired disabilities were more acceptable (DePoy & Gilson, 2004). Individuals injured during wartime were given special consideration. In Europe, blind persons especially were afforded higher status; this resulted from the wartime practice in which prisoners of war were blinded by their captors and allowed to return to their homes. This practice was considered a humane alternative to executing prisoners that still neutralized the threat they posed. The vestiges of this unique position for the blind continue contemporarily. For example, in Spain, one of the national lotteries is staffed and managed by—and proceeds are dedicated to—blind citizens.

The Belgian social statistician Adolphe Quetelet (1796–1874) was influential in framing a new overall view of disability. Quetelet applied the mathematical concepts of the bell curve and normal distribution to human beings, presenting the average man as society's ideal. Thus, the typical became defined as desirable, and deviations from the norm were considered undesirable mistakes. This provided a framework from which to view people born with physical and mental differences from the norm collectively rather than as distinct entities or groups (DePoy & Gilson, 2004; Snyder & Mitchell, 2006). Normal became a standard to strive for, providing justification for systematic efforts to fix those considered abnormal.

By the mid-1800s there were two distinct but overlapping societal models of disability. The moral model, present from earliest recorded history, viewed disability as a moral defect resulting from factors such as sin or the disorder of nature. The emerging medical model viewed disability as an innate deviation from the normal and desirable that could be treated by medical and scientific interventions. Both models labeled disability an undesirable condition to be prevented. Since both the medical and moral models maintain prominence in contemporary life, we will discuss them in greater detail in chapter 3.

As scientific inquiry increasingly supplanted moral explanations for disability, moral and supernatural explanations for disability began to be replaced by physical and scientific explications, increasing the emphasis on curing, or at least treating, biological inadequacies. The increased industrialization and urbanization that corresponded with the Enlightenment contributed to changing perceptions of disability. More and more, the worth of individuals was measured by their ability to work and contribute to the economy. Whereas agrarian and rural communities cared for people with disabilities through family, church, and community, industrial society led to the proliferation of institutions to house the unproductive, including those with disabilities. Although the stated intent of many of these institutions was to cure or serve people with disabilities, segregation and the dearth of resources often turned them into warehouses with subhuman conditions.

The height of the Industrial Revolution, concomitant with the Victorian era in the 1800s, brought increasing modernity and scientific advances in architecture, photography, health, and science, as well as changing social and political sensibilities. Charles Darwin's observations challenged perceptions about the nature and development of humanity. Inventions and advances produced optimism, and professionals held great hope that "deviants" could be molded and changed to be more acceptable to society (Rothman, 1971). However, as the century progressed, a new philosophy of social Darwinism gained prominence. Social Darwinists argued that just as competition promotes biological evolution, social evolution occurs in human populations and government policies can be instrumental in fostering desired social and societal development. These beliefs gave rise to the eugenics movement, which became prominent from the late nineteenth century through much of the twentieth century. Thus, by the turn of the twentieth century, intellectual elites were campaigning for the elimination of the poor, non-productive, and undesirable while advocating the procreation of those with desirable traits (Wiggam, 1924). Whereas Darwin advocated natural selection, eugenicists implemented draconian social engineering measures to promote the survival of the fittest and discourage the reproduction of undesirables in an attempt to purify society. Eugenics was used to justify laws forbidding interracial marriage and mandating the sterilization of disabled people and led to the proliferation of large institutions with degrading living conditions (Longmore, 1987). In a portend of things to come, Alexis Carrel, a French 1912 Nobel Prize winner in medicine and active eugenicist, advocated the "humane" disposal of mentally defective, insane persons and other undesirables through the use of lethal gas in small euthanasia institutions (Carrel, 1935; Szasz, 1977).

In the first half of the twentieth century, both the moral and medical models were firmly entrenched in Western culture, and people with disabilities were segregated from society. Parents of children born with disabilities were expected to institutionalize their children. Institutions for the "retarded" and the insane proliferated. Public access was denied people with mobility disabilities. The 1924 *Buck v. Bell* decision of the Supreme Court of the United States legitimized the forced sterilization of disabled persons. Longmore (2003) recounts the history of Randolph Bourne (1886–1918), a brilliant and articulate antiwar intellectual and feminist who had a "highly visible disability, a twisted mouth, face, and ear from a difficult birth, a severely curved spine and stunted growth from childhood tuberculosis" (p. 35). He was denied jobs and educational opportunities, was isolated socially, and was forced into economic dependence. His critics equated his "deformed" body with a "deformed" mind. A Chicago ordinance forbade people like Bourne from appearing in public, warning, "No person who is diseased, maimed, mutilated, or in any way deformed so as to be an unsightly or disgusting object or improper person to be allowed in or on the public ways or other public places in this city, shall therein or thereon expose himself to public view" (qtd. in Longmore, 2003, p. 36).

Eugenicists distinguished people born with disabilities from those who acquired disabilities. Acquired disabilities, especially when acquired from injury or accident, were more tolerable. For example, World War I produced hundreds of thousands of persons with disabilities in Europe and the United States, and responses to their needs reinforced and strengthened the disability role of the worthy poor (British Broadcasting Corporation, 1999). Franklin D. Roosevelt was elected president of the United States in spite of his experience with polio; however, he went to great lengths to hide his physical disability from the public. Increased survival rates of persons who were born with or acquired disabilities, public responsibility to care for veterans disabled by wars, and technological advances led to increased awareness of and attention to the need to "treat" disabled persons.

Nazi Germany used the eugenics philosophies to justify the T4 program and the genocide of between 75,000 and 200,000 physically and mentally disabled people in Germany. Franz Stangl, commandant of the infamous extermination camps at Sobibor and later Treblinka, gained his expertise using gas to exterminate people while serving as an administrator at Hartheim, a hospital that was converted into an extermination center for disabled people (Garscha & Kuretsidis-Haider, 1997). Joseph Goebbels, Hitler's propaganda minister, who was disabled from polio, nevertheless led the publicity effort portraying disabled persons as subhuman and incurable, justifying the T4 program that defined their murders as mercy killings and release by comfortable death. And while Hitler and his minions justified the genocide of Jews and Gypsies because they viewed them as inferior races, they also justified killing racially "pure" but otherwise "defective" Aryans such as disabled people, and later gay men and women, whom they also labeled defective. In fact, disabled people were used to perfect the extermination techniques later used in the camps.

Early in the twentieth century, the seeds of disability rights were being germinated. For example, in 1935 the League of the Physically Handicapped, a small group of mobility-disabled persons and their supporters, protested against job discrimination against those with disabilities (Longmore, 2003). In the 1940s, the research of people such as Roger Barker and Beatrice Wright began showing similarities between the experiences of disabled persons and other groups who experienced discrimination. The turbulent climate of the 1960s that gave rise to the civil right movements for racial minorities and the women's movement also provided a genesis for a disability civil rights movement. Activists such as Ed Roberts and Judy Heumann, both polio survivors, argued that they were denied the right to education and employment because of discrimination, and they rejected arguments that they were unemployable because of their disabilities. The demand for civil rights promulgated the independent living movement, established with the assertion that society is comprised primarily of the nondisabled and that persons with disabilities are a minority who have been subjected to discrimination and lack of opportunity. Societal barriers, not individual characteristics, present the greatest challenge to full participation for people with disabilities.

DISABILITY IDENTITY AS MINORITY IDENTITY

Negative perceptions of disability have been predominant throughout history, resulting in deeply felt beliefs, often unconsciously held. As we have discussed, ancient texts and scripture, upon which modern societal values are based, treat disability as pathological and immoral. These values have been found in cultures throughout the world in all ages. Often feelings such as pity, fear, and revulsion are unconsciously and automatically experienced. Bryan (1996) observes that "Although rooted in superstition and ignorance, the bias against persons with disabilities is generally not meant to be malicious or segregate the population into a caste system. Regardless of the intentions, many 'nondisabled' persons exhibit feelings of frustration, uncertainty, and bigotry when encountering a person with a disability, especially if the disability is severe. . . . These attitudes served to separate the 'nondisabled' from the 'disabled,' which further disenfranchised persons with disabilities" (pp. 6–7).

Wolfensberger (1972) illuminates common attitudes held toward persons with disabilities. He contends that people with disabilities are frequently labeled deviant and assigned societal role expectations based on these stereotypes. He also observes that people internalize these societally imposed roles. Wolfensberger states: "When a person is perceived as deviant, he is cast into a role that carries with it powerful expectancies. Strangely enough, these expectancies not only take hold of the mind of the perceiver, but of the perceived person as well. It is a well-established fact that a person's behavior tends to be profoundly affected by the role expectations that are placed upon him. . . . Unfortunately, role-appropriate behavior will then often be interpreted to be a person's 'natural' mode of acting, rather than a mode elicited by environmental events and circumstances" (pp. 16–17). Wolfensberger's ideas aid us in addressing the complex issues of the identity of persons with disabilities, the place of disability in society, and the development of Disability culture. Historically, people with disabilities have been perceived as deficient and have been expected to fill roles foisted on them by larger society. For example, persons with intellectual and mental health disabilities have routinely been institutionalized. When their behavior has displayed signs of institutionalization, it has reinforced stereotypes and justified the perception that they need to be institutionalized. Thus, society creates the environment that reinforces its expectations: in these instances, dysfunctional behaviors and limited social functioning. With limited opportunities, persons with disabilities have little choice for anything else.

Let's look at comparisons between people with disabilities and racial and ethnic minorities. For example, people of color in the United States, blacks who lived under apartheid in South Africa, Arabs in some areas of northern Europe, and biracial and non-Japanese individuals in Japan have been subjected to pervasive negative societal images. Lesbian, gay, bisexual, transgender, and questioning (LGBTQ) persons have been subjected to negative images of LGBTQ people. Women have been denied opportunities based on their perceived limitations. Similarly, persons with disabilities have formed their social and personal identities based on the negative stereotypes placed upon them by history and the societies in which they have found themselves (Riddell & Watson, 2003). Like other minorities, persons with disabilities find themselves devalued, objectified, and subject to oppression.

Societal attitudes have tended to separate people with disabilities, denying them full societal participation. Isolation and unfamiliarity have, in turn, in a pernicious cycle, led to stereotypical attitudes toward persons with disabilities and ableism. We use the term *ableism* to describe the belief that people with disabilities are inferior to nondisabled people because of their differences. (Others use the term *disableism* to mean the same thing.) Ableism is similar to other isms such as racism and sexism, wherein the dominant segment of society defines the minority or non-dominant segments of society in stereotypical and/or negative ways. Ableism devalues people with disabilities and results in segregation, social isolation, and social policies that limit their opportunities for full societal participation. Just as with the other isms, when ableism is operationalized into policy and practice, professionals such as government officials, educators, social workers, and health care providers underestimate capabilities, limit self-determination, and behave oppressively toward the people subjected to the ism.

Unfortunately, persons with disabilities are also susceptible to internalizing stereotypes and negative beliefs. This process, which we call *internalized ableism*, is similar to internalized racism and sexism. The concepts of ableism and internalized ableism were developed in the disabled community and have become recognized by scholars and researchers. These isms perpetuate, and are in turn reinforced by, stereotypes. In the next section, we discuss the stereotypes most commonly encountered in today's society.

COMMON STEREOTYPICAL ATTITUDES TOWARD PERSONS WITH DISABILITIES

Disability stereotypes embedded in the medical and moral models continue to be common today. In this section, we discuss commonly held stereotypes.

Perpetual Children

The stereotype of the person with a disability as a perpetual child is embedded in terms such as *handicapped* and *crippled* (Bogden & Biklen, 1993). Charles Dickens's 1843 story *A Christmas Carol* presents Tiny Tim as a cute but powerless and ineffectual child whose primary reason for existence is to remind nondisabled folks how well off and fortunate they are in not being crippled.

Contemporarily, the annual March of Dimes telethon perpetually describes people with disabilities as "Jerry's kids," whether their age is one day or one hundred years. Wolfensberger (1972) labels this the stereotype of the "eternal child." Rather than being expected to go through developmental processes, perpetual children have few expectations placed on them; thus few opportunities for growth and development are provided for them. Low expectations result in the expenditure of fewer resources that would help them reach their potential.

An Object to Be Pitied

A common societal image of persons with disabilities is that of pitied or pitiful individuals: people whom no one would envy, persons no one would want to be (Shapiro, 1993). Wolfensberger (1972) identifies the common view of persons with disabilities as objects of pity, which is displayed in a variety of ways. Contemporarily, public pity is consistently used to raise money for organizations that work with people with disabilities. Posters, billboards, and telethons depict people with disabilities as brave but pitiable. Shapiro (1993) reveals the feelings of Evan Kemp Jr. regarding telethons. An advisor to George Bush Sr., a prime mover of the Americans with Disabilities Act, and a person with a disability himself, Kemp believes that "by arousing the public's fear of the handicap itself, the telethon makes viewers afraid of handicapped people." Kemp goes on to say, "Playing to pity may raise money, but it raises walls of fear between the public and us" (qtd. in Shapiro, 1993, p. 22).

The pity stereotype is born out of ignorance. Even when intentions are altruistic, fund-raisers such as telethons create pity, exploit guilt, and pigeonhole the supposed beneficiaries of charity. Bogdan and Biklen (1993) state: "Thus, the crippled child becomes a poor soul whose disability evokes pity and guilt and the spirit of giving, but also lessens the possibility that disabled people can be regarded as people with personalities, with individual aspira-tions, and with an interest in being perceived as ordinary people" (p. 74).

This pity is manifest in other ways. The 2004 Clint Eastwood film *Million Dollar Baby*, which garnered Academy Awards for Best Picture, Best Direc-tor, Best Actress, and Best Supporting Actress, provides a graphic example. Hilary Swank plays an aspiring boxer who, after sustaining a spinal cord injury, seeks to end her life. Ultimately, her trainer, played by Clint East-wood, mercifully euthanizes her, thus putting an end to her misery. In other words, life with a serious physical disability is considered worse than death. In the 1981 film *Whose Life Is It Anyway?* Richard Dreyfus's character begs for the right to end his life after an automobile accident leaves him with quadriplegia and needing renal dialysis. The film intends for the audience to be relieved when this likable, charismatic character is granted his wish. Again, life with a disability is portrayed as worse than death, a message that is loud and clear to the audience. In another example, Morris (1986) recalls that opposing forces debating the abortion issue often find agreement that abortion is acceptable when a fetus has a severe disability. Prior to acquiring a disability herself, Morris, like many others, was unaware of the embedded societal assumption that disability is a horrible fate.

A Menace or Threat to Society

Yet another stereotype centers on persons with disabilities as menaces or threats to society—people to be feared (Wolfensberger, 1972). Literature, films, and television persistently present persons with disabilities in the roles of criminals, monsters, and villains. Thus, persons with disabilities are por-trayed as deviant. They may be perceived as immoral, if not criminal. They are seen as unworthy and deserving to be shunned because of the way the media portrays them in the movies, television, and literature (Bogden & Biklen, 1993). Persons with mental health disabilities are often portrayed as violent criminals. Most monsters are in fact persons with disabilities, whether the disability is a deformed face, another physical atypicality, or a mental health condition.

One of the authors found these attitudes strongly displayed in his per-sonal life when, on separate occasions, he was asked to become involved in community efforts to keep two group homes out of his neighborhood. One of the group homes was to serve persons with developmental/intellectual disabilities; the other was for people with mental health disabilities. The rationales expressed for keeping them out were similar. There was a strong plea to "protect our children." People were terrified that their children would be sexually molested and physically attacked by "retarded" and "crazy" peo-ple. Neighborhood activists believed group home residents would prey on the community. The rhetoric expressed in door-to-door contact and commu-nity meetings included calls for violence, if necessary, to protect the commu-nity from these people. The group homes were eventually located in the neighborhood. However, even though problems failed to materialize, some community residents continued to shun people living in the group homes.

The perception that people with disabilities are a menace to society has been documented by Rhodes (1993), who recounts how societal fears have led to institutional segregation, marriage restrictions, and sterilization. Draconian measures have been taken to prevent contamination of the gene pool and to protect persons without disabilities.

Sick

Another common stereotype portrays people with disabilities as being sick, thus creating an additional negative identity. This stereotype, which is commonly internalized, portrays those with disabilities as persons to be taken care of. They are believed to need special treatment just because they are disabled. They may be excused from commitments and responsibilities. They may be seen as incapable of contributing to society and as entitled to be served. The internalized stereotype of sickness may leave persons with disabilities dependent on others, prevent them from taking the risks necessary for development, and leave them with self-images as people who do not take risks. In return, they are expected to be grateful for services they receive, even though the system that provides their services punishes them if they try to be independent and exercise self-determination (Bryan, 1996; Devore & Schlesinger, 1999; Mackelprang & Salsgiver, 1996; Zola, 1993).

People with physical disabilities who need attendant care are often forced into the sick role. Rather than having the opportunity to manage their own care, they are forced to rely on physicians to write orders and on nurses who provide care. Instead of directing their own care, they are forced to rely on home health agencies that control purse strings and personnel.

A language of sickness is endemic in popular and professional language relative to people with disabilities. People with disabilities are "confined" to wheelchairs or "wheelchair-bound," just as sick people are confined to bed. Language such as "*afflicted* with cerebral palsy" and "mental *illness*" conveys widely accepted attitudes that persons with disabilities are sick.

Making sickness synonymous with disability maintains a power imbalance that victimizes persons with disabilities. The health care industry has massive financial incentives for placing people with disabilities in the sick role. Health care providers maintain status, professional worth, and income by exercising control over those who are forced to rely on them for services. Professional control creates a conflict of interest in which increased client or patient autonomy would reduce jobs and incomes, thus threatening the status of health and human service professionals. For example, the physician's status is maintained when people must rely on physicians to obtain medications, durable medical equipment, therapy, or attendant care. Individual autonomy in obtaining these needs would decrease the need for, reduce the role of, and reduce the income of physicians, nurses, pharmacies and pharmacists, medical equipment providers, social workers, psychologists, and others.

A Burden to Society

The sick role perpetuates the myth that disabled persons are a burden to society, therefore justifying their isolation and segregation. Many persons with disabilities feel isolated. They never quite fit in. They are forced to see themselves as different from everyone else (Gill, 1993). Not only are they different, but their differences are abnormal and costly to society. The institutionalization of persons with disabilities adds to this identity, along with the segregation that is promoted by group homes and other "special" accommodations. In addition, segregating people with disabilities furthers the perception that societal resources directed to them are costly to society.

Ugly and Sexless

Another common stereotype portrays persons with disabilities as ugly and sexless, an ableist identity internalized by many. How can persons who internalize and adopt the belief that they are "damaged goods" consider themselves beautiful and sexy? In the history of human civilization, there is a dearth of examples of persons with disabilities portrayed as beautiful. In the current media, aside from a few television commercials featuring actors with a disability, beauty and disability or sexuality and disability are rarely combined (Hahn, 1993). The 1928 D. H. Lawrence novel *Lady Chatterley's Lover* portrays a wealthy woman who takes a laborer as a lover because of her husband's paralysis and subsequent impotence. The multi-award-winning 1996 film *Breaking the Waves* tells the story of a woman whose husband coerces her to engage in sex with multiple partners after he is paralyzed in an industrial accident. Rendered asexual himself, he derives vicarious satisfaction by compelling her to tell him the specifics of her sexual encounters. In both stories, the husbands' disabilities are portrayed as having completely robbed them of their sexuality.

Incompetent

Another common stereotype is that of incompetence. Innumerable wheelchair users have felt the sting of this stereotype in restaurants and other establishments when they have been with companions who do not use wheelchairs. Rather than taking the wheelchair user's order, servers ask their companions what the wheelchair user wants to eat, the assumption being that the user is incapable of ordering and needs the help of someone else.

One of the authors, who uses a wheelchair, attended a conference in Washington, D.C., with a colleague who did not. At the airport while they were together, the ticket person asked his colleague whether or not he needed to be pushed to the airplane. The ticket person assumed that because the author used a wheelchair, he could also not talk or respond intelligently to questions. After a quick and articulate response, the ticket person became very much aware of the intellectual ability and verbal skills of someone with a disability.

The perception of incompetence is manifest in various ways and to various degrees. In health settings, these assumptions may be covert, but the meaning can still be clear, as recounted one person who had experienced a spinal cord injury:

> [In rehabilitation] they really blew it. They told me when to get up, when to go to bed, when and what to eat. They told me when I had to take my medications and didn't always bother to tell me why I was taking them. I had to go to therapy at 9:00 a.m. It didn't matter that I've always been a late sleeper. They even told me when I could and couldn't take a crap. Then after three months of this, I was told that I was ready to go home and live completely independently. Hell, what a joke. (qtd. in Mackelprang, 1986, p. 43)

McRuer (2006) discusses the impact of the stereotype of incompetence on rehabilitation services. Social Darwinism and its social ideology of the "survival of the fittest" are manifest in vocational rehabilitation programs wherein funding and programs are cut back, and in assessment and the medical model diagnosis, which are used as a means of solving the "problem of disability" by determining who can compete and who cannot. Proponents of this perspective argue that those who cannot function in competitive employment should not receive rehabilitation services.

Assumptions of incompetence are often displayed when professionals take control of the lives of persons with disabilities. When professionals wrest control over the lives of persons with disabilities, these assumptions can be proved correct because people do not develop the skills to manage their lives. In the situation described in the quote above, for example, the individual was ill prepared to manage his medications because he was uninformed as to their uses and side effects. His capabilities were limited because of a dearth of opportunity to develop and assert independence.

Cursed by God

Another stereotype is that disabilities are the result of a curse from God. This attitude was displayed in the New Testament when the disciples of Jesus assumed that a man was born blind because either he or his parents had sinned. By logical extension, people with disabilities are less worthy and are less favorable in God's eyes than people without disabilities. Contemporarily, AIDS was ignored by the U.S. government for years because it affected gay men and was perceived as resulting from immoral lifestyles. Eventually, in 1996 Congress enacted the Ryan White Care Act, the first concerted federal effort to provide funding for care of low-income people living with HIV/ AIDS, which was intentionally named after a hemophiliac teenager, an "innocent victim" who contracted HIV from the transfusion of contaminated blood products and died of AIDS.

Individuals with disabilities and their families experience much guilt and shame as a result of this perception. Parents blame themselves and each other. Internalized ableism can lead people with disabilities to believe that God views them with disfavor. An example of this occurred with an individual with whom one of the authors worked for several years. Upon learning that he had been diagnosed with a progressive neuromuscular disorder, he sought religious help. He received a blessing that he would be healed if he had "faith and live[d] a worthy life." Initially, he refused to believe his condition was permanent, even refusing all treatment. However, his condition steadily progressed. Three years later, he was depressed and maintained little self-worth. He could not understand what he had done in his life to deserve this "curse from God." He blamed himself for his unsuccessful faith healing. He knew God was punishing him and held him in disfavor. He stated that the only reason he did not commit suicide was that suicide led to "eternal damnation, not just the damnation on this earth" caused by his disability. Parenthetically, members of his religious community also questioned his worthiness and wondered what he had done to deserve God's curse.

A Gift or Test from God

Conversely, disability can sometimes be perceived as a gift or test from God. Some individuals and families find divine purpose when events such as the onset of disability enter their lives. Religious and spiritual beliefs should be respected and can be great sources of strength. However, divine explanations can also lead people to ignore the larger picture. As Condeluci (1995) states, "If raising a child with cerebral palsy is seen as being more difficult than raising any other child then we need to look, not at God, but at people and society. Why is it harder for a family with a child with a disability? One reason is that people have not understood, nor accepted. Another is because our society has not adjusted to welcome someone who might move, talk, or think differently. These don't seem to be God's problems but ours" (p. 22). We acknowledge the value of people finding spiritual meaning to events in their lives. However, there is danger in establishing an identity primarily based on speculations about God's interventions or intentions.

Freaks

People with disabilities have often been treated as freaks. Circuses exploit this through freak sideshows, in which people pay to gawk at people with unusual appearances, many with disabilities. Similarly, grand-rounds presentations, in which naked or nearly naked people are paraded in front of large groups of medical professionals, may have some educational value, but the practice dehumanizes people with disabilities. Quasimodo, the mythical subject of Victor Hugo's *The Hunchback of Notre Dame*, written in 1831, illustrates the long-standing perception of people with disabilities as freaks. Pregnant women were cautioned not to look upon him out of fear for their unborn children. His "ugliness" was equated with evil, and he was mocked without mercy. As a freak, Quasimodo was dehumanized; his life and feelings were unimportant.

Stereotypical attitudes are pervasive in society. Close monitoring of personal reactions to people with disabilities can help people identify and deal with their personal attitudes based on stereotypical beliefs. It is important to acknowledge that stereotypes are not always born of negative presuppositions. Some are born of compassion and sympathy. However, even these stereotypes have negative results. Negative societal attitudes and stereotypes may adversely influence the self-image and future independence of newly disabled individuals. Human service professionals, who may have a vested interest in the dependence of their "clients" and "patients," have a direct effect on the general public's view of disability. Their attitudes are also perpetuated as they influence their students, the future human service professionals. They can reinforce the perception that problems rest exclusively with individuals and small systems, ignoring meso and macro impacts on people's lives.

The stereotypes discussed above arise directly from pejorative social constructions of disability harbored in pathology-based models and paradigms of disabilities. These stem from and are perpetuated in the aggregate society by the moral and medical social constructions of disability.

DISABILITY AS DIVERSITY

Clearly, throughout the ages, in Eastern and Western cultures, and in ancient and contemporary times, disability and persons with disabilities have primarily been perceived as negative, abnormal, and to be avoided. Disabilities have been explained as being out of order with nature and/or God (the moral model). In recent centuries, scientific inquiry and knowledge have produced new explanations of disability as deviation from what is considered normal and desirable (the medical model). Contemporarily, a new perspective on disability has arisen that explains disability as a variation of the human condition, another characteristic among the broad range of traits present in society. We call this approach the *social/minority model* and contrast it with the traditional pathology-based models of disability. We introduce the three models here, and in chapter 2, we will discuss them in detail.

Traditional moral and medical paradigms define the nature of disability in terms of individual deficiencies and the biology of the disability. For example, customary justifications for keeping disabled children out of regular public schools have centered on their impairments. In contrast, the social/minority model focuses on society, its beliefs, and resulting discrimination. The social/minority model rejects traditional justifications for denying disabled children access to education. It contends that children with disabilities have not been allowed to go to regular schools because they have not been allowed in. As a group, as a minority, they have been denied their rights to education (Meyerson, 1990). This approach calls for disability policies based on a civil rights rather than a social services perspective.

The social/minority model offers a constructive alternative to traditional ways of viewing persons with disabilities. The paradigm shift from individual incapacity to environmental discrimination is in itself empowering. Society can only understand the behavior, the self-concept, the educational achievement, and the economic success of persons with disabilities by looking at people with disabilities as a minority group, one that is subjected to discrimination found in the social environment (Fine & Asch, 1993). This perspective encourages persons with disabilities to begin to assert their capabilities, personally and politically, rather than remain objects of pity. It encourages persons with disabilities to see themselves as part of the great mosaic of diversity that makes up our society. Rather than remaining passive objects of service and service providers, people with disabilities become active and capable consumers. Rather than organizing their lives around their deficits and problems, they begin to acknowledge and build upon their strengths and take control of their lives. Personal decision making replaces passivity; empowerment replaces powerlessness. This awareness of strength and control has resulted in significant social and political change.

THE POWER OF LANGUAGE

Language is a system of representation that people use to communicate such concepts as ideas, emotions, and beliefs (Thomas, Wareing, Singh, Peccei, Thronborrow, & Jones, 2004) and that provides a foundation for social identity (McGroarty, 1996). Language reflects the larger society in which we live, while concomitantly social and political forces influence language use (sociology of language) (McKay & Hornberger, 1996). Words and phrases shape our realities, the ways in which we perceive the world.

We examine the meaning of a few words to illustrate the ways in which language is used to describe our thoughts and feelings. From antiquity, the term *patriarch* has been used to describe those who are revered and respected. Ancient patriarchs were considered prophets and benevolent leaders, icons to be exemplified in religious and family life. However, in recent decades, gender studies has reevaluated the meaning of patriarchy, often concluding that it is a system of male dominance that perpetuates the subjugation of women and children. Thus, contemporarily there are highly contrasting perceptions of the concept of patriarchs and patriarchy.

The 1934 musical comedy *The Gay Divorcee* portrays Fred Astaire searching for love interest Ginger Rogers. Other movies such as *Gay Desperado* (1936), *Gay Caballero* (1940), and *Es war eine rauschende Ballnacht* (*It Was a Gay Ballnight,* 1939) all portrayed heterosexual characters and themes. But in 1969 the film *The Gay Deceivers* portrayed heterosexual men who pretend to be gay in order to avoid military service. Of forty-seven films listed by the online *Movie Review Query Engine,* all twenty-five films released after 1969 that had *gay* in the title referred to homosexual orientation, whereas none of the films before 1965 did. Ninety-nine of the first one hundred sites netted by a Google search of the word *gay* referred to homosexual orientation. The meaning of *gay* changed dramatically in the second half of the twentieth century. Today, terms such as *gay rights* and *gaydar* affirm the lives of gays and lesbians. *Homophobia* and *heterosexism* describe negative opinions about and discrimination against gays, while terms such as *the gay agenda* and *the gay lifestyle* are used to conjure negative and dangerous images of homosexual persons.

Historically, the language used to describe disability has been negative and exclusionary. Terms such as *invalid, crippled, deformed, crazy, spastic, insane, mad, retarded, defective,* and *handicapped* are used pejoratively and raise negative images. Common words and phrases used to describe the conditions of people with disabilities include *confined* and *bound* (e.g., "confined to a wheelchair" and "wheelchair bound"), *retarded* (e.g., "You are soooo retarded"), *crazy* (e.g., "That's just crazy"), and *tragic* and *tragedy* (e.g., "tragic accident" and "It's a tragedy that she was born retarded").

Let's analyze the meaning of the term *disability.* The prefix *dis-* has meanings such as "no," "not any," and "apart from." *Able* means competent or capable. Thus, to have a disability literally means to not be able, or to be without ability. Being disabled literally means to be without capability or competence. The dominant group defines disability as pathological. In discussing language, power, and disability, A. G. Johnson (2006) observes:

> Disability and nondisability are also constructed through the language used to describe people. . . . Reducing people to a single dimension of who they are separates and excludes them, marks them as "other," as different from "normal" [white, heterosexual, male, nondisabled] people and therefore as inferior. . . . There is a world of difference between using a wheelchair and being treated as a normal human being [who happens to use a wheelchair to get around] and using a wheelchair and being treated as invisible, unintelligent, frightening, passive, dependent, and nothing more than your disability. . . . And the difference is not a matter of the disability itself but how it is constructed in society. . . . What makes socially constructed reality so powerful is that we rarely if ever experience it as that. We think the way our culture defines something like race

or gender [or disability] is simply the way things are in some objective sense. (pp. 19–20)

The perception perpetuated by the nondisabled majority is that the pathology of disability is objective reality. Few people, including disabled persons who have internalized ableist views, have challenged this socially constructed belief that people with disabilities are uni-dimensionally defined by their deviance from normalcy. Out of this environment came the move to modify language to reflect the multidimensional lives of people with disabilities.

DISABILITY LANGUAGE IN CONTEMPORARY SOCIETY

The last three decades of the twentieth century witnessed the rise of *person-first* language to describe disability. Person-first language places the person first rather than defining people by their disabilities, their perceived pathological characteristics. Person-first language assumes that the characteristics that lead to the label of "disabled" are a part of the individual but do not define the person. This approach is summarized in "Together We Will Make It," a song by Clyde Lambourn (1993) from People First of New Zealand.

> Put the people first
> That's how it's going to work
> When thinking up your schemes
> When dreaming up your dreams
> When planning all your plans
> When governing our lands
> Listen to our verse
> And put the people first
>
> We want to live in the real world
> We want a share of the pie
> But we need you
> And you need us too
> And together we will make it
> You and I.

Kathie Snow (2008), the mother of a child with a disability, echoes these sentiments with the statement:

Contrary to conventional wisdom, individuals with disabilities are not:

- People who *suffer* from the *tragedy* of *birth defects*.
- *Paraplegic heroes* who *struggle* to become *normal* again.
- *Victims* who *fight* to *overcome* their *challenges*.

Nor are they *retarded, autistic, blind, deaf, learning disabled,* etc.—*ad naseum!*

They are *people:* moms and dads; sons and daughters; employees and employers; friends and neighbors; students and teachers; scientists, doctors, actors, presidents, and more. People with disabilities are people, *first.*

Given the traditionally derogatory nature of terms such as *handicap* and *disability,* person-first language has become widely adopted. Person-first language views terms such as *person with a disability* as more acceptable than *disabled person* because of the belief that disabled persons are not defined by their disability; rather, disability is a characteristic they live with. Person-first language was an important sociolinguistic step in changing societal and personal perceptions about disability. Whereas disability language was once almost universally used to exclude people and characteristics, person-first language reflects an inclusive perspective. Person-first language acknowledges the basic humanity of individuals with disabilities irrespective of their individual traits and characteristics.

Increasingly, life with a disability is being perceived as different, not deficient (Gerber, Ginsberg, & Reiff, 1992). People are not "confined to wheelchairs." Instead, they use wheelchairs for mobility. The *Disability Rag,* an early militant disability newspaper, portrayed persons with disabilities as having "disability cool." Its successor, the online publication the *Ragged Edge,* advocates freeing disabled people from the tyranny of "nursing *facilities,*" not "nursing *homes.*" Ed Roberts defined himself on national television when he corrected Larry King's reference to him as a "victim" of polio. He acknowledged his disability but refuted the "victim" label applied by King, a label readily accepted in an ableist society. *Disability Rag* editor Mary Johnson embraced the term *disability* and rejected terms such as *differently abled* and *physically, emotionally,* or *mentally challenged,* stating that such words are used by nondisabled "do-gooders" who "wouldn't understand disability culture if we ran over their toes with a wheelchair." She describes such words as having "no soul" and "no power. They're like vanilla custard" (qtd. in Shapiro, 1993, p. 33).

The closing years of the twentieth century and first decade of the twenty-first century have seen further developments in the use of disability language. For one, disability advocates and activists are increasingly eschewing person-first language in favor of disability identity language. We refer you to the personal narrative of Judy Heumann at the end of this chapter as an example. Notice how Heumann uses terms like *disabled people* as opposed to *people with disabilities.* Heumann explains that person-first language is euphemistic and serves to hamper the political agenda of disability civil rights activists. DePoy and Gilson (2004) argue against person-first language based on their belief that person-first language is almost always used when descriptors (e.g., disability, cancer) are undesirable, and that person-first language implies that disability is located within individuals rather than a societal construction. In her book on increasing disability awareness, Mary

Johnson (2006) embraces disability-first versus person-first language, stating, "In this book, you'll find us more often using the term 'disabled person' or 'disabled people.' Many disability studies scholars prefer using 'disabled person.' . . . Instead of able-bodied, we use non-disabled" (p. 2).

In September 2006, an extensive discussion on disability language was initiated on the Listserv for the Society for Disability Studies, an international organization of disability academics.

> Friday, September 01, 2006 12:05 PM
> Subject: [SDS] people first language?
>
> I feel this is an old issue but I've been getting a lot of flack lately for using the term "disabled people" in grant applications and manuscripts. One recent grant review launched into a long diatribe about "disabled people" conveying a lack of respect for the community and serving as a barrier to full social inclusion. I always try to frame and explain my use of language but invariably someone (usually a non-disabled health or rehab science researcher) will demand that the terms be changed to people first language. I'd like an insider perspective on this, including pros and cons of various language choices, tips on phrasing from people who have been successful in justifying the use of disabled people.
>
> Thanks, Susan

The ensuing discussion revealed that disability scholars from all over the world are split on the use of person-first language. This discussion reflects current international realities.

In some countries such as New Zealand, disability rights advocates have adopted disability-first language, as evidenced by the New Zealand Disabled Persons Assembly, which avers that disabled people live in a "disabling society." However, People First of New Zealand, an organization for people with intellectual disabilities, still advocates the use of person-first language. The United Kingdom's Disabled People's Council, comprised of more than seventy groups run by disabled people, has adopted disability-first language in their name and communications, as have leading English disability scholars such as Tom Shakespeare and actress Liz Carr, a self-described crip activist. However, in much of the world, activists, scholars, and advocates are split.

People who are culturally Deaf have always rejected person-first language. In the United States, those who identify with Deaf culture use American Sign Language as their primary language and method of communication, identify Deafness as a cultural characteristic, and identify with other Deaf people as their primary sources of socialization. Culturally Deaf persons use language such as *Deaf person* with a capital *D* to connote a person who identifies with Deaf culture and *deaf person* with a little *d* to signify deafness as an auditory condition.

Similarly, many blind people also eschew the use of person-first language. For example, the National Federation of the Blind took serious umbrage with a 1993 U.S. Department of Education Office of Civil Rights memorandum that directed employees to use person-first disability language only instead of terms such as *blind people.* In reference to the memorandum, the National Federation of the Blind's Resolution 93–01 states, "A differentiation must be made among these euphemisms: some (such as hard of seeing, visually challenged, and people with blindness) are totally unacceptable and deserving only ridicule because of their strained and ludicrous attempt to avoid such straightforward, respectable words such as blindness, blind, the blind, blind person, or blind persons" (qtd. in Jernigan, 1999), and calls for straightforward language reflecting respect for the blind.

Interestingly, we ourselves are conflicted on the use of language as well. On one hand, we acknowledge that person-first language is respectful and that the pervasive and almost universal negative perceptions of disability throughout history have produced a contemporary environment that is so imbued with ableism that person-first language promotes the basic humanity of persons with disabilities. Conversely, however, we acknowledge that person-first language may foster a belief that disability is inherently pathological rather than a characteristic of diversity, as illustrated by the application of person-first language to other characteristics. Blacks and whites do not want to be called "persons with blackness," or "persons with whiteness." Women and men do not want to be called "persons with femaleness" or "persons with maleness." Similarly, disability-first language (e.g., *disabled man, disabled woman,* and *disabled persons*) embraces disability as a characteristic and identity. On one point the authors agree: people, disabled or not, have the right to be called by whatever names they choose. Currently, both person-first and disability-first language are acceptable.

A challenge for listeners and readers is to be aware of the way people use language beyond the words spoken, written, or signed—to be cognizant of embedded meanings and underlying intent. A second challenge is to be aware of the evolution of language over time. Concomitantly, we should avoid the pitfall of "presentism," that is, applying today's sensibilities to the past. For example, the term *handicapped,* eschewed today by disability activists, was common lexicon in past generations. Similarly, the person-first versus disability-first debate will continue to evolve over time. To accurately comprehend historical events, including the use of language, one must try to understand the sensibilities and contexts at the time of those events.

As for language in the current edition of this text, we acknowledge that our thinking has evolved in the years since the first edition. You will find us using multiple forms of disability language. When referring to disability from pathology-driven perspectives such as the moral and medical models, we primarily use person-first (e.g., "person with . . .") language. Similarly, we primarily use person-first language when discussing impairments concomitant with disability. For example, a "person with paraplegia" may need a new wheelchair for mobility every few years or may require medications to control spasticity. At times, such as when referring to disability as a social construct, we use person-first and disability-first language interchangeably. When referring to disability as an element of diversity (e.g., when discussing disability rights or a disabled athlete), we will primarily use disability-first language. As an example of interchangeable language, let's consider the celebrity Josh Blue, winner of NBC's 2006 *Last Comic Standing*. Josh has cerebral palsy (person-first language), is a disabled comic (disability-first language), and is also a disabled soccer player (disability-first language) who competed in the 2004 Paralympics in Greece.

One form of language we avoid is the use of terms such as "*the* disabled," "*the* physically disabled," and "*the* sensory disabled." While we acknowledge commonalties, we reject this language as lumping people into a one-dimensional group. Just as there is no such thing as *the* black man or *the* white woman, we believe there is no *the* disabled. We also avoid using terms such as *able-bodied*. Since this book is about disability, we use terms such as *nondisabled* to describe departures from disability. Further, many disabled persons are also able-bodied; thus using the term as the opposite of disability is a non sequitur.

Finally, when we write about Disability culture and disability identity, we use disability-first language. Furthermore, we borrow from Deaf culture by using "big *D*' *Disability* when writing about the culture of Disability. This text is our first foray into big *D* Disability language, and we will be interested in the reactions of disability scholars and other readers to this use. We are aware that there are people who question the presence of a "disability culture" or "culture of disability." We suggest that Disability culture is a burgeoning phenomenon and further assert that those in the disability community, including scholars, activists, humorists, sons, daughters, fathers, mothers, athletes, nerds, geeks, couch potatoes, and other disabled people, can all actively contribute to the development of an evolving Disability culture in which we view ourselves and our life experiences as inherently valuable to ourselves, our loved ones, our communities, and society. Thus, we are unabashed advocates for the strengthening of a culture of Disability. More important than the specific wording we use, our embedded intent is to imbue value and a sense of respect for disability, those who live with disabilities, and disabled people.

SUMMARY

Disabilities have been present in all societies and cultures from the beginning of recorded history. In most societies throughout history, disabilities have been viewed as abnormal, and people with disabilities have been marginalized. From ancient Greece to twentieth-century Western societies, disabled people have even been considered so objectionable that they have been deemed unworthy of life. However, there have also been times at which disabled people have been incorporated into the fabric of society. This has been particularly true for those with acquired disabilities, especially when acquired during times of armed conflict.

During most of recorded history, disability has been primarily perceived as morally objectionable or contrary to the natural nature of existence. Explanations for disability often involved the displeasure of God. With industrialization and the modernization of society, disability became increasingly explained in scientific terms, but still with a pathological and deficiency orientation. Important to this characterization was the belief that people with disabilities were a burden to society's economic productivity. The Enlightenment era produced a belief that physical abnormalities could be treated, ameliorated, or cured through scientifically applied strategies. However, by the end of the nineteenth century, a new and pernicious philosophy of social Darwinism and eugenics sought to eradicate disabled people from the face of the earth. Most eugenicists limited their actions to stopping the reproduction of people they considered defective; however, others advocated—and the Nazis ultimately carried out—the murder of thousands of disabled people under the guise of merciful euthanasia. Even today, we find common portrayals of disability as a condition worse than death, as evidenced by the 2004 Academy Award–winning film, *Million Dollar Baby*, among others.

In the twentieth century, disability stereotypes continued to pervade societies throughout the world. However, in the second half of the century, sporadic attempts to redefine disability gained steam, and the disability rights movement was born. Disabled people have gained rights and access to society. An alternative to pathology-driven explanations for disability has been developed. A new philosophy locates the problems disabled people face externally—as resulting from discrimination, devaluation, and lack of opportunity. A new Disability identity and culture are gradually gaining recognition.

Language is a powerful tool that frames our worldviews and perceptions, often without our realizing it. Language is also constantly evolving. Person-first disability language arose to counter the perception that people with disabilities are defined by their disabilities. As the meaning of disability evolves, so does disability language. Contemporarily, in some circles we are witnessing the embracing of disability-first language as a way to demonstrate disability identity, pride, and Disability culture. We fully expect that disability language will continue to evolve, possibly rendering obsolete the language we use today.

DISCUSSION QUESTIONS

1. How have disability and people with disabilities been perceived throughout history?

2. How have perceptions of disability influenced the treatment of disabled persons in society?
3. What are the similarities between ableism and other isms such as racism and sexism?
4. How did historical views and perspectives of disability, sexual orientation, and race contribute to the Holocaust?
5. The unemployment rates of disabled persons exceed 50 percent in many countries. How do traditional moral and medical models explain the causes of high unemployment rates? How does the social/minority model explain this?
6. What has been the historical reciprocal relationship between the isolation of people with disabilities and ableism?
7. What stereotypes of disability have you witnessed in your life? How have the mass media reinforced this?
8. What are the advantages and disadvantages of the use of person-first language to describe disability? Disability-first language? What are your opinions on person-first versus disability-first language?

PERSONAL NARRATIVE: JUDY HEUMANN

Judy Heumann was assistant secretary for the Office of Special Education and Rehabilitation Services under President Clinton. She has also worked as the World Bank Group's adviser on disability and development. She acquired a disability from polio in 1949 when she was a young girl. She has been a leader in the disability civil rights movement since its early years in the sixties.

As far as disabled people are concerned, I didn't have a lot of role models as I was growing up. That was part of the problem. There weren't a lot of disabled role models out there; we didn't know them. The truth of the matter is from elementary to high school and even through college, I had one teacher with a disability. She was an elementary school teacher, and she had one leg that was four or five inches different in length from the other. Outside of that, I don't remember any disabled people in special positions.

I had one teacher, Mrs. Malikoff; she was a speech pathologist in my elementary school. She didn't have a disability, but she was the only professional who ever really talked to me about a career. I remember her very vividly, saying, "You can be a speech therapist."

President Roosevelt was an important person in my life because I knew that he was disabled and my parents always made sure that I knew that he was. You couldn't get a higher role model than at that level.

As I was growing up, I realized a lot of people influenced my life in different ways. Many were nondisabled civil rights leaders and women's leaders. They were challenging themselves and challenging the system. They had beliefs that they fought for. These role models have ranged from local people in the community to more famous people known at the national and international levels.

As far as disabled people are concerned, I have learned a lot over the years from people like Mary Lou Breslin and Ed Roberts and Kitty Cone and Denise McQuade and Justin Dart. In my lifetime, there has been a very strong emerging movement of disabled individuals who feel common problems and common solutions and feel an identity among each other as a group of disabled people. We have a common agenda, a common vision for what we hope to accomplish, and I think that's been critically important.

When you consider the 49 million disabled people in the United States, I do not know how many of them identify with Disability culture. For those of us who have felt the need to come together and work together, we definitely feel this is a very important part of our lives that has really helped us to improve our individual lives as well as the collective lives of disabled people.

Problems still exist in the United States, and they are many and varied. We don't have a national health care policy, which would guarantee that all individuals, disabled or not, can get health care. Work disincentives exist in policy that result in disabled individuals who are capable and who wish to work being unable to do so. Various policies also make it more difficult for children to be integrated into schools. For example, I personally wish personal attendant services were much easier for people to obtain and that people could get money directly to hire their own personal attendants. I wish personal attendant services were available on a twenty-four-hour-a-day basis. I wish the government would provide easy and direct assistance for things like technology at school and in the workplace. Those types of barriers still limit opportunities for too many people.

I think we're certainly moving ahead on implementing laws like the Individuals with Disabilities Education Act, section 504 of the Rehabilitation Act, and the Americans with Disabilities Act. We're seeing some major structural changes in this country as far as physical barriers are concerned, and I think those changes are quite remarkable and are having a profound effect on both disabled and nondisabled people.

SUGGESTED READINGS

Foucault, M. (2006). *History of madness* (J. Murphy & J. Khalfa, trans.). London: Routledge.

Johnson, A. G. (2006). *Privilege, power, and difference* (2nd ed.). New York: McGraw-Hill.

Johnson, M. (2006). *Disability awareness: Do it right.* Louisville, KY: Avocado Press.

Lifton, R. J. (1986). *The Nazi doctors and the psychology of genocide.* New York: Basic Books.

Longmore, P. K., & Umansky, L. (2001). *The new disability history: American perspectives.* New York: New York University Press.

McRuer, R. (2006). *Crip theory: cultural signs of queerness and disability.* New York: New York University Press.

Riddell, S., & Watson, N. (Eds.). (2003). *Disability, culture and identity.* London: Pearson/Prentice Hall.

Snyder, S., & Mitchell, D. (2006). *Cultural locations of disability.* Chicago: University of Chicago Press.

REFERENCES

Albrecht, G. (1992). *The disability business: Rehabilitation in America.* London: Sage.

Bogdan, R., & Biklen, D. (1993). Handicapism. In M. Nagler (Ed.), *Perspectives on disability: Text and readings on disability* (2nd ed., pp. 69–76). Palo Alto, CA: Health Markets Research.

British Broadcasting Corporation. (1999, May 26). *Health: War transformed attitudes to disability.* Retrieved October 9, 2008, from http://news.bbc.co.uk/2/hi/health/353682.stm

Bryan, W. V. (1996). *In search of freedom: How people with disabilities have been disenfranchised from the mainstream of American society.* Springfield, IL: Charles C. Thomas.

Carrel, A. (1935). *Man, the unknown.* New York: Harper & Brothers.

Condeluci, A. (1996). *Interdependence: The route to community* (2nd ed.). Winter Park, FL: GR Press.

DePoy, E., & Gilson, S. (2004). *Rethinking disability: Principles for professional and social change.* Belmont, CA: Brooks/Cole.

Devore, W., & Schlesinger, E. G. (1999). *Ethnic-sensitive social work practice* (5th ed.). Columbus, OH: Merrill.

Fine, M., & Asch, A. (1993). Disability beyond stigma: Social interaction, discrimination, and activism. In M. Nagler (Ed.), *Perspectives on disability: Text and readings on disability* (2nd ed., pp. 61–74). Palo Alto, CA: Health Markets Research.

Garscha, W., & Kuretsidis-Haider, C. (1997, September). *War crimes trials in Austria.* Presented at the twenty-first annual conference of the German Studies Association, Washington, DC.

Gerber, P. J., Ginsberg, R., & Reiff, H. B. (1992). Identifying alterable patterns in employment success for highly successful adults with learning disabilities. *Journal of Learning Disabilities, 25,* 475–487.

Gill, C. J. (1993). Isolation: Confronting the painful social realities that come with disability. *Mainstream, 18*(1), 18–25.

Hahn, H. (1993). Can disability be beautiful? In M. Nagler (Ed.), *Perspectives on disability: Text and readings on disability* (2nd ed., pp. 217–226). Palo Alto, CA: Health Markets Research.

Jernigan, K. (1999). *The pitfalls of political correctness: Euphemisms excoriated.* Retrieved August 18, 2008, from http://www.blind.net/pg000005.htm

Johnson, A. G. (2006). *Privilege, power, and difference* (2nd ed.). New York: McGraw-Hill.

Johnson, M. (2006). *Disability awareness: Do it right.* Louisville, KY: Avocado Press.

Lambourn, C. (1993). *Together we will make it: People First of New Zealand's song.* Retrieved December 13, 2006, from http://peoplefirst.org.nz/downloads/downloads.htm

Livneh, H. (1980). Disability and monstrosity: Further comments. *Rehabilitation Literature, 41,* 280–283.

Livneh, H. (1982). On the origins of negative attitudes toward people with disabilities. *Rehabilitation Literature, 43,* 338–347.

Longmore, P. (1987). Elizabeth Bouvia, assisted suicide and social prejudice. *Issues in Law and Medicine, 3*(2), 141–168.

Longmore, P. (2003). *Why I burned my book and other essays on disability.* Philadelphia: Temple University Press.

Mackelprang, R. W. (1986). *Social and emotional adjustment following spinal cord injury.* Unpublished doctoral dissertation. University of Utah, Salt Lake City.

Mackelprang, R. W., & Salsgiver, R. O. (1996). People with disabilities and social work: Historical and contemporary issues. *Social Work, 41*(1), 7–14.

McGroarty, M. (1996). Language, attitudes, and standards. In S. McKay & N. Hornberger (Eds.), *Sociolinguistics and language teaching* (pp. 3–46). New York: Cambridge University Press.

McKay, S., & Hornberger, N. (1996). Language and society. In S. McKay & N. Hornberger (Eds.), *Sociolinguistics and language teaching* (pp. 1–2). New York: Cambridge University Press.

Metzler, I. (2006). *Disability in medieval Europe: Thinking about physical impairment during the High Middle Ages, c. 1100–1400.* London: Routledge.

Meyerson, L. (1990). The social psychology of physical disability: 1948 and 1988. In M. Nagler (Ed.), *Perspectives on disability: Text and readings on disability* (pp. 13–23). Palo Alto, CA: Health Markets Research.

Miles, M. (2002). *Community and individual responses to disablement in south Asian histories: Old traditions, new myths?* Stockholm-Johanneshov, Sweden: Independent Living Institute.

Morris, R. (1986). *Rethinking social welfare: Why care for the stranger?* New York: Longmore.

Plato. (1991). *The republic* (Benjamin Jowett, Trans.). New York: Vintage Books.

Rhodes, R. (1993). Mental retardation and sexual expression: An historical perspective. In R. W. Mackelprang & D. Valentine (Eds.), *Sexuality and disabilities: A guide for human service practitioners* (pp. 1–27). Binghamton, NY: Haworth Press.

Riddell, S., & Watson, N. (Eds.). (2003). *Disability, culture and identity.* London: Pearson/Prentice Hall.

Rothman, D. (1971). *The discovery of the asylum: Social order and disorder in the new republic.* Boston: Little, Brown.

Shapiro, J. P. (1993). *No pity: People with disabilities forging a new civil rights movement.* New York: Times Books.

Snow, K. (2008). *To ensure inclusion, freedom, and respect for all, it's time to embrace people first language.* Retrieved August 19, 2008, from http://www.disability isnatural.com/peoplefirstlanguage.htm

Snyder, S., & Mitchell, D. (2006). *Cultural locations of disability.* Chicago: University of Chicago.

Szasz, T. (1977). *The theology of medicine.* New York: Syracuse University Press.

Thomas, L., Wareing, S., Singh, I., Peccei, J., Thronborrow, J., & Jones, J. (2004). *Language, society, and power* (2nd ed.). New York: Routledge.

Wiggam, A. E. (1924). *The fruit of the family tree.* Indianapolis, IN: Bobbs-Merrill.

Wolfensberger, W. (1972). *The principle of normalization in human services.* Toronto: National Institute on Mental Retardation.

Wright, B. (1983). *Physical disability—a psychological approach* (2nd ed.). New York: Harper & Row.

Zola, I. K. (1993). Self, identity and the naming question: Reflections on the language of disability. In M. Nagler (Ed.), *Perspectives on disability: Text and readings on disability* (2nd ed., pp. 15–23). Palo Alto, CA: Health Markets Research.

2

Human Development and Disability

STUDENT LEARNING OBJECTIVES

1. To understand theories of human behavior used by human service professionals
2. To recognize the place of disability in the context of traditional theories of human experience and behavior
3. To understand the impact of disability on human development and human behavior
4. To identify general tasks of people with disabilities in the developmental process
5. To understand some of the implications of disabilities on human development through the life span
6. To recognize that how one understands human identity and behavior influences one's perceptions of disability
7. To be familiar with the social-ecological model of human development

All persons develop as they go through life, and disabilities, whether present from birth or acquired later in life, strongly influence people's lives. Traditional approaches to explaining human behavior, growth, and development of disabled people have focused on (1) the problems people face in coping with disabilities and/or (2) the problems disabled people create for families and as members of society. In this chapter, we briefly review major theories of human development and the place of disability within those approaches. We provide readers with an alternate conceptual framework for understanding life with a disability, introducing you to the *social-ecological model* of human development. We do not assume that disabilities are innately problematic; rather we assume that disabilities are a part of the broader human fabric of society.

TRADITIONAL DEVELOPMENTAL THEORIES

Developmental theories are most commonly used by human services professionals to explain human experience in the social environment. Table 2.1

TABLE 2.1 Developmental Theories

Theorist	Theory Description	Theory Focus
Freud	Psychoanalytic theory	Psychosexual development throughout childhood
Erickson	Ego psychology	Psychosocial stage development from birth through old age
Piaget	Cognitive development	Cognitive rather than emotional development from birth to adulthood
Kohlberg/Gilligan	Moral development	The use of cognition and reasoning involved in moral judgments from childhood to adulthood
Fowler	Spiritual development	Stages of faith development through the life span

summarizes some of the major developmental theories that we explain in detail below.

Psychoanalytic Theory

Freud (1964) believed all development was sexual and tension reducing in nature and focused on the intrapsychic elements of human development. He outlined five stages of development. The oral phase occurs during the first year, when the mouth is the primary source of pleasure. He believed sucking is a primary source of sustenance and satisfaction. The mother's breast, sucking and oral pleasure, and exploration are major libidinal foci during this stage. In the second year, during the anal phase, control becomes important, with a focus on retention and expulsion of feces. Toilet training and regulating reflexive bowel impulses are libidinal foci as the child learns to control the bowel in order to receive parental approval. From years three through six, in the phallic phase, the focus switches to the genitals. The child learns that stimulation of the genitals produces pleasure. Freud believed that female feelings of inferiority to males and penis envy originate in this stage as females learn males have a penis. During this stage, Oedipus and Electra complexes, castration anxiety, and the development of the superego or conscience are key elements. In Freud's fourth phase, latency, occurring in the preadolescent years, the child is seemingly uninterested in sexual matters. Sexual energy is sublimated and directed toward socially acceptable activities. The final stage of development, the genital phase, begins at the onset of puberty as libido dramatically rises. Oedipal and Electra conflicts resurface, and the person directs sexual impulses toward persons of the opposite sex. The person needs to develop new defenses and may become rebellious and withdraw from family to meet psychosexual needs (Newman & Newman, 2006; Rappaport, 1972).

Psychoanalytic theory accents the tensions between intrapsychic and interpersonal worlds and the ways in which people cope with these conflicts (Newman & Newman, 2006); it emphasizes biological processes and internal conflicts. Psychoanalytic theory has been criticized because of its gender bias and devaluation of women (Alpert, 1986; Ellenberger, 1970; Fast, 1984).

Psychoanalytic theory uses persons without disabilities as templates for development. If persons with disabilities are addressed in the context of developmental tasks, they are viewed as the consequence of abnormal development. For example, those whose disability delays bowel and bladder control will experience arrested development. Similarly, persons whose parents provide physical care during the genital phase are susceptible to serious Oedipus and Electra complexes.

Cognitive Theory

Jean Piaget's focus on human development lay within the cognitive realm. He believed people develop cognitive schemas that guide them in organizing their lives and perceiving the world (Piaget, 1985). People are always striving for equilibrium, which allows them to interact effectively with the environment. Adaptation occurs as individuals' thinking evolves in response to new experiences. Piaget viewed cognitive development as occurring in four progressive stages in which children develop new thought structures and integrate them with old competencies. Critical to development are *cognitive schemes* out of which people develop life meanings and organize their worlds. Schemes evolve through assimilation and accommodation. *Assimilation* occurs when problems are solved through the utilization of existing schemes. For example, an infant who cries because it is cold is employing a preexisting schema used to signal hunger. *Accommodation* is the process of developing new schemes out of old ones in response to new problems. Walking and tricycle and bicycle riding are progressive schemes in which new schemes develop and elaborate on preexisting schemes (Rappaport, 1972).

Like Freud's, Piaget's stages of development are confined primarily to the childhood years. In Piaget's first stage, sensorimotor intelligence, which lasts until about one-and-a-half years of age, infants learn to organize and control elements of their environment as they develop increasingly complex sensory and motor schemes. This is manifest in a hungry infant who learns to spit out a rubber pacifier because it has learned that nourishment will not be forthcoming. Stage 2, preoperational thought, begins with language development and continues until about age six. The use of symbolic schemes such as language and "make believe" play are important elements as the child organizes its world. Concrete thinking is prominent at this stage, in which children view things arbitrarily and immediately (for example, "This toy is mine because I have it and I want it"). Children are self-oriented and lack the ability to analyze their thinking processes. Stage 3, concrete operational thought, begins at about age six, continuing to early adolescence. Increasing understanding of causal relationships leads to improved problem solving. Problem solving is concrete rather than abstract and hypothetically related. Stage 4, formal operational thought, begins in adolescence, continuing into adulthood. The ability to understand interconnected variables allows people to develop complex rules and laws to use in problem solving (Newman & Newman, 2006; Rappaport, 1972).

Complementing and building on Piaget, Vygotsky emphasized the social, contextual, and interactional nature of development. In particular, he emphasized the importance of culture and language in shaping thoughts and ideas. A critical cultural element in shaping cognition, according to Vygotsky, is the development and use of tools of human invention. Physical tools include advances such as automobiles and weapons. Psychological tools include languages, alphabets, and coding systems (Miller, 1993; Vygotsky, 1978). Although Vygotsky's work does not specifically focus on disability, the concepts of culture elucidated in this framework are especially important, as persons with disabilities establish language and symbols to enhance culture. Tools are particularly important, as technological advances such as wheelchairs, telecommunication devices, and drugs change the context in which persons with disabilities live and interact with their environment. However, like other developmental theorists, cognitive theorists primarily address problems arising from disability that delay or prevent successful completion of stages and tasks.

Ego Psychological Theory

In ego psychological theory, development occurs in psychosocial stages. Erik Erickson (1963) described eight stages of psychosocial development and ego tasks. Erikson's theories are epigenetic in nature; that is, each stage is dependent on the successful completion of the previous stage (Kail & Cavanaugh, 2004). In the first year the infant experiences the stage of trust versus mistrust. Trust is developed when parents provide a safe and nurturing environment. From one to three years is the stage of autonomy versus shame and doubt. Children begin to forge individual identities and control. The third stage, initiative versus guilt, occurs at age four to five years. In this stage, children exercise increased environmental control. Industry versus inferiority occurs from age six to eleven. School, peers, and an expanding world are important elements of this stage. Identity versus role confusion occurs during adolescence. Dramatic physical and emotional changes occur as people attempt to find meaningful identities as they begin to separate from family. Beginning at about age eighteen to twenty years is stage 6, intimacy versus isolation, which lasts until about age twenty-five. Successfully developing strong intimate relationships is important in this life stage. Generativity versus stagnation comprises the adulthood years from age twenty-five to sixty-five. Success in raising children and developing satisfying work and community activities and relationships is important at this stage. Stage 8, ego integrity versus despair, occurs at sixty-five years and older. In this stage of life, people review their lives and strive for meaning in their retirement years. Erickson believed that stages follow an epigenetic or biological pattern and that development is progressive as people transition from one stage to the next.

Erikson and other ego psychological developmental theorists developed role expectations for women and men heavily based on Western culture and traditional European and American lifestyles. For example, Erickson's stage 8, ego integrity versus despair, was developed in the context of a Western first-world environment, life expectancies, and retirement age. Originally from Germany, Erikson moved to the United States at age thirty-one and developed his theory in the United States, where children began school at age five and adults were expected to retire and receive Social Security benefits at age sixty-five.

Other developmental theorists have expanded on and modified Erikson's work. Following his death, his wife posited a ninth stage of development reflecting increased longevity. Newman and Newman (2006) expanded his psychosocial stages of development from eight to eleven stages by adding a prenatal stage occurring from conception to birth, and a very old stage from seventy-five years of age to death. In addition, they divided adolescence into early and late adolescence. Influenced by Erikson, Maas (1984) developed a nine-stage contextual-developmental-interactional approach to human development throughout the life span that focuses on the "interaction between personal social development and contexts" (p. 4). He acknowledges the negative impact of racism, discrimination, segregation, and lack of community resources on development. Though Maas refers to people with disabilities as patients and in terms of lost competencies, he discussed the need for supportive environments to maximize their capabilities. Luciano L'Abate is a recent theorist who describes human development as the unfolding and development of competencies in home, work, and leisure. He identifies the family as the major explanation for typical and acceptable development in all three contexts (Thomas, 2001). L'Abate (1998, 1999) contends that families and social contexts are the primary determinants of human behavior, arguing that seemingly internal processes such as physiology and psychology are more the outcomes than causes of human behavior.

Ego psychological theorists have primarily viewed development in a nondisabled context, while the healthy development of persons with disabilities has been neglected. They tend to portray people with disabilities in the context of missed or unresolved stages of development arising from their individual pathologies. Though more recent theorists have attended to the importance of external and environmental influences on development, they continue to focus on the problems wrought by disability and the gaps between disabled persons needs and the resources available to them.

Moral Development Theory

Lawrence Kohlberg (1984) was a developmental psychologist who was influenced by Piaget and moved from psychology to the education field. Like Piaget, Kohlberg taught that children advance through developmental stages that are heavily socially influenced; however, unlike Piaget, Kohlberg emphasized moral development and reasoning. He described three levels of development, each with at least two stages (Kohlberg, 1984, 1986; Rich & DeVitis, 1994).

I. Preconventional Level. This level, which is primarily observed in young children, is divided into two stages of moral development. However, Kohlberg also described a third stage, stage 0, in which the child's judgments are egocentric. Subsequent stages are characterized by their social contextual nature.

- Stage 0. The child's judgments are egocentric; right and wrong are determined by what feels good or bad.
- Stage 1. This stage is characterized by "heteronomous morality," in which the moral significance of an act is seen as real and unchanging. Rules are absolute, defined by authority figures, and to be followed to avoid punishment.
- Stage 2. This stage is characterized by individualistic thinking, instrumental morality, and exchange. Individuals are motivated by their own interests, but there also arises awareness that others may have different but equally valid interests. Moral rightness or wrongness is relative and contextual, depending on the situation and actors involved.

II. Conventional Level. Kohlberg believed that this is the level of moral development at which most adults in society typically operate. Moral judgments are made relative to social contexts such as family, in-group, community, and country. Loyalty to others and maintaining social order are valued on their own merits.

- Stage 3: Kohlberg described this stage as characterized by "interpersonally normative morality." Personal morality is determined by one's actions relative to being a good citizen and engaging in pro-social roles and altruistic behavior, and by how positive or negative motives determine one's actions.

- Stage 4. Kohlberg described this stage as involving "social system morality." It has a "law and order" mentality. Morality is based on the premise that social systems have impartially applied rules and procedures that people are obligated to follow to maintain order and consistency.

III. Post-conventional Level. Kohlberg believed this level is achieved by only a minority in society. Moral values are not defined by those in authority, nor by one's standing or identification within a group. Individuals who achieve this level believe that even those who are in the minority or those whose ideas are unpopular or whose status are not valued are to be afforded fundamental rights and opportunities.

- Stage 5. In this stage, the individual values "human rights and social welfare morality." Society is evaluated on how well it promotes the welfare and preserves the rights of its members. Rules and laws are evaluated by how well they promote social good, equality, equity, and reciprocity.
- Stage 6. Kohlberg described this as the final stage of development, in which people adopt the stance that all people are free, equal, and autonomous. The position of the least advantaged is considered in accordance with principles of universality, comprehensiveness, and consistency.

Kohlberg's associate Carol Gilligan developed a moral schema similar to Kohlberg's; however, she departed from him in that she asserted that his approach was male driven and that women's voices are different from those of the dominant male paradigm. She asserts that moral development is gender influenced (though not gender specific) and that females are more likely to be attuned to social responsibility and care for others than to individual rights and justice. Her criticisms of Kohlberg also apply to other theorists such as Piaget, Freud, and Erikson, whose theories, she averred, silenced feminine perspectives in favor of male ways of knowing and thinking. Gilligan believes that theorists' emphases on the individual and on separation rather than on relationships and connection have produced models wherein the apex of moral development is unattainable by the majority of women. Furthermore, she suggests, as do others with similar views, that these theorists' explanations are inadequate and, especially for women, convoluted. Given this perspective, for example, Kohberg's stage 5 is in line with Gilligan's highest stage of moral development (Gilligan, 1982; Gilligan & Attanucci, 1986; Hall, 2002; Rich & DiVitis, 1994).

This feminist critique of traditional developmental theory has implications for disability as well. Traditional developmental theory was developed based on nondisability assumptions and contexts. For example, Irwin (2001) observes that a trio of life-course expectations guides life span theory:

schooling in childhood, independence in adulthood, and later-life retirement. To her three elements, we add a fourth: the expectation that infants and young children are primarily influenced in the context of a family structure. These assumptions have not historically applied to disabled people. Children with developmental disabilities have been removed from family homes and institutionalized from infancy. Deaf children were once sent to deaf boarding schools, which became a source of cultural development, however, one without biological family. Consider the experience of one of the authors as a disabled youth who was institutionalized during his adolescence.

> My parents were convinced that, as an adolescent, I should be institutionalized so they could perform the surgeries and therapy to make my CP-affected limbs function normally. One winter night I organized a group of residents for a "campout" for which we opened a window and slept on the floor. For so doing, I was severely punished.

Moral developmental theory suggests that interpersonal and rule-based morality are important developmental tasks at this stage. However, given an oppressive institutionalized context, breaking rules in an attempt to generate "normal" adolescent experiences may trump any moral responsibility based on social contract or authority.

Spiritual/Religious Theory

Drawing on the work of theorists like Erikson, Piaget, and Kohlberg, Fowler (1981) proposes six stages of faith development. Infants first develop primal faith, which allows them to experience the relative safety of the environment.

- Stage 1. Intuitive-projective faith: From ages two to six, children learn the spiritual language and symbols, such as stories, prayers, and songs, upon which they base their faith.

- Stage 2. Mystic-literal faith: During preadolescence, children learn about collective, communal truths. Myths are accepted as literal truth based on external authority.

- Stage 3. Synthetic-conventional faith: During adolescence, faith conforms to conventional ideology of one's group. Adolescents do not critically evaluate the basis of their faith. Fowler believes most people remain at this level.

- Stage 4. Individuative-reflective faith: Individuals begin a self-reflective process, in which the location of authority is repositioned internally rather than externally. Spiritual beliefs are not defined by one's reference group.

- Stage 5. Conjunctive faith: There is continued reliance on internalized beliefs and acknowledgement of discrepancies between personal and conventional beliefs. Individuals are more tolerant of others' beliefs and extend relationships and service to those who are different.
- Stage 6. Universalizing faith: Fowler teaches that this stage is rare. Individuals search for universal values and embrace altruism and justice over self. Examples include Mother Theresa and Mahatma Gandhi.

In the decades since Fowler first proposed his stages of faith development, others have further developed faith- and religious-based explanations of spiritual development and have developed instruments to measure different levels of attainment (Streib, 2001, 2005); however, most are based on a Western and often Christian frame of reference. A significant limitation of such spiritual conceptualizations for disabled people arises in the place that disability has in cultural views of disability and faith.

As we have discussed, the moral model of disability is rooted in spiritual and religious beliefs. These beliefs are not limited to Western religious and spiritual traditions. Kiev (1969) suggests that disability had a universally negative connotation in early religions. Bryant (1993) avers that Buddhist beliefs suggest that disabled people help nondisabled people to be in touch with mortality, and some Muslims believe that disability arises from the acts of demonic spirits, while Taoism teaches people to honor disabled people because of their effacement and meekness. These creeds all juxtapose disabled people with nondisabled people. When a disabled individual is a member of a community that views disability as resulting from sin, as being out of harmony with nature, as a curse or trial, or as a test for the nondisabled, he or she may be forced to reject or devalue a portion of him- or herself in order to accept the orthodoxy of the church, synagogue, mosque, or other faith community. Conversely, however, spirituality and religion can be a great source of strength and fulfillment for both disabled (Salsgiver, Watson, Cooke, & Madison, 2004) and nondisabled persons alike.

A unique religious disability perspective is described by Bryant (1993), who discusses the creation of L'Arche communities, in which disabled and nondisabled individuals live and work together with dignity. Founded in 1964 by Jean Vanier, a Canadian, to create Christian communities in which people with and without disabilities coexist on equal terms, these communities have expanded to countries like India and welcome people of any faith. L'Arche communities work to liberate disabled people who have been oppressed and rejected by society as well as the nondisabled people who live with them.

THEORIES OF ADAPTATION TO DISABILITY

In contrast to theories that address overall human development throughout the life span, several theories hypothesize time-limited processes focusing specifically on adjustment to disability. Three themes emerge in writings about the adjustment to acquired disability: first, disability and chronic illness are viewed as one construct; second, the literature focuses on the internal psychological processes involved in individual adjustment; and third, adjustment to disability is always a process of overcoming or dealing with loss.

One of the first to write on the subject, Crate (1965) outlined five stages of adaptation to an acquired chronic illness or disability. In stage 1, disbelief, the person denies the disability or minimizes its effects. Stage 2, developing awareness begins as denial cannot be maintained. Anger and depression are common reactions. In stage 3, reorganization, the person further accepts limitations and begins to modify relationships with loved ones. Stage 4, resolution, occurs as the individual comes to grips with loss of function, grieves, and begins to identify with others with the same disability. In stage 5, identity change, the person accepts the disability and modifies behavior accordingly. Subsequent writers have elucidated stages of adjustment that are similar to Crate's (Bray, 1978; Lawrence & Lawrence, 1979). These stages have been developed to help individuals, families, and professionals deal with the "trauma" of disabilities and have focused on psychosocial problems in adjusting. It is important to note how closely these stages of adaptation to chronic illness and disability parallel the stages of adaptation to death and dying formulated by Kübler-Ross (1969): (1) shock and disbelief, (2) anger and resentment, (3) bargaining, (4) depression and sorrow, and (5) acceptance.

Stewart and Rossier (1978) discuss seven dominant personality types that can be used to guide interventions with persons with disabilities, specifically spinal cord injuries. The dependent, overdemanding patient needs boundless care and attention. The orderly controlled patient uses much self-discipline but needs extensive explanations for his or her condition. The dramatic and emotionally engaging patient is warm and well liked but feels easily slighted by lack of attention. The long-suffering and self-sacrificing patient derives self-worth and comfort from suffering. The paranoid patient's belief that others are out to get him or her is validated by the disability. The patient with feelings of superiority is self-centered and feels all powerful. The unloved and aloof patient needs an isolated lifestyle. Human service professionals using this typology would expect problems in adjustment and personality with all patients, as all are defined by their pathology. Healthy, non-pathological personality traits are absent from their descriptors.

Other authors have focused on other aspects of work with persons with disabilities. Rolland (1988, 1989) places chronic illness and disability in three categories: progressive (e.g., diabetes, arthritis), constant (e.g., spinal cord injury, blindness, deafness), and relapsing or episodic (e.g., multiple sclerosis, systemic lupus erythematosis). He also discusses three time phases to which individuals with illness and disabilities and their families must adjust: the initial crisis phase, the chronic phase, and the terminal phase. Rolland focuses on losses, incapacities, and family struggles experienced when people experience illness and disabilities. Again, his focus is on the struggles of life with a disability. Patterson (1988) articulates many difficulties experienced by family members of children with illness and disability. She also discusses the hardships that disabilities produce in the contexts of Piaget's cognitive stages and Erickson's psychosocial stages of development. Though Patterson's focus is primarily on the negative aspects of illness and disability, she concludes that far more is known "about the hardships and demands in families of chronically ill children and how they develop problems than . . . about how they successfully adapt. . . . This focus on successful adaptation is clearly needed" (p. 106).

The last decade of the twentieth century brought an expanded focus on disability and chronic illness adjustment. For example, Kendall and Buys (1998) contend that linear sequential stages of adaptation to disability do not sufficiently address the complex process of disability adjustment that is characterized by recurrent reactions. They suggest that individuals strive for optimal functioning and should be respected as experts on themselves and that both internal and external environmental resources are critical to adjustment. They describe adjustment as a process "characterized by ongoing sorrow" (p. 16); however, their emphasis on environmental resources acknowledges the external factors involved in life with a disability.

Livneh (2001) suggests that the process of adaptation to chronic illness and disability involves three distinct classes of interacting variables. First, antecedents involve triggering events precipitating disability (e.g., trauma, disease, aging) and contextual variables in which the disability occurs (e.g., sudden versus gradual onset, gender, ethnicity). Second, the process of psychosocial adaptation involves personal reactions (e.g., anxiety, depression, and acceptance) and contextual influences (e.g., personality attributes, environmental factors). Third, outcomes are determined by three quality-of-life domains: intrapersonal functioning (e.g., biological and psychological health), interpersonal functioning (e.g., family, peers), and extrapersonal functioning (e.g., work, school, living environment).

Bishop (2005) connects psychosocial adaptation to chronic illness and disability to overall quality of life. Because disability can affect perceived quality of life, people should seek to overcome perceived personal and situational deficits. Responses usually take the form of changes in central life activities, values, roles, and resources. First, Bishop suggests that adaptation and quality of life are positively influenced when people reorder the importance of life domains. For example, an acquired disability can result in the loss of ability to engage in highly valued activities, for instance, when hearing loss makes it impossible to listen to music. Increasing the value of alternate activities such as reading and art can improve quality of life and enhance adjustment. Second, Bishop avers that adaptation is influenced by the amount of control people perceive they have over their lives. For example, some physical impairments may require individuals to rely on attendant care; however, people can retain control over who provides their care, and how and when care is provided. By focusing on overall quality of life, authors like Bishop broaden the focus of life with a disability beyond the problems associated with disability to overall life satisfaction.

The preponderance of adjustment literature focuses on the problems, incapacities, and adjustment problems facing persons with disabilities and their families. While it is important to understand the individual, social, and family dynamics of disabilities, a strong pathological focus creates a number of problems. First, people automatically assume that disability and pathology are synonymous. Disabled people and their families are expected to experience emotional problems such as depression and anxiety. If they do not manifest these psychological problems, they are not perceived as adjusting well. In other words, if emotional difficulties are absent, the person has psychological difficulties. Trieschmann (1980) observes: "Have professionals in clinical interactions placed disabled persons in a 'Catch 22' position? If you have a disability, you must have psychological problems; if you state you have no psychological problems, then this is denial and that is a psychological problem" (p. 46).

Second, when individuals, families, and human service workers focus exclusively on problems and incapacities, they neglect acknowledging and cultivating people's inherent and/or potential strengths. In addition, if persons with disabilities and their loved ones do not adopt the views of professionals, they are at risk of being labeled problematic, in denial, or resistant. They are pressured to internalize pathological views of themselves. When everyone around them views their situation as a tragedy, it is difficult for them to view their situation any differently.

Third, in the tradition of the medical model, most authors view chronic illness and disability as synonymous. Therefore, people with disabilities are sick. Sickness implies a need for professional guidance and control. It implies lack of health. People who are sick deserve sympathy and pity (Mackelprang & Salsgiver, 1996).

While we do not want to minimize the impact of disability on the lives of individuals and families, we approach disability and adjustment from a different perspective. First, we recognize that illness and injury often cause disabilities. However, rather than defining the disability in terms of illness or disease, we define disability by the meaning the disability carries for the individual. People with disabilities are people who experience a disability as part of their lives—not the definition of their lives. Having a disability means difference, not tragedy. Given the opportunity and the resources to perceive disability as difference, families can provide nurturing and validating environments for children with disabilities (Affleck, Tennen, & Gershman, 1985; Summers, Behr, & Turnbull, 1989).

Therefore, as we discuss disability through the life span, we approach developmental processes without assuming there are problems. In presenting these processes, we discuss the psychological-emotional, cognitive, and social tasks and implications of development. Although having a disability influences these processes, it does not define the processes.

DEVELOPMENTAL THEORY IN THE CONTEXT OF DISABILITY

Historically, persons with disabilities have been pathologized or neglected in the developmental literature. When included, they have typically been addressed from an ableist perspective in that the focus is on their individual problems and their impact on families (Gaylord-Ross & Browder, 1991). In contrast, we address the implications of acquiring and/or living with a disability at different times in life given people's social contexts. Rather than proposing a distinct set of stages, we draw on the works of developmental theorists and apply those concepts to people who are living with disabilities in various life stages.

Birth to Three Years of Age

Many disabilities are acquired at birth or soon thereafter. Children with disabilities that are present from infancy or toddlerhood experience their lives differently than persons who acquire disabilities later in life. One of the major implications of disabilities acquired at birth or acquired early in life is that the disability is present before individuals have the cognitive skills to be aware of their disability. Their first experiences are from a disability perspective. Families are aware of the disability from infancy and integrate them. Their earliest memories will be of being treated and perceived as a child with a disability.

Families who are heavily influenced by a medical model approach to caring for their children are likely to treat their child with a disability differently than nondisabled children. Other children grow up in families and communities in which they are treated similarly to children without disabilities rather than as special or deficient. When these children are supported in developmental tasks, they may not perceive their differences as they develop cognitively (Wright, 1983). For these children, increased awareness of disability may come later when their world expands. Some may be surprised by the societal ableism in school and community.

Children with early-onset disabilities may experience more protectiveness than children without disabilities. In infancy, there may be increased contact with parents and other nurturers because of increased needs (Affleck et al., 1985). According to Erickson's framework, this may lead to a strong sense of trust in the environment. On the other hand, if contact with others is painful, as may occur with physical disabilities requiring therapeutic physical touch or surgeries, contact with parents and others may be perceived as unsafe. Mistrust can be especially problematic when separations from family occur due to events such as hospitalization or institutionalization.

Children with sensory disabilities such as deafness and blindness need nurturing that takes into account their disabilities. For example, deaf children may require visual nurturing cues, such as a playpen placed in easy view of the parent to compensate for the lack of auditory cues that let the child know that a nurturer is nearby. Blind children may benefit from increased auditory and verbal stimuli in the environment.

An early developmental task common to all theories is infants' need to gain physical and cognitive control over their environments (Pillari, 1998). Infants with disabilities may have greater difficulty learning to manipulate and control their environments than youngsters without disabilities. Physical limitations may hamper the efforts of some; for example, a child with cerebral palsy may have difficulty shaking a rattle or holding a bottle. Children with intellectual or cognitive disabilities may have cognitive delays that constrain development of language abilities (Longres, 2000). Informed and supportive families and social environments facilitate their development. For example, children in countries that have recently enacted laws that mandate early educational interventions for disabled children in their first three years are showing far greater capabilities than previously thought possible. Vygotsky's (1978) emphasis on tools helps us understand the development of young children with disabilities. Wheelchairs, TTYs, and other adaptive devices are critical tools for children with disabilities as they learn to control their environment at this stage.

Persons with early-onset disabilities and their families are susceptible to environmental problems not faced by children without disabilities (Gallagher, Beckman, & Cross, 1983; Valentine, 1993). First, some parents become protective, sometimes to the extent that their children are unable to successfully meet cognitive and physical developmental tasks appropriate for their ages. With the best of intentions, and often the advice of professionals, parents may do things for their children to the extent that they are not allowed to struggle and to learn from failure and success in controlling their environments. Parents may lack knowledge and skills. It is critical that parents learn the developmental needs of their children with disabilities, develop skills, and obtain the tools to help them successfully meet developmental tasks and learn to control their immediate environments (Davis, 1993).

Second, children with disabilities are at greater risk for experiencing their environment in unpleasant ways. Surgeries, injections, physical therapy, and medications are examples. The touch of others can become frightening and unpleasant. Parents may be forced to restrain their children while they are undergoing unpleasant procedures. Separations from family for hospitalizations may be required. Therefore, efforts to compensate for unpleasant procedures may be needed. Parents may need support in making sure their children receive additional safe contact with others. Environments can be modified to minimize children's fears, and treatments limited to those with maximal value.

Third, children with disabilities may have higher susceptibility to being mistreated and abused than those without disabilities (Garbarino, Brookhouser, & Authier, 1987). Several factors contribute to this. Some children require higher levels of physical contact from others who may exploit them. Some may be less capable of understanding abuse or explaining it when it occurs. Still others may not be believed when abuse occurs.

Fourth, low expectations have traditionally limited children with disabilities significantly. For example, in the past, parents of children with Down syndrome were routinely advised to institutionalize their children in institutions such as training schools, where they were segregated and warehoused. Even the most caring professionals could not compensate for the lack of individual attention and nurturing provided in home environments. Today, children with Down syndrome are reared from birth in family homes, attend mainstream schools, live independently or with support, and work in adulthood.

Increased expectations and opportunities have resulted in vastly improved lives. In homes and living with families, there are more opportunities for bonding and for environmental stimulation and control, which assist children in developmental tasks. It is critical that parents and caregivers understand legal protections and opportunities that are available to their children with disabilities. In the United States, federal legislation such as the Equal Education for All Handicapped Children Act of 1975 and the 1990 Individuals with Disabilities Education Act make services available to children with disabilities from birth, and families can use these resources to access technology, interventions, and supports to aid them in helping their infants and toddlers with disabilities in developing. Other countries have implemented similar laws and policies, as we will discuss in chapter 5.

Three to Six Years of Age

By age three, children's understanding of their symbolic world is increasing rapidly. Words are primary symbols in their lives as language development expands their understanding of the world. Language provides a cognitive scheme for vastly increased communication with others and for increased cognitive sophistication (Lenneberg, 1967; Nelson, 1973; Pillari, 1998). Children begin to develop a sense of right and wrong and begin to shape behaviors in response to others' expectations and needs. Nonverbal language, such as tone of voice, facial expressions, and gestures, which are meaningful from birth, continue to be important. The scope of relationships expands to friends and others past parents, family, and caregivers.

Disabilities can significantly affect this time of development. For example, language development is often different in children with disabilities. Children with intellectual disabilities may experience delays in verbal language skills. They may rely on alternate ways of communicating, such as gestures, nonverbal vocalization, and pictures, developing verbal mastery later than children without intellectual disabilities. Deaf children are responsive to language, but not the verbal language predominant in hearing culture. Visual communication and early attention to sign language are critical to language development for these children (Spencer, Bodner-Johnson, & Gutfreund, 1992). Language comprehension develops visually rather than auditorally. Language articulation is manual rather than verbal. Thus, while language development is different for children with disabilities, supportive environments, sometimes including technological aids, can help them gain skills in symbolic scheme development that Piaget considered important. Their sense of industry in relationship to their environment is enhanced as they learn that their world will respond to their efforts to control their lives. Though traditional developmentalists focus on speech development as the critical task at this age, in reality it is language and communication that are important, not this one form of expression.

Expanding the environment for disabled children is as important as it is for nondisabled children. It is critical that they have the opportunity to interact with others with and without disabilities. To experience their expanding world at this age, children with physical disabilities may require technology such as wheelchairs and physical assistance to go into public. Due to the reactions of others, they may also be compelled to learn how to cope with being different. Successfully doing so permits them to control their lives. Contact with others who have disabilities provides them with the chance to be with others who have similar social experiences and physical perspectives on the world. For example, wheelchair-using children share commonalties that those without disabilities cannot understand. Exposure to peers and role models with disabilities can permit the sharing and cultural development upon which they can build throughout their lives. Playing and interacting with children and others with and without disabilities can provide a foundation for later in life, when disability takes on increased meaning.

Relationships between parents and children at this time of life are changing as children gain independence and increased separateness from others. Children with disabilities may be forced into increased physical closeness with caregivers because of greater physical or other needs; however, they still have these developmental tasks. Therefore, independence and autonomy may be gained in alternate ways. Children needing physical assistance in activities of daily living may develop a sense of separateness by controlling the time and methods of their care. It may be necessary for others to physically assist them, but they can learn about and begin to direct and exercise control over their personal care. They develop a sense of personal separateness as they establish personal body space boundaries.

Two practices that were common in the past severely limited the development of children with disabilities. The institutionalization of children with disabilities isolated them from the larger world and hampered their abilities to develop skills to interact with the larger world. Others were isolated in family homes for protection. These practices deprived children with disabilities of the environments that allow them to develop skills and denied them the opportunity to learn how to meet challenges in society. Fortunately, in recent decades, the deinstitutionalization movement has led to the closure of institutions and to the creation of community resources not available to past generations of disabled children.

Six to Twelve Years of Age

For most children, their world expands greatly at this age. Schools and increased numbers of peers expand their world socially and geographically. Increased concrete problem-solving skills help children deal with new situations. Many children with disabilities are already accustomed to having more people in their lives, especially when they have had ongoing professional involvement. However, now their expanding environment is different. With medical and other professional interactions, they are placed in the passive roles of patients and clients who are needful of remediative interventions. As they enter school settings, they encounter the roles of students and learners. The number of potential peers expands greatly as they come into contact with other students (Pillari, 1998). Relationships with educators may be a new experience (Galbo, 1983). This is a time for much opportunity and for potential problems.

Supportive environments are especially critical at this stage as children take their first major steps away from their families. Educational environments that provide resources to meet the needs of students with disabilities without segregating or stereotyping them are important (Newman & Newman, 2006). Children with learning disabilities may benefit from educational plans that address their specific learning capabilities. Children with physical disabilities may require alternate but equivalent physical education opportunities. It is important to balance the need for integration with other nondisabled students without sacrificing educational needs.

Whenever possible, meaningful contact with other disabled peers is important at this age. Traditionally, young school-aged children with disabilities have been inculcated with a culture that views them as deficient. Because thinking at this age is still concrete, children are susceptible to internalizing messages that they are bad and undesirable. Opportunities to socialize, interact, and learn as equals of peers without disabilities can help dispel some of these misperceptions and prevent internalized ableism. In addition, increased exposure helps nondisabled children perceive children with disabilities as peers and friends rather than tragedies or as "special" people.

A common manifestation of internalized ableism that people with physical disabilities experience at this time of development is body images that are not consonant with their reality. Because they have been subjected to pervasive negative messages about disabilities, it is common for children with disabilities to perceive themselves as nondisabled, denying the presence of the disability. For example, one of the authors dreamed about himself without his disability during childhood. He was sometimes surprised to see himself in a wheelchair in full-length mirrors. The negative connotations of disability influenced him to view himself without his disability. Children who use wheelchairs may visualize themselves as great runners. Some experience the shock of body image dissonance when they see reflections of themselves because their self-images are not the images reflected in mirrors. This is a response among children who may otherwise, with their burgeoning but limited cognitive abilities, be forced to see themselves as undesirable and defective because of society's attitudes toward disability. This phenomenon is similar to children of color who try to wash dark skin white to be acceptable. These are healthy responses in ableist or racist environments. These children see themselves as acceptable; however, their characteristics are unacceptable. Therefore, to develop and preserve a positive self-image, they try to mold themselves to conform with approved images.

A challenge for providing supportive environments for children with disabilities at this age is determining the optimal exposure to people from different backgrounds. Contact with others with disabilities can be extremely critical. For example, deaf people have been greatly aided in developing culture and solidarity from contact with each other. For some, early contact occurred in deaf schools and residential centers for deaf and hard-of-hearing people. These contexts allowed them to experience lives in which deafness was the norm, not inferior. However, "special" programs can isolate people and deny them other opportunities. For example, nursing homes and institutions for people with physical and intellectual disabilities as well as mental health disabilities have been closing down in large numbers. Once commonplace, they are now seen as archaic and isolating. More children with disabilities are living in homes and are being educated in regular schools and classrooms. The isolationist wisdom of the past has been replaced by wisdom of considerable integration.

An important issue for children with disabilities at this time of development is the age of onset of disability. Children with early-onset disabilities know nothing else. By the time they reach this age, families have generally organized their lives and adjusted emotionally to the child's disability. Onset of disability at this time of life can be especially confusing. For example, some forms of muscular dystrophy may not be diagnosed until this age.

Children can become confused and frustrated at changes taking place in their bodies. For example, children with muscular dystrophy may face progressive physical limitations and physical restrictions that are distressing. Families experience the crises of uncertainty during evaluations and diagnostic procedures. Self-concept is modified in response to disability. Family and social relationships are altered. Grief and mourning can be experienced by the child and family. Financial resources can be strained, and support systems taxed (Valentine, 1993).

Onset of disability at this age presents children with cognitive, emotional, and social changes that those born with disabilities do not experience. On the other hand, children who acquire disabilities during childhood have advantages. They have not been limited by discriminatory attitudes and practices from birth. Thus, early personality development and positive self-concepts can be valuable as they cope with changes brought about by disability. For example, Ed Roberts reported that the street skills he developed before becoming disabled by polio provided life skills he drew on after the onset of his disability (Shapiro, 1993).

Twelve to Eighteen Years of Age

The search for personal identity and the meaning of life is a major element in the lives of adolescents. Physical, emotional, and social changes, beginning with puberty, must be coped with by adolescents. Sexual development and feelings burgeon during this time of life (Brooks-Gunn & Reiter, 1990; Tanner, 1990).

Adolescents with disabilities experience the same changes as those without disabilities; however, development is sometimes complicated by the social environment. A common adolescent developmental task is the need to separate from family and find one's own sense of unique identity (Pillari, 1998). Individuals whose parents provide physical care can be hampered in this separation. Ambivalence and conflict can result between parent and adolescent when adolescents need parents to assist with activities of daily living but resent the need for parents to provide intimate care. Technological aids and attendants can sometimes alleviate the need for intimate physical parent-child contact, but attendants can complicate family relationships. Their assistance may be appreciated, but they may also usurp traditional family caregiving roles and produce ambivalent responses.

Identity development for disabled persons is sometimes complicated by the problems concomitant to disability. For some, the extra time and effort needed to get through the day can deplete energy they might otherwise expend in age-appropriate activities. Ongoing relationships with disabled peers and role models, non-ableist portrayals of persons with disabilities, and an environment that values their disabilities can be critical to their development of disability-affirming self-images and rejection of shame-based identities (Longres, 2000). People in the lives of all adolescents, including families, friends, counselors, and teachers, can all be resources in helping adolescents with disabilities reject the images, stereotypes, and limitations of an ableist society. Supports that facilitate future educational, employment, and living options can provide a sense of hope for the future.

Cognitively, adolescents develop an increased understanding of complex and interconnected societal rules and norms. Historically, people have been forced to accept their disabilities as the cause for the limitations imposed on them by society. With supportive environments and positive identities, they can be better equipped to acknowledge that limitations are often externally imposed rather than internally caused. The sense of right and wrong, developed at earlier ages, also expands to a fuller understanding of right and wrong, justice and injustice. Positive self-identity can help adolescents with disabilities recognize injustices rather than accepting societally imposed ableism.

Developing a positive sexual self-image is an important part of adolescence. As for all youths, this can be problematic for disabled adolescents who do not meet the artificial standards of beauty and physical prowess set by today's media and mainstream culture. Adult role models can help provide a more realistic understanding, and social opportunities facilitate normal sexual development. In families without similarly disabled adults, these role models may need to be found outside the family. Adolescents view themselves as sexual beings when parents and others relate to them assuming they will marry or develop other long-term relationships as adults. Overprotectiveness and avoidance of sexuality and relationships can lead adolescents to internalize messages that they are asexual. Finally, sexual knowledge is critical—both knowledge about sexuality in general and the specific implications of the disability on sexuality. Adolescents need opportunities for self-exploration. In addition, group and educational programs about sexuality and disability can aid positive psychosexual development. For example, one of the authors volunteered with his local center for independent living by writing "Ask Dr. Sex" articles for their newsletter and providing educational groups for disabled youths. The questions and concerns raised by youths with all types of disabilities were very similar to questions typically asked by nondisabled youths of comparable age.

Some adolescents have intimate physical contact with personal care attendants, physicians, nurses, and therapists, and burgeoning sexuality can be influenced by contact with these people. They may experience romantic or sexual feelings toward caregivers and providers. If their bodies are objectified by others during care, therapy, examinations, and other procedures, they may come to view their bodies as asexual. Adolescents (and others) with disabilities are also more susceptible to sexual abuse by providers and others who may take advantage of their vulnerabilities (Andrews & Veronin, 1993; Rhodes, 1993; Sigler & Mackelprang, 1993). Sexual abuse can occur at any age, and environments that discourage victimization and help adolescents (and others) exercise sexual self-determination are important for personal and sexual growth.

People who acquire disabilities as adolescents face added challenges that those who enter adolescence with disabilities do not have. They often carry pre-disability stereotypical ableist attitudes that can hamper acceptance of a disability. Families can be thrown into crisis. Sometimes pre-disability friendships are lost, and they may be forced to find alternate peers and activities. For example, listening to music may be impossible for people who lose their hearing, and adaptive sports may be required for persons who acquire physical disabilities. Developing an identity with a disability can be difficult and produce confusion, especially in the months following onset. Therefore, supportive environments that account for adolescent developmental needs and that are disability affirming are important. Opportunities to maintain friendships and family relationships as well as develop new peer and mentor relationships can aid significantly in this process.

Young Adulthood

Transitions from adolescence to adulthood can be influenced by laws and policies. For example, in the United States, once people graduate from high school or reach age twenty-two, they are no longer covered by laws that mandate schools to provide services to which disabled individuals are entitled. In a study of disabled youths and young adults up to age twenty-two years, respondents reported life satisfaction similar to that of the nondisabled reference group. However, post–high school respondents who were no longer entitled to benefits mandated by the Individuals with Disabilities Education Act reported dramatically lower levels of employment than the nondisabled group (Altshuler, Mackelprang, & Baker, 2008; Mackelprang & Altshuler, 2004).

Disability can present other challenges as people move into adulthood. Families of origin lose legal and often physical control and responsibility. This is a time when primary intimate relationships shift from families of origin to families and loved ones in the making. Young adults' abilities to successfully meet the challenges of this time of life can depend on how successfully families have prepared them to launch adult lives. Individuals whose disabilities necessitate ongoing care and support find that independence may mean that they take control of from whom, what, and how care is provided. For some, it means that they become employers of caregivers. Adequate supports are critical to this transition. Too often, adults with disabilities have been relegated to large institutions such as nursing facilities because less restrictive environments are unavailable. Social structures and priorities are especially important for adults with disabilities who rely on social supports for independence. Allocating resources to communities rather than institutions provides greater access to a variety of living options. Deprofessionalizing services and redirecting resources to the control of individuals allows people who use attendants to hire and direct personal attendants rather than being dependent on others to control how and from whom they receive care. Directing resources for people with mental health, intellectual, and physical disabilities to isolated, self-contained settings fosters dependence, whereas directing resources to the community provides more options and greater self-determination.

At this time of life, people search for intimacy with others. Historically, people with disabilities have been denied opportunities for intimate relationships. For example, people with intellectual disabilities have been legally enjoined from marrying (Rhodes, 1993). Some have been forcibly sterilized, sometimes without their knowledge. People with disabilities living in institutions, including persons with mental health and physical disabilities, have been denied access to intimate relationships with others. To successfully meet the challenges at this time of life, barriers to intimacy must continue to be removed. Given the opportunity, persons with disabilities are increasingly entering into intimate relationships with both disabled and nondisabled people. These include persons with mental retardation who are marrying, and with adequate supports, they can successfully raise children (Whitman & Accardo, 1993).

To prevent isolation, young adults depend on adequate resources. For persons with disabilities, job and education opportunities and access to transportation and technology may be especially important (Murphy & Murphy, 1997). Without these, dependence and lack of control are likely to result. For example, unemployment among persons with disabilities is rampant in large measure because of current laws. For instance, young people with spinal cord injuries are often unable to work because employment income would terminate federal medical benefits that are critical to their ongoing health. Entering the workforce would raise their income to a level that would disqualify them for benefits such as Medicaid. Thus, if they work, they lose medical coverage for expenses that can cost hundreds of dollars per month. Consequently, they are forced to live on Supplemental Security Income and/or Social Security Disability Insurance rather than enter the workforce.

Young adulthood is a time during which disabled persons can continue to use role models to develop Disability culture and pride. At the same time, they are shapers and developers of Disability culture for those who follow. In addition, given the opportunity and right, they can help dispel common myths that perpetuate ableist societal views. This further prepares them for the roles of parents of children with and without disabilities who, in turn, have parents with disabilities who are capable of providing love and nurturing.

People who acquire disabilities in young adulthood generally have the majority of their lives to live. Most have already developed personalities and self-images. A new disability, however, can force changed self-image and modify intimate relationships. Newly formed intimate relationships such as recent marriages can be especially vulnerable if one of the partners acquires a new disability. Community supports such as centers for independent living, equal educational and employment opportunities, and professional and peer supports can help people who acquire disabilities successfully integrate changes personally and can assist families who undergo the changes precipitated by an acquired disability. Accepting the disability and embracing the social and cultural elements of one's new life situation can help make this time of life successful.

Middle Adulthood

Middle adulthood is a time of expanded interests and options. Persons with disabilities in their forties and fifties with families continue to invest time and energy in them, but their focus can extend outward to community and others. Generating legacies and contributing to society are elements of this time of life. As people journey through middle adulthood, they are more likely to have the stability to expand their interests outward than previously (Erickson, 1963; Maas, 1984).

Persons with disabilities in their middle years have been instrumental in developing a burgeoning Disability culture and in changing the political and legal landscape for those who follow. Some persons with disabilities in middle adulthood are contributing at the local level by influencing entities such as school boards, municipal governments, and community organizations. Others, such as Mary Lou Breslin, Evan Kemp Jr., and the late Justin Dart, have contributed on a more sweeping scale by influencing national and international policies. Whatever the scope of their influence, disabled persons in middle adulthood can receive personal satisfaction by acting as role models and using their influence for the benefit of future generations. In addition, national leaders with disabilities, such as Franklin Roosevelt and Bob Dole, have contributed to enhancing positive perceptions of people with disabilities. Finally, disability advocates, especially disabled activists, have also contributed to society by leading the move to expanded rights and opportunities (Shapiro, 1993).

Middle adulthood is a time of life when large numbers of people begin to acquire age-related disabilities as a result of conditions such as diabetes or heart disease. Traditionally, people who acquire disabilities at this age usually have not identified with a general culture of Disability. If they have maintained their identities as nondisabled persons who have problems, they can benefit from an accurate understanding that acquiring a disability need not be shameful or tragic. Learning to live with and integrate changes into their lives is important. Finding meaning and growth from acquiring a disability may be helpful. Networking with others who are successfully living with similar disabilities can be an excellent way to facilitate this.

Persons with disabilities, whether newly acquired or long term, can be a great asset to the community. The maturity and stability that come at this time of life provide them greater opportunities to influence communities and society. As the number and visibility of persons with disabilities in middle adulthood increase, so can their societal contributions and legacies to the disability community as well as society in general.

Older Adulthood

A common label in the U.S. disability community for persons without disabilities is "TAB," an acronym for "temporarily able-bodied." By old age, most people have acquired impairments from a variety of conditions that may lead to disabilities. Visual, hearing, and physical disabilities are common. Anyone who lives long enough will acquire some type of disability in life. Most who acquire late-life disabilities do not identify with Disability culture; however, resources and supports are important to persons in the last stages of their lives. Ageism as well as ableism can endanger full lives when they manifest in attitudes and social policies. Without supports, the risks for despair and hopelessness increase (Erickson, 1963; Maas, 1984).

Persons who have lived lives with disabilities can be better prepared for the problems attendant to old age than those who acquire them late in life. Their life experiences may have prepared them to deal with social systems that are important to meeting their needs. However, they may also be more susceptible to a myriad of problems as a result of their long-term disabilities. For example, people who have had polio are susceptible to post-polio syndrome, which significantly diminishes strength and endurance. Long-term wheelchair users may experience shoulder deterioration from wear and tear as a result of pushing their chairs.

As people enter older adulthood, self-determination and the opportunity to contribute are important (Newman & Newman, 2006). Independence, whether physical or in directing others who provide care, is important to help maintain ego integrity. As in other stages, supportive environments are critical to successful lives in older adulthood.

Social policies can be critical to the well-being of older persons who acquire disabilities and their families. Policies that allow people who need physical assistance to live in the community rather than being relegated to nursing facilities are important. Too many older Americans are institutionalized because resources that could help them live in the community are targeted for high-cost institutional care that allows residents little self-control. Policies that foster independent living contribute to high-quality lives.

Other social supports that allow people to acquire physical aids such as therapies and durable equipment (e.g., wheelchairs, walkers) without impoverishing them are critical in helping maintain independence. Adequate access to tools that promote independence and allow older persons with disabilities to control their lives and exercise self-determination can help change the meaning of older adulthood. At no age is this more important than in older adulthood.

End-of-life decisions and policies are especially important for older persons with disabilities. Older persons need to maintain control over decisions; however, there is much controversy in society regarding these end-of-life decisions. For example in 1997, the state of Oregon legalized physician aid in dying. Shortly thereafter, the Netherlands formally legalized euthanasia, which had been practiced for decades. Other countries have enacted similar measures. These measures have been advocated to ensure self-determination; however, they have been formulated in a society that devalues old age and disability. Supportive environments can help people find value in their lives and make end-of-life decisions, consider health care directives, and complete living wills based on their needs and not out of any duty to "get out of the way" or reduce their burden on society (Mackelprang & Mackelprang, 2005).

Contemporary developmental theories have generally either ignored disability or conceived of disability from a pathology framework. To affirm lives with disabilities, a shift in perceptions that considers the implications of living with a disability as a normal part of life is needed. We recognize the fact that acquiring a disability may require adjustment; however, we eschew focusing exclusively on the problems that disabilities cause for individuals and families. The developmental tasks and needs of persons with disabilities and their families mirror the needs of persons without disabilities. However, as with all diversity, there are considerations and needs that are more typical for disabled persons than nondisabled persons.

THEORIES OF HUMAN DEVELOPMENT RELATED TO IDENTITY

The disability movement has much in common with other social justice and diversity movements based on group identity. Many of these groups have been subjected to devaluation and discriminatory practices, in part based on their perceived inferiority or deficiencies. Theoretical approaches to group identity include feminism, which bases its analyses on gender; Marxism, with its emphasis on social and economic class; racially based theories; and queer theory. The emphasis of these approaches attends to devalued and underclass groups in society, which thus have much in common with disability activists. However, a review of these theories suggests that they share a tendency to define disability as a pathological condition rather than a form of diversity. These attitudes have been present from antiquity, as evidenced by Plato's (1991) assertion that disabled children should be put out to die. Groce (1999) contends that all known societies have developed complex, and often pathology-based, systems of beliefs and practices concerning disability. In this section, we discuss a variety of theories that categorize people by their characteristics. We begin with a brief review of evolutionary and economic theories, then focus on theories based on categories such as gender, ethnicity, and sexual orientation.

Evolutionary Theory

Charles Darwin's groundbreaking nineteenth-century work on evolution posited that conditions such as natural selection lead to ever-adapting and evolving species. Darwin believed that natural processes lead to evolutionary gains and used primitive cultures and intellectually disabled individuals as lesser-evolved examples of development, and white males as the apex of the evolutionary chain (Darwin, 1859, 1871; Snyder & Mitchell, 2006). Though Darwin believed in natural selection, eugenicists of the nineteenth and twentieth centuries advocated active social engineering, in which classes and races designated inferior were to be controlled through the discouragement of reproduction, and through policies such as race laws. In addition, disabled people were to be eliminated by measures such as the outlawing of marriage; institutionalization; forced sterilization; and, in the case of Nazi Germany, genocide.

Economic Theories

Industrial societies of the eighteenth through twenty-first centuries determined that people's value is directly related to their contributions to society, most often in the form of economic outputs. Marxism can be considered a liberation-based ideology that views the bourgeois as oppressing the proletariat in the pursuit of economic gain. *The Communist Manifesto* states, "The modern bourgeois society that has sprouted from the ruins of feudal society has not done away with class antagonisms. It has but established new classes, new conditions of oppression, new forms of struggle in place of old ones. . . . It has simplified class antagonisms. Society as a whole is more and more splitting up into two great hostile camps, into two great classes directly facing each other—bourgeoisie and proletariat" (Marx & Engels, 1848, p. 1). Marx asserted that a high number of disabled people in industrial society was indicative of the corruption inherent in capitalism. Marx and his colleagues argued that the abolition of capitalism would help eliminate the tragedy of disability wrought by poor and inhumane working conditions.

Capitalists argue with Marxism that they value and reinforce the economic contributions of the wage-earning class, as evidenced by their pay and benefits. For example, in capitalist economies, employees have contributed to retirement benefits, and in the United States, wage earners have been provided health insurance through employment (though this practice is eroding and lack of insurance is becoming an ever greater problem). Working for wages earns people status and provides monetary benefits that non-workers are denied. Parents who choose to work in the home rather than in the competitive workforce are ineligible for Social Security benefits and Medicare should they become disabled and unable to work. Disabled people who have not had the opportunity to work and pay taxes are also ineligible. To qualify for these benefits, one must have a substantial work and tax-paying history. One's value is directly related to one's history as a taxpayer, while the contributions of those who are not members of the workforce are devalued. Of course, the upper classes are afforded the greatest value in capitalist society, as they are afforded special privileges and status as a result of their perceived contributions. In contrast, the high unemployment rate and low income of disabled persons places them in the most vulnerable of socioeconomic positions.

Feminism and Gender-Related Theories

Feminism, which views the human condition through the lens of gender, has contributed the foundations for the empowerment of women. However, feminism has traditionally distanced itself from disability. Early feminists such as Charlotte Perkins Gilman and Margaret Sanger equated disability with corruption and scourge and posited that women who were forced into the domestic sphere and denied education produced deteriorating and infe-rior—that is, disabled—offspring (Snyder & Mitchell, 2006). Much of the feminist and disability discourse has come from Europe. Morris (1993) discusses her experiences in Great Britain and how nondisabled feminists have ignored women with disabilities or have taken anti–disability rights stances relative to the pro-choice/pro-life debate. Waldschmidt (2006) addresses disability and feminism in Germany. She points out that feminists have argued for women's rights for reproductive control while ignoring problems such as genetic selection. Disabled women have recently added to the discourse, albeit with controversial voices. For example, they have argued for women's right to choose but have criticized as naive feminists who do not understand that medical advances such as the routine use of genetic diagnostics are invasive for women and are anti-disability as well. She cites the 1992 work of Degener and Kobsell, who argue that prenatal genetic testing is a form of eugenics and that choosing to terminate an unwanted pregnancy is funda-mentally different from choosing to terminate a pregnancy based on prenatal diagnostics.

Morris (1992) states that feminism needs to add the voices of disabled and older women to its discourse. She suggests the mantra that "The personal is political" is an impediment to including disabled voices in feminist dialogue. "Disabled people—men and women—have little opportunity to portray our own experiences within the general culture—or within radical political movements. Our experience is isolated, individualised; the definitions which society places on us centre on judgements of individual capacities and personalities. This lack of voice, of the representation of our subjective reality, means that it is difficult for non-disabled feminists to incorporate our reality into their research, their theories, unless it is in terms of the way the non-disabled world sees us" (p. 161).

In recent years, disability has become increasingly incorporated into women's and feminist dialogues (Smith & Hutchinson, 2004; Waldschmidt, 2006). Lloyd (1992) argues that the women's movement has neglected disabled women and that the disability movement has attended to men's issues while neglecting women. She draws upon the experience of black feminism and the social model of disability to provide a model for disabled women to reframe their disability and gender experiences. Overall (2006) discusses how the social constructions of characteristics such as gender, old age, and disability perpetuate the mechanisms used for discrimination. Garland-Thomson (2002) articulates four civil rights–based domains for integrating feminist disability theory into feminist theory based on parallel mechanisms of devaluation. First, females and disabled persons in contemporary society are considered non-normative and deficient. In fact, she points out that all women's bodies have been portrayed as handicapped in a sexist society. The second area of analysis is the body and the politics of appearance. This involves two components: the politics of appearance and the medicalization of the bodies of women and disabled persons. The third area of consideration is identity. Feminism has increasingly emphasized the multiple characteristics and identities that women hold. Cultural stereotypes often consign women to dependent roles and further define disabled women as asexual, removing them from the spheres of femininity and beauty. The fourth domain is activism, including traditional feminist disability activism, such as breast cancer awareness as well as the protests of groups such as Not Dead Yet, which opposes assisted suicide. She also notes that the contributions of disabled people in areas such as fashion are a form of activism and illustrates her point by discussing Aimee Mullins, an athlete and fashion model who is also a double amputee. Mullins makes no attempt to hide her prosthetic legs yet was voted one of *People Magazine*'s fifty most beautiful people in 1999. Recent scholars and feminist activists are leading to evolving perceptions about disability that are dramatically different from the ideas of a century ago.

Queer Theory

Unlike homosexuality, which has been accepted and celebrated in some societies such as ancient Greece, disability has rarely had similar societal acceptance. Conversely, in countries such as the United States, gays and lesbians are often denied basic civil rights. Even so, disability and homosexuality share much in common relative to their places in Western civilization and contemporary society. The moral model of disability and homosexuality is shared by Christianity, Judaism and Islam, and Baha'i. In several Middle Eastern countries, homosexual relations are a capital offense. As discussed in chapter 4, disability has also been considered morally repugnant. The medical model has permeated beliefs about both disability and homosexuality. Controversies abound relative to how to prevent and "cure" both characteristics. Some consider homosexuality to be an impairment or disability. Some gays and lesbians intentionally distance themselves from disability; likewise, some disabled people carry heterosexist attitudes. When LeVay (1991) published research about brain differences between homosexual and heterosexual men, he was criticized by religious conservatives, who claimed he was sanctioning sinful behavior. Concomitantly, he was condemned by gay rights activists, who accused him of legitimizing the argument that homosexuality is a biologically based disability and felt that his research would promulgate attempts to prevent or cure homosexuality. Friess (2000) provides evidence of heterosexism in the Deaf community by describing some of the pejorative signs deaf people use for gays and lesbians.

In some ways the gay/lesbian and disability communities have commonalities that make them distinct from other groups. Unlike members of other groups, disabled and homosexual youths are usually raised by nondisabled and heterosexual parents and families, who can also have ableist and heterosexist attitudes. Disability is described, especially by nondisabled persons, with euphemisms such as "differently abled" and "physically/mentally challenged." Thus, adopting a disability identity becomes even more difficult when disabled people are not exposed to disability-affirming language. The terms *gay* and *lesbian* have been adopted as descriptors for homosexuals who embrace their sexual orientation. Terms such as *queer* and *cripple*, previously used as negative descriptors, are now commonly used by gays and lesbians and by disabled people, respectively. However, some organizations, such as the North American Association of Research and Therapy of Homosexuality, are devoted to "curing" homosexuals. Some religious groups refuse to acknowledge homosexuality as an attribute, choosing euphemisms such as "same-sex attraction." Some who acknowledge that homosexuality may have a biological component equate it with congenital disabilities and suggest that intrauterine medical treatment can be used to cure both (Associated Press, 2007).

Disability and queer activists, educators, and theorists are increasingly bridging the gaps and finding connections between the two groups. The research of Mackelprang, Ray, and Hernandez-Peck (1996) describes similarities in acceptance of the two groups in higher education. Onken and Mackelprang (1997) discuss the similarities in the process of coming out that gays and lesbians share with people who are born with or acquire disabilities at a young age. Colligan (2004) addresses the intersections between disability studies, sexual identity, and queer theory. Fox (2004) investigates disability and queerness in the arts. Sandahl (2006) discusses the intersection between gay, disability, and feminist performance art. McRuer (2006) contends that queerness and disability share cultural connections. He also contends that disabled people share with gays and lesbians the invisibility that arises when people assume they are able-bodied and heterosexual. His chapter "Crip Eye for the Normative Guy" invites readers to imagine how the popular television show *Queer Eye for the Straight Guy* might play out if five disabled people helped inept nondisabled persons navigate the world.

Racial/Ethnic Theory

Multiple, sometimes conflicting perspectives currently guide conceptualizations of race and ethnicity. At one end of the spectrum, race and ethnicity are defined as distinct biological classifications. At the other end, physical anthropologists and social scientists aver that race and ethnicity have little biological relevance but are primarily social cultural constructions. We believe that, like disability, race and ethnicity are multifaceted and fall along a biological-social continuum. While all societies have established beliefs and rules relative to disabled persons (Groce, 1999), our discussion focuses on the intersections between dominant and minority racial/ethic groups and disabled persons.

Eugenicists viewed non-white racial groups as genetically inferior and defective—in essence, disabled. Wiggam (1924) discusses a common early twentieth-century belief that poor "blood" "has cost the lives of families and empires. It has cost America a large share of its labor troubles, its political chaos, many of its frightful riots and bombings—the doings and undoings of its undesirable citizens. Investigation proves that an enormous proportion of its undesirable citizens are descended from undesirable blood overseas. America's immigration problem is mainly a problem of blood. For over a generation America has been changing her blood" (p. 6).

Wiggam makes it clear that the blood of defective non-northern European whites is the cause of woes—and that being non-white is a de facto impairment or disability. He considers racial minorities and disabled persons threats to society—stereotypes that exist contemporarily. Colonialist European practices were based on a racist foundation that considered colonized people and cultures inferior to white attributes and values. Kipling's 1899 "White Man's Burden" portrays non-whites as sick, unhealthy, and slothful savages. Non-whites and disabled persons have been stereotyped as hypersexual and likely to engage in rape and promiscuous sexual behaviors (Snyder & Mitchell, 2006; Wiggam, 1924). Racist and ableist connections of "inferior" races to disability have motivated a disconnection between ethnic identity and disability. Lukin (2006) discusses the parallel natures of racism and ableism, while acknowledging that the U.S. civil rights movement ignored black disabled people as a group, while disabled activism has ignored disabled people who are non-white. Thus, Lukin contends, disabled blacks have had little context to claim dual identities. We suggest that others considered to be racial minorities have experienced similar ethnic-disability identity disconnections.

Gould (1996) traces the numerous ways in which common nineteenth- and twentieth-century biological explanations have been used to diminish and discriminate against many racial groups, such as the measurement of skull size and the use of facial characteristics to determine the genetic inferiority of non-whites attempting to immigrate to the United States. Contemporary geneticists explain genetic differences with more caution than eugenicists of the past, not equating difference with deficiency. Cavalli-Sforza (2000) explains that there are genetic differences in populations arising from the African diaspora 50,000–100,000 years ago, and that the world's population can be divided into five genetic groups: African, Oceanic, Asian, European, and American. However, Cavelli-Sforza and others also contend that the magnitude of genetic differences is far greater within populations than between populations—that all populations carry the same genes, but in differing proportions (Foster & Sharp, 2002; Krieger, 2005).

Social constructionists reject biologically based explanations of race. For example, the position statement of the American Anthropological Association (1988) states:

> Historical research has shown that the idea of "race" has always carried more meanings than mere physical differences; indeed, physical variations in the human species have no meaning except the social ones that humans put on them. . . . [Race] subsumed a growing ideology of inequality devised to rationalize European attitudes and treatment of the conquered and enslaved peoples. Proponents of slavery in particular during the 19th century used "race" to justify the retention of slavery. The ideology magnified the differences among Europeans, Africans, and Indians, established a rigid hierarchy of socially exclusive categories underscored and bolstered unequal rank and status differences, and provided the rationalization that the inequality was natural or God-given. The different physical traits of African-Americans and Indians became markers or symbols of their status differences.

Let us consider the intersection of biological and social conditions. The amount of melanin, which affects skin color and provides the body protection from the sun's damaging rays, is directly related to proximity to the equator. Darker skin protects people from the harmful effects of the sun, while lighter skin allows for greater synthesis of vitamin D, which became increasingly important as populations migrated toward the poles. (In addition, the diets of people who live nearer the poles have traditionally consisted of greater amounts of meat, which also provides the body with vitamin D.)

Skin color and ethnic identity, even contemporarily, have far greater social than biological significance. Similarly, the social perceptions of disability are primary in defining disabled lives. In the United States, blacks were at one time considered to have 60 percent of the worth of whites. Disabled persons have often been consigned to institutions and isolated in homes. People have struggled to win the rights of minority peoples—often those of color—while the independent living movement has been fought for disability rights. Much of the unrest in countries around the world today is racially and ethnically motivated. Apartheid in South Africa was abolished only in this generation, and inequities are still abundant. The 1994 Rwandan genocide of more than 500,000 Tutsis by ethnic Hutus was based ostensibly on racial differences. Though genetically indistinguishable, the slaughter of the Tutsis (often referred to as "cockroaches" by the Hutus) was justified by what are believed to be their inferior attributes. In 2005, demonstration and civil unrest in Paris, France, and Sydney, Australia, and in other countries were directly tied to social conditions and economic depression of people from North Africa, who are easily distinguishable by their skin color and Muslim beliefs. Today, the ethnic cleansing of blacks in the Darfur region of Sudan is being perpetrated by the Sudanese Janjaweed militia. Several studies demonstrate that health disparities, traditionally explained as arising from race, are much better explained through a lens of poverty and discrimination (Krieger, 2005; Krieger, Chen, Waterman, Rehkoph, & Subramanian, 2005; Mustillo, Krieger, Gunderson, Sidney, McCreath, & Keafe, 2004).

Racial, ethnic, and cultural identities are influenced by a combination of biological and social factors. During the last three hundred years, populations have become much less isolated and less distinct. Culture arises from a combination of the interaction between common progenitors, the communities and societies in which people reside and develop identities, and the processes by which people come to see themselves as members of specific groups. Disabled persons are members of all racial and ethnic groups.

We now introduce you to one conceptualization of value development based on culture. Based on the research of Kluckholm and Stodtbeck (1961) on ethnic and cultural groups in the United States, it was developed as a lens for viewing ethnic families in therapy (McGoldrick, 1982; McGoldrick, Pearce, & Giordano, 1982). Labeled value orientation theory, it is posited by McGoldrick as an ecologically based taxonomy by which people from one ethnic background can gain an understanding of the orientations of people from differing backgrounds based on the five life dimensions listed below.

I. Time: the temporal focus of human life
    1. Past: importance of personal and family history and prior learning
    2. Present: importance of here and now (one need not worry about tomorrow)
    3. Future: sacrificing today for an enhanced tomorrow

II. Activity: preferred pattern of action in interpersonal relations
   1. Doing: emphasis on working hard, achieving to attain goals and rewards
   2. Being: taking life as it comes (it is enough to exist)
   3. Being in becoming: develop one's inner self, achieving self-actualization

III. Relational: the preferred way of relating in groups
   1. Individual: self-determination and independence in thought and action
   2. Collateral: connecting with significant others to deal with life's issues
   3. Lineal/hierarchical: vertical, relying on leaders and followers

IV. Humanity/nature: the ways people relate to nature or supernatural environments
   1. Harmony with nature: coexistence of people and nature
   2. Mastery over nature: seeking challenges to overcome or conquer
   3. Subjugation to nature: influence of external forces such as karma or a deity on life

V. Basic nature of humanity: attitudes about the innate good or evil of human behavior
   1. Neutral/mixed: One is not born good or bad but is influenced by environment and life choices.
   2. Good: People are born inherently good and have a good basic nature.
   3. Evil: People are basically born corrupt and need redemption to change.

Fernandez and Marini (1995) and Fernandez and Freer (1996) further expanded the values orientation framework to posit choices across ethnic groups and disabled persons in U.S. society. This framework was developed in the United States and influenced by the societies of ancestral origin. On the time dimension, they suggest that African Americans' present orientation is related to the lack of life control they have experienced historically, beginning with slavery and continuing with racism and lack of opportunity. They suggest that Asian Americans' past orientation is related to spiritual traditions of ancestral worship, while Latino Americans' past orientation is influenced by a strong attention to family tradition and honor. In contrast, Native Americans' present orientation is connected to a cultural emphasis on the cyclical and rhythmic nature of life. The disability present orientation is based on the need to survive in the present. This taxonomy suggests that culture affects first-, second-, and third-order choices for groups. The first-order choices of value orientations of these groups are illustrated in table 2.2.

TABLE 2.2 First-Order Choices across Ethnicities and Cultures

	European American	African American	Asian American	Hispanic American	Native American	Disabled Individuals
Time	Future	Present	Past-Present	Past-Present	Present	Present
Activity	Doing	Doing	Doing	Being in becoming	Being in becoming	Being
Relational	Individual	Collateral	Collateral	Collateral	Collateral	Individual
Humanity/Nature	Mastery	Harmony	Harmony	Harmony	Harmony	Subjugated
Basic Nature	Neutral	Neutral	Good	Neutral	Good	Good

The values orientation model provides a framework for understanding similarities and differences between the cultural values of different groups of people. It was developed using experiential rather than empirical evidence. It is a social and contextual approach using ethnicity and disability as an independent variable. Though developed for specific groups in the United States, these value dimensions may also be applicable to others. For example, a present-time orientation may be generalizable to groups anywhere that are compelled to live in the present, with little or no control over their future as a result of social policies and economic uncertainties. Readers should consider the applicability and relevance of these explanations in light of the methodology used and societal contexts, as well as evolving societies in which value orientations may change over time.

SOCIAL-ECOLOGICAL MODEL OF HUMAN DEVELOPMENT

Thus far in this chapter, we have discussed multiple ways people describe and explain human development and behavior. Each of these is based on the assumptions that observers or theorists bring to the situation. In this section we discuss the social-ecological model, which examines the assumptions we use to understand human diversity and how our understandings influence our explanations based on characteristics such as race, sexual orientation, chronological age, and gender.

The social-ecological model is a grounded approach that includes multiple elements of human existence and experience and combines them into a cogent structure with discrete but overlapping domains. It consists of three spheres of influence: the biosocial, psychosocial, and social structural domains. The *biosocial* domain is concerned with (1) biological attributes and functioning and (2) the social contextual meanings of biological traits and conditions. The *psychosocial* domain consists of (1) people's cognitive, emotional, and psychological traits and conditions and (2) the interactions and reciprocal relationships within people's social and environmental contexts. The *social structural* domain focuses on reciprocal relationships between people's immediate social environments and the larger social and cultural systems around them. Societal structures such as governments, educational institutions, religious organizations, social policies, and industry are indicative of the values and priorities of societies. As figure 2.1 illustrates, each of these domains is distinct, yet they overlap.

Let's consider the biological and social elements of the biosocial domain on the dimensions we have discussed. Biological sex is determined by chromosomal makeup at conception. An XX structure leads to female development, and an XY structure leads to male development—complete with corresponding physical characteristics and capabilities. For example, only women can become pregnant and bear children. However, the social contexts in which people live also determine the life course of men and women.

FIGURE 2.1   Social-Ecological Model

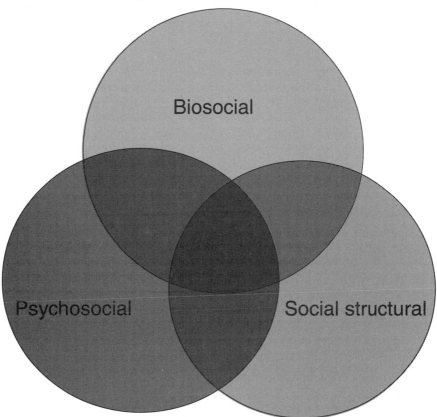

To illustrate, we ask you to reflect on the impact of differing social contexts for a female living in the following circumstances: the eighteenth-century United States, Taliban-led Afghanistan in 2000, and the Netherlands in 2008.

In twenty-first-century United States, women have voting, property ownership, reproductive, and other rights that were unavailable a few generations earlier in the United States. Yet in the twenty-first century in some countries, genital mutilation (e.g. clitoridectomies) is routinely performed on young girls. The killing of women who have been raped is acceptable because they have dishonored their families.

The psychosocial implications and interactions with the biosocial domain are pervasive. Men's and women's self-images, self-determination, opportunities, family relationships, place in society, and general quality of life are psychosocial elements influenced by how gender is defined. We can assess the biosocial and psychosocial implications of gender by looking at the social structural components of society. For example, in 2000 Afghanistan, schools for girls were nonexistent, and women were not allowed uncovered or alone in public. In 2000 in the United States, women made up more than half of college students, while a century ago, U.S. societal structures discouraged women from being educated, and it was not until 1920 that the Nineteenth Amendment to the U.S. Constitution was ratified, giving women the right to vote.

South Africa provides an example of the biosocial implications of race. For more than three hundred years, black Africans were subjected to the rule of whites, predominantly Afrikaners of Dutch origin, who justified their actions based on the philosophy that the "preservation of the pure race tradition of the [Afrikaner people] must be protected at all costs in all possible ways as a holy pledge entrusted to us by our ancestors as part of God's plan with our People" (qtd. in "South Africa," 2000). Blacks were subjugated and denied basic civil rights because of racial differences. A biologically based difference in skin color was used to invoke a "divine" justification to deny basic human rights to 70 percent of the people who resided within the borders of South Africa. The psychosocial implications of apartheid are self-evident. Afrikaners were raised to believe they were superior to blacks in every way. For the majority of blacks, daily survival was a challenge. Blacks who fought for rights were at risk of incarceration or death. Biological determinism justified apartheid; however, the social structural elements of South Africa were far more influential, as laws and institutions ensured its perpetuation. Only upon international pressure and sanctions was apartheid abolished as social policy. Even so, the biosocial, psychosocial, and social structural vestiges of apartheid remain, in large measure because of three hundred years of social policies and structures that defined blacks as inferior.

Sexual orientation is multifaceted, having biological and nonbiological causalities, and the biosocial interpretation of homosexuality varies greatly depending on one's context. Beliefs range from homosexuality being biologically predetermined to homosexuality being an immoral choice or psychological pathology. The psychosocial impacts, including poor self-image, depression, and suicide risk, for gay and lesbian youths are greater than for heterosexual youths—a result that occurs in multiple countries (Fergusson, Horwood, & Beautrais, 1999; Hegna, 2007). Contemporarily, we are seeing increased understanding that the social structural responses such as discrimination and violence, not the individual characteristics associated with homosexuality, are the primary obstacles facing gays and lesbians today. For example, as recently as 1986, the U.S. Supreme Court upheld the constitutionality of laws criminalizing consensual homosexual sex. Today, homosexual intercourse carries the death sentence in Saudi Arabia, Pakistan, Iran, Mauritania, Sudan, Somalia, and Yemen. Only recently have the rights of gays and lesbians been acknowledged in some countries. For example, Belgium and Spain legalized gay marriage in 2003 and 2005, respectively. Several other European countries have legalized same-sex domestic partnerships, affording rights similar to marriage. In Canada, a series of court cases beginning in 2003 led to the legitimization of same-sex marriage, culminating in the 2005 Civil Marriage Act, which formalized it nationwide.

The biosocial implications of disability also vary dramatically, as illustrated by the fate of people born with Down syndrome. Biologically, Down syndrome is characterized by an extra twenty-first chromosome—thus its designation as trisomy 21. Down syndrome results in intellectual disabilities and distinctive physical characteristics. Psychosocially, in the nineteenth and twentieth centuries, individuals born with Down syndrome were likely to be removed from families, institutionalized, and warehoused—thus subjected to isolation and environmental deprivation. Opportunities and psychosocial development were severely limited, yet the lack of development was blamed exclusively on biology. The deplorable conditions to which Down syndrome–affected people have been subjected have arisen out of the social structures and policies that led to the construction of institutions and warehouses for the developmentally disabled. In Nazi Germany the social structures went one step further when institutions were used to routinely euthanize people with Down syndrome. However, in the last decades of the twentieth century, people with Down syndrome began to be afforded education, integrated into society, and given opportunities previously denied. The biological traits with which they were born have not changed; however, biosocial conditions differ dramatically. And while their biological characteristics do mean they live with some limitations, the social structural changes have allowed them to maximize their biosocial and psychosocial functioning and have dramatically improved their quality of life and allowed them to make contributions to society.

SUMMARY

Human development, the human condition, and human behavior in social contexts have been the subject of numerous lines of inquiry. Longitudinal development theories have been used by multiple theorists to explain individual human development over the life span. Other theories have investigated the human condition based on characteristics such as gender, ethnicity, and economic structure.

In contemporary life, the social constructions and meanings of race/ ethnicity, gender, sexual orientation, disability, and other characteristics have at least as much significance as real or perceived biological differences. Non-whites have been treated as inferior in North America, much of Europe, and previously colonized nations and still face the remnant influences of the racist and colonialist past. Women, who have been portrayed as the "weaker" sex, generally reject this characterization. Gays, lesbians, bisexuals, and transgender persons have been labeled mentally ill and biologically deficient and have vigorously fought against such characterizations. Like disabled people, these groups have characteristics that are atypical of those who have traditionally held power. Like disabled people, GLBT individuals and racial-ethnic minorities have characteristics that are considered atypical. As for disabled people, societal reactions to these characteristics are the primary limiters of their full participation in society. The fight for civil rights is a common thread for all these groups that have been subjected to discrimination and devaluation.

We have discussed longitudinal human development from a disability perspective. We have provided information on the intersections of disability with multiple identity groups. Finally, we have presented the social-ecological perspective, which addresses three domains of the human condition: the biosocial, psychosocial, and social structural domains. We encourage you to continually assess your assumptions about the human condition and how those beliefs influence your conclusions relative to individual characteristics, the place of different groups in society, and the reasons for that placement. We believe that, like other groups, disabled people are, and will always be, a part of society. Societal beliefs and policies can be used to benefit all people universally. Conversely, they can be used to devalue individuals and groups with supposedly undesirable or inferior characteristics. Social policies and societal structures based on inclusiveness and access for all people benefit all people—those in the minority and the majority.

DISCUSSION QUESTIONS

1. How do traditional theories of human development and human behavior explain the place of disabled people in family life and in society?
2. Choose a traditional developmental theory and describe how it compares the development of nondisabled people with the development of people with one of the following: physical disability, intellectual disability, deafness, or blindness.
3. How have feminism and economic theories defined the roles of disabled persons in society?
4. How do the childhoods and family lives of youths who grow up in ethnic minority homes and families compare with the lives of GLTB youths? With disabled youths?
5. What are the similarities and differences between growing up disabled and growing up gay?

PERSONAL NARRATIVE: BILL HYATT

Bill Hyatt has lived with a disability since birth. At the time he provided this narrative, he was working as a resource developer for the California Central Valley Regional Center in Fresno, California.

I was born with cerebral palsy. It took my parents awhile to figure out that there was something different about me. My family was a migrant working family, so they kept going from doctor to doctor, each one giving various diagnoses. It wasn't until I was three that there was a correct diagnosis. Since I was the youngest of five and had a disability, my parents tended to be overprotective of me. I think they had lower expectations of me than they did of my brothers and sister. I think that in their minds, the scenario was that I was going to grow up and live in a wheelchair forever and ever and they were going to take care of me.

As a child, I went to a "special" school. This school had a wide range of kids. We had a high incidence of people with mental retardation but had people with low IQ, normal IQ, and above-normal IQ. Eventually, they started transitioning me from special schools to regular schools.

I discovered that there was a difference between me and most boys I was around when I was about eight or nine years old. I figured out that I wasn't going to be a policeman or a fireman. It was around that age that I began to see some differences between me and the other kids at the special school. In a lot of ways, I seemed like a fish out of water because I didn't fit in totally with the kids at the special school, and I didn't fit in totally with the kids at the regular school. I feel that way even today.

When they transitioned me from the special schools to the regular schools, they did two things. First, they started me off with short periods of time in the regular school and each year increased the periods of time I was there. Second—and this is what I don't understand—they put me in remedial classes instead of with kids who were more capable. They assumed that because I had a disability, I was academically best suited to the lower-level classes.

When they began integrating me in junior high, it was terrible. Other kids did not accept me; they would call me names and hurl insults and that sort of thing. When it came time to hurl the insults, I would hurl them back, and they couldn't catch them because they would just go over their heads. But I still didn't feel accepted.

High school was a little bit better for me in that I didn't have so much of that. When it came time to go to high school, they gave me a choice of staying in the special school or going full-time to the regular one—I chose the regular one. I always wanted to go to my high school. That was where all my brothers went, and that was where I wanted to go. It was also pretty accessible.

In high school, I found my niche, which happened to be in journalism. I was a part of that for four years. I got along pretty well with the kids in high school and made some friends there, but I didn't date. I couldn't take behind-the-wheel training in driver's education because they didn't have any cars with handicap equipment. So I adapted a golf cart and took my behind-the-wheel training in that. But it's kind of hard to date in a golf cart. I actually got a driver's license when I had the golf cart.

I attribute a lot of my drive and success to my therapist. My physical therapist was a very big man, about six feet tall. Interestingly, he had a disability himself: he had had polio as a child. In some ways he was like a third parent because, for me, growing up in a special school where I had therapy about 70 percent of the day, he was a very significant adult in my life. While my parents had low expectations of me, he, on the other hand, had very high expectations. I remember one incident very clearly. When I was just about to graduate from junior high, I started talking about working in a special workshop because that was what we disabled people did back then. He responded that if I did, he would kick my butt. He'd had a lot of experience observing differences in people, and he saw that I had more abilities than others saw.

My first two years at Bakersfield College were a really great time for me. I loved it. Sometimes I wish I could go back. I didn't get a real car until I went to college. I got my first student aid grant for $800 and went right out and bought an $800 car. For the four years I was in high school, I was the only person there with a significant disability, but at Bakersfield there were lots of disabled students from all around. Because I had a car, I got involved with other disabled students. There were a whole lot of interesting things going on in college life.

I also started dating in college. I didn't date a whole lot, but I did date a mix of disabled and nondisabled students. I wound up getting semi-serious about one particular young woman who happened to have epilepsy. I remember vividly that whenever she would have a seizure at the mall or elsewhere, she would turn toward a window in order to hide it, and she never even remembered doing it. It was her coping mechanism, but she had no memory of it after.

The term *Disability culture* has particular significance to me. It's a shared experience that people with disabilities have. Not every disability is the same, but the reactions that the greater society has toward us are very similar. So even though I don't have mental retardation or epilepsy or those other things, I've shared experiences with people who do. The commonality I have with other people with disabilities is very important to me. It helps keep me balanced.

I'm on the Internet a lot, and I find it's a great source of strength. It has become a place I can go to connect with others with disabilities. For example, it's one of the few places I can tell a disability joke and they get it.

I grew up in the late sixties and early seventies, so the civil rights movement was very important to me. People like Robert Kennedy and Martin Luther King Jr. were great role models for me. I don't really recall disabled role models from my youth. When I was growing up, the only one I remember that had a disability was President Roosevelt, and I didn't really have much of a desire to be president. And we know he wasn't too open about having a disability either. But when I was growing up, I remember people were always mentioning Roosevelt's disability to me. I do remember one TV show, *Ironside*. It really wasn't a very good show, but the star was a wheelchair user. So, as for disabled role models, I really didn't have too many.

I think the number one issue facing people with disabilities is society's recognition of how people with disabilities are treated. The greater society needs to recognize that people with disabilities have been treated differently and negatively by society. Laws to protect us are in place; now it's a matter of people honoring the law, and understanding why laws are there in the first place.

I have personally experienced discrimination in my life because of my disability. Sometimes, though, discrimination is so subtle or hidden that it's hard to figure out when it's happening. I've applied for jobs that I didn't get because of my disability. At the time it really hurt. Sometimes I have felt like an outsider in work situations too. It's not because other employees were bad people or anything like that, but that's the way it's been. My presence has made them feel uncomfortable, or they just haven't been accepting of me.

ADA and other laws have been helpful to people with disabilities. Disability laws have prompted people to do things, not because they were the right things to do but because the law said they had to. In spite of the fact that some say people can't be changed legislatively, I think we have to begin somewhere. The laws are getting people's attention.

The issue is important not only for the greater society but among ourselves as people with disabilities. People with disabilities are sometimes slow to identify with a disability, especially in these times, when it is not OK to be outside the norm. Too often we believe that we must overcome our disability rather than live with it. Too often people feel shame or embarrassment at being disabled.

I want to be very clear in my own mind about what success means. I'm a success because I have the capability to do the things that I enjoy doing. I feel successful because I have a job I enjoy, but people who don't have jobs can be successful as well. Most people do not have the ability to be happy all the time, but having choices in my life is really important to feeling successful.

One of the biggest obstacles to success, I think, is other people's expectations about me. They don't know me, but they have preconceived ideas about what somebody with CP in a wheelchair can and can't do. That's one of the biggest problems for me. I can deal with the physical barriers, but the other barriers are much harder to contend with. It's people's attitudes, their stereotypes, and their assumptions that create barriers.

We've got to remember that everybody is an individual. Don't make assumptions about people with disabilities. Some people are very good people and some people are jerks—people with and without disabilities. I think if people can begin to see people as people, the rest will follow.

SUGGESTED READINGS

Chilman, C. S., Nunnaly, E. W., & Cox, F. M. (1988). *Chronic illness and disability.* Newbury Park, CA: Sage.

Mackelprang, R. W., & Valentine, D. (1993). *Sexuality and disabilities: A guide for human service practitioners.* Binghamton, NY: Haworth Press.

Myer, L. H., Peck, C. A., & Brown, L. (1991). *Critical issues in the lives of people with severe disabilities.* Baltimore: Paul H. Brooks.

Newman, B. M., & Newman, P. R. (2006). *Development through life: A psychosocial approach.* Pacific Grove, CA: Brooks/Cole.

Shapiro, J. P. (1993). *No pity: People with disabilities forging a new civil rights movement.* New York: Times Books.

REFERENCES

Affleck, G., Tennen, H., & Gershman, K. (1985). Cognitive adaptations to high-risk infants: The search for mastery, meaning, and protection from future harm. *American Journal of Mental Deficiency, 89*(6), 653–653.

Alpert, J. L. (1986). *Psychoanalysis and women: Contemporary reappraisals.* Hillsdale, NJ: Analytic Press.

Altshuler, S. A., Mackelprang, R. W., & Baker, R. L. (2008). Youth with disabilities: *A standardized self-portrait of how they are faring. Journal of Social Work in Disability and Rehabilitation, 7*(1), 1–18.

American Anthropological Association. (1998, May 17). *American Anthropological Association statement on "race."* Retrieved March 28, 2007, from http://www.aaanet.org/stmts/racepp.htm

Andrews, A. B., & Veronin, L. J. (1993). Sexual assault and people with disabilities. In R. W. Mackelprang & D. Valentine (Eds.), *Sexuality and disabilities: A guide for human service practitioners* (pp. 137–159). Binghamton, NY: Haworth Press.

Associated Press. (2007, March 16). Homosexuality may be based on biology, Baptist says. *New York Times.* Retrieved March 29, 2007, from http://www.nytimes.com/2007/03/16/us/16baptist.html?ex = 1175313600&en = bfc0538cdbc61991&ei = 5070

Bishop, M. (2005). Quality of life and psychosocial adaptation to chronic illness and acquired disability: A conceptual and theoretical synthesis. *Journal of Rehabilitation, 71*(2), 5–13.

Bray, G. P. (1978). Rehabilitation of spinal cord injured: A family approach. *Journal of Applied Rehabilitation Counseling, 19,* 70–78.

Brooks-Gunn, J., & Reiter, E. O. (1990). The role of pubertal processes. In S. S. Feldman & G. R. Elliott (Eds.), *At the threshold: The developing adolescent* (pp. 16–53). Cambridge, MA: Harvard University Press.

Bryant, M. (1993). Religion and disability: Some notes on religious attitudes and views. In M. Nagler (Ed.), *Perspectives on disability: Text and readings on disability* (2nd ed., pp. 91–95). Palo Alto, CA: Health Markets Research.

Cavalli-Sforza, L. L. (2000). *Genes, peoples, and languages.* New York: Farrar, Straus and Giroux.

Colligan, S. (2004). Why the intersexed shouldn't be fixed: Insights from queer theory and disability studies. In B. Smith & B. Hutchinson (Eds.), *Gendering disability* (pp. 45–60). Piscataway, NJ: Rutgers University Press.

Crate, M. A. (1965). Adaptation to chronic illness. *American Journal of Nursing, 65,* 73–76.

Darwin, C. (1859). *On the origin of the species.* London: John Murray.

Darwin, C. (1871). *Descent of man and selection in relation to sex.* Retrieved January 4, 2008, from http://www.infidels.org/library/historical/charles_darwin/origin_of_species/

Davis, H. (1993). *Counselling parents of children with chronic illness or disability.* Baltimore: Paul H. Brooks.

Ellenberger, H. (1970). *The discovery of the unconscious.* New York: Basic Books.

Erickson, E. (1963). *Childhood and society* (2nd ed.). New York: Norton.

Fast, I. (1984). *Gender identity: A differentiation model.* Hillsdale, NJ: Analytic Press.

Fergusson, D., Horwood, J., & Beautrais, A. (1999). Is sexual orientation related to mental health problems and suicidality in young people? *Archives of General Psychiatry, 56,* 876–880.

Fernandez, M., & Freer, R. (1996). Application of an integrated model for counseling persons with spinal cord injury across ethnicities. *SCI Psychosocial Process, 9*(1), 4–9.

Fernandez, M., & Marini, I. (1995). Cultural values orientation in counseling persons with spinal cord injury. *SCI Psychosocial Process, 8*(4), 150–155.

Foster, M., & Sharp, R. (2002). Race, ethnicity, and genomics: Social classifications as proxies of biological heterogeneity. *Genome Research, 12*(6), 844–850.

Fowler, J. (1981). *Stages of faith: The psychology of human development and the quest for meaning.* San Francisco: Harper & Row.

Fox, A. (2004). "But Mother—I'm—crippled!": Tennessee Williams, queering disability, and dis/membered bodies in performance. In B. Smith & B. Hutchinson (Eds.), *Gendering disability* (pp. 233–250). Piscataway, NJ: Rutgers University Press.

Freud, S. (1964). *The standard edition of the complete psychological works of Sigmund Freud: Vol. 22. New introductory lectures on psychoanalysis.* London: Hogarth.

Friess, S. (2000, November 21). Seen but seldom heard. *The Advocate,* pp. 27–32.

Galbo, J. J. (1983). Adolescents' perceptions of significant adults. *Adolescence, 18,* 417–428.

Gallagher, J. J., Beckman, P., & Cross, A. H. (1983). Families of handicapped children: Sources of stress and its amelioration. *Exceptional children, 50*(1), 10–19.

Garbarino, J., Brookhouser, P. E., & Authier, K. J. (1987). *Special children, special risks: The maltreatment of children with disabilities.* New York: Aldine de Gruyter.

Garland-Thomson, R. (2002). Integrating disability, transforming feminist theory. *NWSA Journal, 14*(2), 1–32.

Gaylord-Ross, R., & Browder, D. (1991). Functional assessment: Dynamic and domain properties. In L. H. Myer, C. A. Peck, & L. Brown (Eds.), *Critical issues in the lives of people with severe disabilities* (pp. 45–66). Baltimore: Paul H. Brooks.

Gilligan, C. (1982). *In a different voice: Psychological theory and women's development.* Cambridge, MA: Harvard University Press.

Gilligan, C., & Attanucci, J. (1986). Two moral orientations. In C. Gilligan, J. Ward, J. Taylor, & B. Bardige (Eds.), *Mapping the moral domain: A contribution of women's thinking to psychological theory and education* (pp.73–86). Cambridge, MA: Harvard University Press.

Gould, S. (1996). *The mismeasure of man.* New York: W. W. Norton.

Groce, N. (1999). Disability in cross-cultural perspective: Rethinking disability. *The Lancet, 354*(9180), 756–757.

Hall, K. (2002). Feminism, disability, and embodiment. *NWSA Journal, 14*(3), vii–xiii.

Hegna, K. (2007). Suicide attempts among Norwegian gay, lesbian and bisexual youths. *Acta Sociologica, 50*(1), 21–37.

Irwin, S. (2001). Disability and the life course. In M. Priestly (Ed.), *Disability and the life course: Global perspectives* (pp. 15–25). Cambridge: Cambridge University Press.

Kail, R., & Cavanaugh, J. (2004). *Human development: A life-span view* (3rd ed.). Belmont, CA: Wadsworth.

Kendell, W., & Buys, N. (1998). An integrated model of psychosocial adjustment following acquired disability. *Journal of Rehabilitation, 64*(3), 16–20.

Kiev, A. (1969). *Magic, faith, and healing: Studies in primitive psychiatry*. New York: Free Press.

Kluckholm, F., & Strodtbeck, F. (1961). *Variations in value orientations*. Evanston, IL: Row Peterson.

Kohlberg, L. (1984). *The psychology of moral development* (Vol. 2). San Francisco: Harper & Row.

Kohlberg, L. (1986). A current statement on some theoretical issues. In S. Mogdil & C. Mogdil (Eds.), *Lawrence Kohlberg, consensus and controversy* (pp. 485–546). Philadelphia: Falmer Press.

Krieger, N. (2005). *If "race" is the answer, what is the question? On "race," racism, and health: A social epidemiologist's perspective*. Retrieved September 17, 2005, from http://raceandgenomics.ssrc.org/Krieger?

Krieger, N., Chen, J., Waterman, P., Rehkoph, D., & Subramanian, S. (2005). Painting a truer picture of U.S. socioeconomic and racial/ethnic health inequalities: The public health disparities geocoding project. *American Journal of Public Health, 93*, 312–323.

Kübler-Ross, E. (1969). *On death and dying*. New York: Macmillan.

L'Abate, L. (1998). Discovery of the family: From the inside to the outside. *American Journal of Family Therapy, 26*(4), 265–280.

L'Abate, L. (1999). Taking the bull by the horns: Beyond talk in psychological interventions. *Family Journal, 7*(4), 206–220.

Lawrence, S. A., & Lawrence, R. M. (1979). A model of adaptation of chronic illness. *Nursing Forum, 18*, 33–42.

Lenneberg, E. H. (1967). *Biological foundations of language*. New York: Wiley.

LeVay, S. (1991). A difference in hypothalamic structure between heterosexual and homosexual men. *Science, 253*(5023), 1034–1037.

Livneh, H. (2001). Psychosocial adaptation to chronic illness and disability: A conceptual framework, *44*(3), 151–160.

Lloyd, M. (1992). Does she boil eggs? Towards a feminist model of disability. *Disability, Handicap and Society, 7*(3), 207–221.

Longres, J. F. (2000). *Human behavior in the social environment* (3rd ed.). Itasca, IL: F. D. Peacock.

Lukin, J. (2006). Black disability studies. *Temple University Faculty Herald, 36*(4). Retrieved March 28, 2007, from http://www.temple.edu/instituteondisabilities/programs/ds/facultyherald2.htm

Maas, H. S. (1984). *People in contexts: Social development from birth to old age*. Englewood Cliffs, NJ: Prentice Hall.

Mackelprang, R. W., & Altshuler, S. (2004). A youth perspective on life with a disability. *Journal of Social Work in Disability and Rehabilitation, 3*(3), 39–52.

Mackelprang, R. W., & Mackelprang, R. D. (2005). Historical and contemporary issues in end-of-life decisions: Implications for social work. *Social Work, 50*(4), 315–324.

Mackelprang, R. W., Ray, J., & Hernandez-Peck, M. (1996). Social work education and sexual orientation: Faculty, student and curriculum issues. *Journal of Gay and Lesbian Social Services, 5*(4), 17–31.

Marx, K., & Engels, F. (1948). *Manifesto of the Communist Party*. New York: International Publishers.

McGoldrick, M. (1982). Ethnicity and family therapy. In M. McGoldrick, J. Pearce, & J. Giordano (Eds.), *Ethnicity and family therapy* (pp. 3–30). New York: Guilford Press.

McGoldrick, M., Pearce, J., & Giordano, J. (1982). *Ethnicity and family therapy*. New York: Guilford Press.

McRuer, R. (2006). *Crip theory: Cultural signs of queerness and disability*. New York: New York University Press.

Miller, P. H. (1993). *Theories of developmental psychology* (3rd ed.). New York: W. H. Freeman.

Minuchin, S., & Fishman, H. C. (1981). *Family therapy techniques*. Cambridge, MA: Harvard University Press.

Morris, J. (1992). Personal and political: A feminist perspective on researching physical disability. *Disability, Handicap, and Society, 7*(2), 152–166.

Morris, J. (1993). *Pride against prejudice*. Gabrioloa Island, Canada: New Society.

Murphy, D. M., & Murphy, J. T. (1997). Enabling disabled students. *Thought & Action: The NEA Higher Education Journal, 13*(1), 41–52.

Mustillo, S., Krieger, N., Gunderson, E., Sidney, S., McCreath, H., & Keafe, C. (2004). The association of self-reported experiences of racial discrimination with black/white differences in preterm delivery and low birth weight: The CARDIA study. *American Journal of Public Health, 94*, 2125–2131.

Nelson, K. (1973). Structure and strategy in learning to talk. *Monographs of the Society for Research in Child Development, 38*(1–2).

Newman, B. M., & Newman, P. R. (2006). *Development through life: A psychosocial approach* (9th ed.) Pacific Grove, CA: Brooks/Cole.

Onken, S. J., & Mackelprang, R. W. (1997). *Building on shared experiences: Teaching disability and sexual minority content and practice*. Paper presented at the annual program meeting of the Council on Social Work Education, Chicago.

Overall, C. (2006). Old age and ageism, impairment and ableism: Exploring the conceptual and material connections. *NWSA Journal, 18*(1), 126–137.

Patterson, J. M. (1988). Chronic illness in children and the impact on families. In C. S. Chilman, E. W. Nunnaly, & F. M. Cox (Eds.), *Chronic illness and disability* (pp. 69–107). Newbury Park, CA: Sage.

Piaget, J. (1985). *The equilibration of cognitive structures*. Chicago: University of Chicago Press.

Pillari, V. (1998). *Human behavior in the social environment* (2nd ed.). Pacific Grove, CA: Brooks/Cole.

Plato. (1991). *The republic* (B. Jowett, Trans.). New York: Vintage Books.

Rappaport, L. (1972). *Personality development: A chronology of experience*. Glenview, IL: Scott, Foresman.

Rhodes, R. (1993). Mental retardation and sexual expression: An historical perspective. In R. W. Mackelprang & D. Valentine (Eds.), *Sexuality and disabilities: A guide for human service practitioners* (pp. 1–27). Binghamton, NY: Haworth Press.

Rich, J., & DeVitis, J. (1994). *Theories of moral development.* (2nd ed.). Springfield, IL: Charles C. Thomas.

Rolland, J. S. (1988). A conceptual model of chronic and life threatening illness and its impact on families. In C. S. Chilman, E. W. Nunnaly, & F. M. Cox (Eds.), *Chronic illness and disability* (pp. 17–68). Newbury Park, CA: Sage.

Rolland, J. S. (1989). Chronic illness and the family life cycle. In E. A. Carter & M. McGoldrick (Eds.), *The changing family life cycle: A framework for family therapy* (2nd ed., pp. 433–456). Needham Heights, MA: Allyn and Bacon.

Salsgiver, R. O., Watson, A., Cooke, J., & Madison, L. S. (2004). Spiritual/religious access for women with disabilities. *SCI Psychosocial Process, 17*(1), 27–32.

Sandahl, C. (2006). More than just funny: Reading Galloway from a disability perspective. *Liminalities: A Journal of Performance Studies, 2*(3). Retrieved March 29, 2007, from http://liminalities.net/2-3/san.htm

Shapiro, J. P. (1993). *No pity: People with disabilities forging a new civil rights movement.* New York: Times Books.

Sigler, G., & Mackelprang, R. W. (1993). Cognitive impairments: Psychosocial and sexual implications and strategies for social work intervention. In R. W. Mackelprang & D. Valentine (Eds.), *Sexuality and disabilities: A guide for human service practitioners* (pp. 89–106). Binghamton, NY: Haworth Press.

Smith, B., & Hutchinson, B. (2004). *Gendering disability.* Piscataway, NJ: Rutgers University Press.

Snyder, S., & Mitchell, D. (2006). *Cultural locations of disability.* Chicago: University of Chicago.

South Africa: Revolution at the ballot box. (2000). *Bill of Rights in Action, 2*(2). Retrieved August 18, 2008, from http://www.crf-usa.org/bria/bria12_2.html

Spencer, P. E., Bodner-Johnson, B. A., & Gutfreund, M. K. (1992). Interacting with infants with a hearing loss: What can we learn from mothers who are deaf? *Journal of Early Intervention, 16,* 64–78.

Streib, H. (2001). Faith development theory revisited: The religious styles perspective. *International Journal for the Psychology of Religion, 11*(3), 143–158.

Streib, H. (2005). Faith development research revisited: Accounting for diversity in structure, content, and narrativity of faith. *International Journal for the Psychology of Religion, 15*(2), 99–121.

Summers, J. A., Behr, S. K., & Turnbull, A. P. (1989). Positive adaptation and coping strengths of families who have children with disabilities. In G. H. S. Singer & L. K. Irvin (Eds.), *Support for caregiving families: Enabling positive adaptation to disabilities* (pp. 27–40). Baltimore: Paul H. Brooks.

Tanner, J. M. (1990). *Fetus into man: Physical growth from conception to maturity.* Cambridge, MA: Harvard University Press.

Thomas, R. M. (2001). *Recent theories of human development.* Thousand Oaks, CA: Sage.

Trieschmann, R. B. (1980). *Spinal cord injuries: Psychological, social, and vocational adjustment.* New York: Pergamon Press.

Valentine, D. P. (1993). Children with special needs: Sources of support and stress for families. In R. W. Mackelprang & D. Valentine (Eds.), *Sexuality and disabilities: A guide for human service practitioners* (pp. 107–129). Binghamton, NY: Haworth Press.

Vygotsky, L. S. (1978). *Mind in society.* Cambridge, MA: Harvard University Press.

Waldschmidt, A. (2006). Normalcy, bio-politics and disability: Some remarks on the German discourse. *Disability Studies Quarterly, 26*(2), 42.

Whitman, B. Y., & Accardo, P. J. (1993). The parent with mental retardation: Rights, responsibilities and issues. In R. W. Mackelprang & D. Valentine (Eds.), *Sexuality and disabilities: A guide for human service practitioners* (pp. 123–136). Binghamton, NY: Haworth Press.

Wiggam, A. (1924). *The fruit of the family tree.* Indianapolis, IN: Bobbs-Merrill.

Wright, B. (1983). *Physical disability—a psychological approach* (2nd ed.). New York: Harper & Row.

3

Traditional Approaches to Disability: Moral and Medical Models

STUDENT LEARNING OBJECTIVES

1. To understand the medical and moral models that attempt to explain disability
2. To understand the components of oppression that directly relate to persons with disabilities, including containment, compartmentalization, the feeling that the lives of people with disabilities are expendable, and blaming of the victim
3. To understand the various impacts of oppression for persons with disabilities
4. To understand the connection between negative social constructs of persons with disabilities and identity formation
5. To understand the process of internalized ableism

As discussed in chapter 1, disability has been present in society from the beginning of recorded history. In this chapter, we delve further into the meanings and definitions of disability. We ask you to consider two recent award-winning movies about quadriplegia to illustrate. The film *Murderball* chronicles the escapades of the U.S. Quad Rugby team, a raucous and highly competitive group of disabled elite athletes. In contrast, the film *Million Dollar Baby*, like so many films and movies before it, justifies euthanizing people with severe disabilities. Mackelprang and Mackelprang (2005) provide several U.S. and European examples of public policies and practices that are guided by the belief that severe physical disability is worse than death.

In this chapter we delve further into traditionally dominant societal models of disability: the moral and medical models that we introduced to you in the first chapter. The moral and medical models have been the most commonly used disability models throughout history. Finally, we discuss the impact of ableism and oppression on people with disabilities.

THE MORAL MODEL

The earliest recorded views of disability explained disability as resulting from immorality or sin. This ancient model is a part of Western culture and is dominant in many other current world cultures (Ingstad & Wyte, 1995). The model perceives disability as the direct result of sin and evil or as being out of order with nature. Longmore (1993) concludes that the moral paradigm portrays disability as a state of existence in conflict with the very moral and spiritual center of the universe. Disability, according to this model, is the result of loss of control of the moral essence of the individual. A person with a disability represents an impaired spirit: a heart that is out of order.

This "moral" view of disability sprang forth from early human cultures and continued to dominate thinking until the end of the Middle Ages. Albrecht (1992) suggests that disability and impairment are as old as the human species itself and that the linkage between disability and impairment and sin and immorality was probably the first way societies had of looking at disabling conditions. Groce (2005) classifies religious and spiritual beliefs about the causes of disabilities into two categories: birth and later life. The reasons for the birth of a child with a disability generally center on sinful acts of the family, incest, or marital infidelity. The reasons that disability occurs in later life may also concern divine punishment of the individual or the community in which the individual resides. Neolithic tribes, believing that the etiology of a disabling condition lay in the disabled person's acquisition of evil spirits, sought remedy by drilling holes in the skulls of persons with disabling conditions.

As discussed in chapter 1, the link between moral degradation and disability remains a part of contemporary society. Persons with disabilities can be ostracized because of their perceived link with evil. Discrimination in all arenas, including employment, education, and housing, can be traced in part to the moral paradigm of understanding disability. Some individuals still believe that people are disabled because they or their parents are or were evil. Even persons with disabilities themselves continue to seek out the answer to the question "Why me?" through understanding their own imagined sins (Salsgiver, 1995).

A primary source of the moral model of disability in Western culture is Judeo-Christian tradition. Within the context of these religious traditions, persons with disabilities are viewed as experiencing disability because of God's wrath and judgment (Livneh, 1982). Bryant (1993) also points out that many Jews and Christians view illness and disability as God's punishment for sins and transgressions. Wright (1983) discusses in detail the connection between Judeo-Christian beliefs and negative attitudes toward persons with disabilities. The ancient Hebrews saw persons who were ill or had physical disabilities as sinners. Characteristics that would keep a priest from the temple included being blind, being lame, having a malformed foot or a misshaped hand, being a dwarf, or having a broken bone. Early Roman Catholic priests had to be free of physical disabilities. Indeed, Tony Coelho, a former member of the U.S. House of Representatives from California and coauthor of the Americans with Disabilities Act, was prevented from becoming a Jesuit priest because of his epilepsy (Fadiman, 1997; Jones, 1995).

Christian thought equates disability with suffering, and suffering with the process of cleansing moral failings (Wright, 1983); as a result, society views persons with disabilities as noble in their pursuit of simple life objectives. They are looked upon as heroes because they seek to function in the same way as everyone else in spite of their disabilities. When David Letterman interviewed Christopher Reeve on *The Late Show* in 1998, he introduced Reeve as a hero. Reeve reminded Letterman that he was lucky in a number of areas, including wealth. Reeve did not see himself as a hero—just as an actor and director. Letterman sadly did not understand that Americans link disability with suffering and believe that within the process of suffering lies nobility (Mackelprang & Salsgiver, 2003).

TenBroek and Matson (1959) discuss the religious link with negative attitudes toward persons who are blind or visually impaired. Judeo-Christian belief holds that blindness is symbolic of death. Within the sacred writings of the Jews, the blind man is a dead man. Visual impairment and blindness as well as mental health disability result directly from not following the rules of behavior set forth by Jewish law.

As a person with cerebral palsy, one of the authors, Richard Salsgiver, has experienced the negative impact of this view of disability in his life. We use his experiences throughout his lifetime to illustrate major points throughout this chapter and periodically throughout the text.

> The moral paradigm of conceptualizing disability affected me in my youth and continues to influence certain aspects of my life as a person with a disability. When I was a child, my parents rarely took me to visit others or out in public. I believe, in part, that their isolation of me was an overprotection, but in part, it centered on their insidious shame that somehow they were responsible for my disability through some sinful act. In fact, when visitors came to our home and were curious about my "crippledness," my father would explain to them that a cure was imminent. He said that he had a vision that if he gave up the sinful act of smoking cigars, I would walk.
>
> I found that the connection between moral degradation and disability followed me in my professional work when I began my first administrative position in a social welfare agency in 1985. During lunch time, for the fun of it, I ran a support group for newly disabled persons. Inevitably the discussion would turn to the cause of each member's disability. For the most part, members settled on some sinful act in their lives. When they couldn't think of a sin that had caused their disability, they conjectured that the sin had occurred in a previous life.
>
> When I held the position of director of diversity programs at the Office of the Chancellor of the California State University in the early 1990s, my duties included presenting trainings on disability and the Americans with Disabilities

Act. After one such training, one of the participants approached me. Disparagingly, he brought up my conclusion presented at the training that the assumed link between sin and disability is part of the deep-rooted societal prejudice around disability. The participant informed me that this was not prejudice, but the reality. Persons with disabilities, particularly alcoholics and drug addicts, brought disability upon themselves because of sinful acts committed either by themselves or their parents!

Dominant Western culture shares the moral model of disability with a variety of nonindustrialized cultures. Nicolaisen (1995) points out that the Punan Bah of Central Borneo in Malaysia connect disability to taboo acts committed by either the father or the mother of the person with the disability. The Maasai of Kenya believe that disability and illness are a sign of cosmic disorder. They believe that God causes disability because of inherited sin (Talle, 1995). The people of southern Somalia believe that the evil eye or the curse causes disability. Disability caused by the evil eye occurs when one has done harm to another person. Disability caused by the curse occurs when one does not return a favor or fulfill an obligation. For Somalians, the most common cause of disability is the evil eye (Helander, 1995). According to Devlieger (1995), the Songyre of Zaire believe that sorcerers, either with or without the authorization of God, cause disability.

Many ethnic groups in the United States, both Christian and non-Christian, hold the beliefs of the moral paradigm concerning disability. Many Latinos believe that disability is a result of the sins of the parents of the person with a disability (Smart & Smart, 1991). Santana-Martin and Santana (2005) point out that many Latinos find physical disability more acceptable than mental/psychological disability. A child with a physical disability in a Latino family is generally looked upon as normal. He or she is basically treated like the other children in the family. African Americans may view disability, particularly mental health disability, as the result of a life of sin. But a sense of spirituality helps many African Americans deal with the experience of disability (Ho, 1987). Native Americans may believe that disability is caused by the loss of the soul, the intervention of evil spirits, or immoral behavior (Farley, 1995).

Peoples of Laos, Thailand, and Vietnam who have settled in Western countries also hold beliefs that are consonant with the moral paradigm. Consider the Hmong, many of whom immigrated as refugees to the United States, Canada, and France as a result of the Southeast Asian conflicts of the 1960s and 1970s. They believe in a direct connection between disability and wrongdoing. Some Hmong people believe that the self is made up of many souls. Disability is caused when one or more souls leave the person. Often this is caused by the individual doing harm to others or doing wrong. Healing with the help of a Shaman or priest seeks to reunite the soul or souls with the person (Fadiman, 1997; Livo & Cha, 1991). Arokiasamy, Rubin, and Roessler (1978) examine the beliefs of Hindus regarding disability. For them, the life of suffering encountered by many people with disabilities is the result of a former life of sin.

Liu (2005) discusses Chinese concepts of disability as punishment for sins in a past life or the sentence of the parents of the person with a disability. Shame and guilt are the centers of the disability experience in China. The family experiences shame from the outside world. The individual experiences guilt for what he or she has brought upon the family.

This description of the connection between cultural beliefs and attitudes about disability is not meant to be an indictment against the religious or spiritual beliefs of any of the described cultural groups. In fact, religion and spirituality can play important positive roles in the lives of persons with disabilities. For example, Salsgiver, Watson, Cooke, and Madison (2004) found in a qualitative empirical study that religion and spirituality provide women with disabilities, in particular, with the support and socialization that allow them to live their lives in a self-fulfilling manner. Not only are religion and spirituality tools for coping with disability; disability reinforces their spiritual and religious lives. Wolfe (1993) notes another two-sided nature of the role of religion in the lives of persons with disabilities. Judeo-Christian religious tradition offers many lessons on the dignity and worth of persons with disabilities that need to be transferred into the aggregate culture. Wolfe analyzes the story of Moses, using contemporary dialectic to demonstrate this. There is strong evidence that Moses had a significant speech impairment. When asked by God to lead his people out of slavery, Moses was hesitant, saying that he was slow of words and speech. God replied that it is He who makes decisions about people and whether they are disabled or not. God implied, in choosing Moses as a leader, that some people with disabilities are worthy and capable of leadership. When Moses remained unconvinced, God provided what we might today term "reasonable accommodation" in Aaron to help Moses speak to his people. This Judeo-Christian lesson demonstrates the compassion of Western thought, and that persons with disabilities can hold roles of responsibility and status. Unfortunately, these values are not the ones that are generalized in dominant Western culture.

The entrenchment of certain religious beliefs often has a negative impact on persons with disabilities. Western society has drawn the equation between sin and disability primarily from Christianity (Mackelprang & Salsgiver, 1996), and this underlying negative value, along with other beliefs, has had a number of negative consequences for persons with disabilities that we will discuss later.

THE MEDICAL MODEL

The medical model grew from the moral model. Unlike the moral model, the medical model of disability is unique to Western culture, with origins in the Enlightenment era in Europe and America. Influenced by thinkers such as John Locke, the Enlightenment dictated social thought and action for hundreds of years in Europe and the United States and indeed remains with us today. Philosophers of the Enlightenment believed that humans are basically good. They believed that human beings can be perfected, and existing failings and limitations can be eliminated not only from individuals but from society in general. In particular, Locke believed that the continued improvement of humanity would never stop (Russell, 1965). Antisocial behavior, disease, mental disability, physical disability, crime, poverty, and war could be eliminated.

Within this environment, the medical model emerged, with its faith that with the correct intervention, all human abnormalities could be corrected (Mackelprang & Salsgiver, 1996). Institutions dedicated to perfecting the imperfect sprang up (Rothman, 1971) with the hope that these inadequacies could be cured by professional intervention. When cure was not possible, persons with disabilities could at least be trained to become functional enough to behave acceptably in social situations (Longmore, 1987).

The medical paradigm of disability that is part of contemporary U.S. culture exhibits certain specific characteristics. First of all, the focus of the problem of disability centers on the individual with the disability (DeJong, 1979). The medical model does not, for the most part, concern itself with factors external to the individual. Even when it acknowledges environmental influences, it does not consider these points of change. The second characteristic of the medical paradigm involves the concept of biological dysfunction. According to the medical model, there is something drastically wrong with the person with a disability. The biological organism is out of sync with the natural order of the universe (Longmore, 1993). The third characteristic of the medical paradigm of disability centers on action. The medical model relies on the intervention of professionals. Solutions to problems are made possible by the knowledge and skills of physicians, physical therapists, occupational therapists, clinical therapists, professional counselors, certified special education teachers, and other professionals (DeJong, 1979). The fourth characteristic of the medical model concerns the issue of who is in control. The medical model assumes professionals are the controlling factor in how persons with disabilities are treated. The fifth characteristic relates to intervention/treatment goals and outcomes. The medical model seeks perfection, cure, the eradication of the physical or mental dysfunction, making the abnormal normal through treatment (Whyte, 1995). The story of Jennie Marsh (pseudonym) illustrates the medical model approach. Born with cerebral palsy, Jennie recalls her relationships with health care professionals as an adolescent.

> I was barely human. One time, as a fourteen-year-old, I was paraded in front of a whole class of doctors so they could see my "abnormal gait." I was wearing only my panties. They would never have done that to a nondisabled girl, but it

was OK to parade me almost naked. And the crazy thing is, it wasn't until years later that I realized they had dehumanized me.

There are several endemic problems with the medical model in relation to disability that lead to oppression. First, the medical model assumes disability is an internal pathology rather than primarily a social construct based on interactions in society. Disability advocates and scholars have concluded that the meaning of disability is, in large measure, socially constructed (Wright, 1983) rather than an individually contained deficiency. Unlike the medical model, the social construction perspective emphasizes looking beyond the individual and the individual's functional capacity and avers that society and culture are the loci in which problems of disability must be addressed. Professional control increases treatment mistakes because practitioners discount input from recipients. Third, the medical model seeks to do the impossible when it comes to most people with disabilities by attempting to mold them to conform with dominant cultural definitions of "normal." The medical model, much like the moral model, sees disability as aberrant. In the case of the moral model, persons with disabilities are out of sync with the spiritual world. According to the medical model, persons with disabilities are out of sync with the logical world and either need to be "fixed" or eliminated (Longmore, 1993). To illustrate, let's consider one of the authors' adolescent experiences with the medical model arising from treatment of his cerebral palsy.

My diagnosis of cerebral palsy at two-and-a-half years old resulted in a series of consultations with specialist physicians in Pittsburgh, Pennsylvania. These consultations resulted in my parents seeking a cure for my "crippledness" through various types of surgical interventions. In our multiple trips to Pittsburgh hospitals, physicians stretched my legs, broke my bones, and cut my ligaments, all under general anesthetic, mostly ether.

The experiences with ether were the worst times. Upon my arrival in the operating room, they rolled me onto the surgical bed under huge green lights. Then someone put a metal screened mask over my mouth and nose and slowly dropped ether on it. Immediately, I gasped for breath. The harder I breathed, the more I gasped, and I would soon begin to lose consciousness. I began to feel as if I were falling, and I would try to repeat the last word I heard someone say over and over and over again in my mind. In later operations, I tried to develop additional ways of coping.

I found at the point where words repeated, that if I shouted something pleasant, the word or phrase would repeat over and over again. Later my mechanisms for coping included wetting myself right before going under anesthesia, which, of course, created havoc in the operation room.

In retrospect, I can't imagine the psychological and emotional damage done to children in the unsuccessful medical attempts to make us physically normal.

The medical model's emphasis on normalcy as defined by the dominant society results in enormous emotional, psychological, and social costs for persons with disabilities. However, the medical industry's attempt to make people with disabilities "normal" is rarely if ever successful. Yet it is a primary objective in the practice of medicine. Situations similar to mine are experienced by hundreds of thousands of other persons with disabilities who have experienced the same kind of objectification at the hands of the medical model. Those experiences bind the disabled community together to form one of the important foundation stones of Disability culture.

ABLEISM AND OPPRESSION

The moral and medical models of disability are the roots that nourish the oppression of persons with disabilities in society. In the aggregate, we label this oppressive value system *ableism*. Ableism is the belief that because persons with disabilities are not typical of the nondisabled majority, they are inferior. Ableism precipitates oppression, while the results of oppression, including exclusion and ostracism, reinforce the attitudes, actions, and policies of those who oppress. Goldberg (1978) identifies four manifestations of oppression that can be used to understand ableism: containment, the feeling that the lives of people with disabilities are expendable, compartmentalization, and blaming the victim. In addition, we delineate a fifth indicator: denial of disability.

Containment

Containment refers to limiting the choices, exposure, and life experiences of disabled persons, as well as the opportunities for disabled persons to fully participate in society, and may be geographical, psychological, or social. This component of oppression of persons with disabilities stems from both the moral model and the medical model. Within the moral paradigm, the linkage of disability with sin tends to result in the ostracism of persons with disabilities. No one wants to associate with a group of people who are abnormal, immoral, and transgressive (Livneh, 1982). In addition, Judeo-Christian teachings see human beings as being made in the image of God. Thus people are superior in the realm of animals and are not really animals. Persons with disabilities remind nondisabled persons of humanity's imperfections, thus separating us from God (Livneh, 1980). This component of the moral model isolates persons with disabilities because no one wants to be reminded that he or she is finite and mortal and that we will all die like animals do. In some Asian societies, a person's disability causes shame to his or her family and ancestors; therefore disabled persons are hidden away.

The medical model offers the greatest justification for the confinement of persons with disabilities. The connection between confinement and the medical model has historical roots. John Locke and other leaders and thinkers of the Enlightenment era expressed great optimism about the possibility of making human beings perfect. In Western societies, this idealistic belief led to the development of institutions dedicated to changing the imperfect human to the perfect human (Rothman, 1971). However, as Longmore (1993) points out, for the majority of persons with disabilities, anything approaching perfection is impossible. Medical science cannot remold people with disabilities in the image of normalcy. Thus the optimism of the Enlightenment was replaced by frustration and fear based on the futility of the enormous energy invested in making persons with disabilities perfect. The fear comes out of the renewed feeling of hopelessness in the face of natural forces and the fear that persons with disabilities will perpetuate their abnormalities (Longmore, 1987). Consequently, institutions that originally offered hope for making persons with disabilities "normal" became warehouses to hide the shame and fear of disability. Richard Salsgiver's early life was directly affected by the oppressive manifestations of the medical model. When he was six years old, his parents, at the urging of several physicians, confined him in an institution for six years—until he was twelve years old.

Although such institutions have been closed in recent years, similar types of institutions such as nursing facilities and convalescent centers and various "special" programs keep disabled people isolated, segregated, and warehoused. In the United States, the 1999 Supreme Court ruled in *Olmstead v. L.C.* that unnecessarily institutionalizing disabled persons is disability discrimination. However, people continue to be warehoused in institutions due to the misappropriation of resources to medical institutions rather than to community resources. In response, the National Council on Independent Living holds an annual march on the Capitol with slogans such as "What do we want? Freedom. When do we want it? Now!" A similar slogan—"Nothing about us without us"—demands the right to self-determination. Yet even today, thousands of disabled people continue to be incarcerated in medical and mental health institutions.

The Feeling that the Lives of People with Disabilities Are Expendable

The second component of oppression that Goldenberg (1978) addresses is expendability. Throughout history, persons with disabilities have always been considered disposable based upon both the moral and the medical paradigms of disability. It is the medical paradigm, with its beliefs centering on the "normal" and "functioning" ideals for humans, that is the model most responsible for the belief that persons with disabilities are expendable. The ancient Greeks, founders of much of Western morality and ethics, believed in abandoning children with disabilities and allowing them to die, for fear of their contamination of others.

Some of the spirit of optimism of the Enlightenment era declined with the rise of the eugenics movement in America and Europe. Eugenicists saw disability, particularly "mental retardation" and "mental illness," as the source of social problems. They could not be allowed to reproduce (Rhodes, 1993). Wiggam (1924) taught,

> Intelligent, wholesome, sane, energetic, moral people have more factors in their germ-cells for these virtues than have the unintelligent, the immoral, neurotic, and stupid. The high injunction of Mendelism to eugenics is then that these good factors can be concentrated in families, and by wise marriages preserved there and handed down to bless the race. The bad factors have a tendency by assertive mating, the attraction of like for like, to become concentrated also in family lines. Where these become positively antisocial the individuals possessing them can be either confined or sterilized, and their strains of pollution weeded out of the race. (p. 60)

Coulter (1993) reminds us of the fact that the Nazi physicians used disabled persons to develop the extermination methods that they would later use with the Jews. He discusses the current belief that the lives of infants born with anencephaly are expendable (see box 3.1).

Issues of eugenics arise in current practices of prenatal testing and genetic counseling. Blumberg (1994) explores in detail the matter of screening pregnant women for fetal "defects" with the objective of aborting unwanted, disabled fetuses. With prenatal screening now routine, women are more likely than ever to be made aware that they may carry fetuses with disabilities. If physicians find increased risks for "abnormalities" in the fetus, they may suggest abortion and/or refer the parents for genetic counseling. Too often health care providers emphasize the negative aspects of disability while minimizing the positives. For example, Skotko (2005a, 2005b) reports on research with more than 1,000 mothers of children with Down syndrome in the United States and Spain. A significant number of these women reported that their physicians emphasized the negatives and minimized the positive aspects of life with Down syndrome. Blumberg discusses the dangers of genetic counseling: "Too often counselors do little more than provide future parents with a dreary laundry list of problems their child could have and express sympathy. Rarely are clients encouraged to discuss disability related concerns with people who are disabled or who are parents of disabled children" (p. 5). He concludes: "Instead, much medical literature seems to assume that the purpose of counseling is to help ambivalent parents to accept giving up the fetus just as they earlier accepted testing" (p. 7).

Fetuses with disabilities are at greatly increased risk of being considered expendable and aborted. Some justify these actions as a compassionate act intended to prevent the birth of children who would be consigned to lives of misery. However, we suggest that this is a specious assumption. For example, Altshuler, Mackelprang, and Baker (2008) found that disabled youths express life satisfaction on par with nondisabled peers. Nondisabled persons may consider the lives of their disabled peers less valuable, but the youths themselves disagree.

> ## Box 3.1 Anencephaly and Organ Donation
>
> Anencephaly is a neural tube defect in pregnancy that often results in fetal death. The skull, scalp, and cerebral cortex are generally partially or completely absent in infants born with anencephaly. Generally what remains is the brain stem. In essence, the conscious part of the brain is missing, but the primitive, life-supporting areas are present and function and can sustain breathing and heartbeat for several hours to several days. Some argue that anencephaly is a condition of brain absence or that anencephalics are not fully living or human. Others argue that brain death occurs with the cessation of all brain function, including that of the brain stem.
>
> Euthanasia of children with anencephaly for the sake of organ donation has become a source of controversy. If anencephalics live to their natural death, their organs become unviable for donation. Therefore, to be viable organ donors, they must be declared brain dead—or brain absent—before brain stem function deteriorates and their organs are destroyed. Some parents and health care professionals argue for prompt removal of organs for transplant. Others, such as the Canadian Medical Association, oppose this practice.
>
> What are your thoughts about the following?
>
> 1. Are anencephalic infants living, brain dead, or brain absent?
> 2. Should the organs of anencephalics be used for transplant if it means removing them while heartbeat and respiration are still functioning?
> 3. Are anencephalic children disabled? Is this a disability issue?

Prenatal testing and disability are difficult and complex issues that create ambivalence in the disability community. For those who oppose abortion rights, the matter would seem simple: fetuses should not be aborted. However, as feminist writer Jennie Morris (1991) states, even ardent nondisabled pro-lifers are likely to make exceptions when a fetus has a severe disability. Most disability rights leaders believe that women have the right to choose whether or not to have an abortion. They consider women's right to reproductive self-determination to be as fundamental a right as the right of disabled people to control their own bodies and lives. On the other hand, it is fair to ask how the disability community can support the eradication of future children with disabilities. For example, the majority of pregnancies in which the fetus is determined to have Down syndrome result in abortion (U.S. Preventive Services Task Force, 1996). Blumberg (1994) succinctly presents the dilemma: "Quite simply put, the movement's dilemma is that abortion is being used to keep people with disabilities from entering the world, and a great number of us want abortion to remain legal" (p. 7).

Asch (1994) probes the source of the dilemma and finds a potential way out. The issue centers not so much on the fact that genetic screening is made available or that women may choose to abort a fetus with a potential disability; the problem lies with the medical model bias of the professionals providing the genetic counseling:

> Our discomfort arises out of the knowledge that when information about life with a disability is described at all, it usually is a description filled with gloom and tragedy and limited opportunities completely at odds with the views of the disability rights movement and of the legislators and professionals whose work supports movement goals. Rather, the whole genetics enterprise is permeated by the medical model of disability—linking every difficulty to the physiological characteristics of the condition and not to any characteristics of the society in which people with the condition live their lives. Many of us repudiate the medical model and call for a virtual overhauling of the way genetics professionals go about their work. (p. 13)

To mitigate these dangers, health care and reproductive health professionals must provide a broad range of information about the lives of persons with disabilities. Families receiving information from health care providers and genetic professionals need to hear about the fact that most persons with disabilities perceive their lives to be positive and rich. In fact, Skotko (2005a, 2005b) found that mothers' positive or negative perceptions of their newborn children's disabilities were directly related to the attitudes their health care providers displayed. On a larger scale, societal attitudes need changing. Families need to know about the history of disability and the victories won by the disability community (Asch, 1994). Families need not start with the assumption that the fetus with a potential disability should be aborted. Thus the likelihood of disability precipitating abortion as a result of ableism and discrimination decreases.

Chestnut (2001) talks about the experiences of Martha Beck, a famous writer and life coach, with the medical profession: "If you read Martha's bestseller, *Expecting Adam* . . . , you know that near her sixth month of pregnancy with her second child, she discovered she was carrying a fetus with Down's syndrome. 'Our obstetrician was absolutely terrified about me having Adam,' she says of the Harvard doctor who desperately tried talking her into aborting. 'Then I looked at him and thought, his whole life is about destroying anything in him that is like a stupid little boy. This child is his monster, the bogeyman under his bed' " (pp. 151–152).

For too many health practitioners, persons with disabilities are those phantoms and bogeymen that they would like to somehow get rid of. If you can't cure them, prevent their births. The issue is a complex one that requires the consideration of a myriad of variables. Box 3.2 places some of these variables in your hands.

Box 3.2   Reproductive Rights and Disability

The issue of women's right to choose to have an abortion is debated worldwide. Below is a list of potential reasons a woman might conceivably use to determine whether or not to terminate a pregnancy. Would you favor a woman's right given the following situations or based on the following characteristics?

Mother-related variables:
- Any time for any reason
- When the mother's physical health is threatened
- When the mother's mental health is threatened

Child's characteristics:
- Eye color
- Sex
- The presence of Down syndrome
- Short stature
- High risk of schizophrenia
- The presence of spina bifida

How absolute versus situational are your beliefs relative to abortion? What are the reasons for your answers? How do your attitudes about various characteristics affect your responses?

In addition to preventing the birth of children with disabilities, many in society and within the medical community support euthanasia and assisted suicide. On October 24, 1993, while the rest of his family worshiped in church, Robert Latimer placed his severely disabled daughter Tracy in his pickup truck in the garage of their home, closed the garage door, started the truck, and left twelve-year-old Tracy to die. Convicted of second-degree murder by a jury of his peers in a Canadian court, his appeals were based on the belief that he was doing her a favor. In his mind, as well as the minds of the many physicians who testified in his defense, Tracy was better off dead (Eckstein, 1996–1997). Harkins (1994) discusses a physician who for three years tried to convince the mother of Corey Brown, a twelve-year-old girl with cerebral palsy and scoliosis, to agree to a do-not-resuscitate order for her at school. Again, the underlying position was that a person with a disability is really better off dead.

The majority of the so-called mercy killings and attempted mercy killings are of adult women with disabilities, whom society views as sexually unattractive, unable to carry out traditional female roles such as bearing and raising children or taking care of the home, and unable to compete in the workplace (Asch & Fine, 1988; Montgomery, 1998). Many in the disability community believe that Terry Schiavo died because of the social construction of people with disabilities that defined her as expendable, while others disagree (Mackelprang, 2005; Salsgiver, 2005).

Many medical professionals are convinced that helping people with severe conditions kill themselves is an act of mercy. Not Dead Yet, a disability rights group, believes that assisted suicide is a way families and society can get rid of people with disabilities who are considered a burden (Goldberg, 1998). Longmore (1997) points out an interesting irony in American beliefs about disability. Many professionals who support assisted suicide believe that individuals are autonomous and have self-determination. They should have the right to end their lives. Longmore questions this argument and sees it as a rationalization: "This is the sort of 'autonomy, self-determination and liberty' society willingly accords people with disabilities: the freedom to choose death. . . . And then it applauds our 'courage' and 'rationality,' all the while ignoring how society itself has battered us and made our lives unbearable" (p. 14).

Expendability is rationalized by the compartmentalization of people with disabilities. Like most issues around disability, there are several points of view based upon values and priorities. Think through the scenarios presented in box 3.3 and answer in your own mind the questions posed.

Compartmentalization

A third element of oppression that Goldenberg (1978) discusses is compartmentalization. Compartmentalization is the stereotyping of persons with disabilities, or placing them in predetermined categories. Both the moral model and the medical model support the compartmentalization of persons with disabilities. Perhaps the most grievous role in which society places persons with disabilities is that of the object of pity, which has origins in the idea that people with disabilities are poor souls; that they are indeed objects of charity; and that when one takes care of them, the caretaker is guaranteed a place in heaven (Bogdan & Biklen, 1993) or at least is involved in the work of the divine. This particular stereotype is particularly insidious. Shapiro (1993) explains pity and its exploitive nature succinctly and powerfully: "The poster child is a surefire tug at our hearts. The children picked to represent charity fund-raising drives are brave, determined, and inspirational, the most innocent victims of the cruelest whims of life and health. Yet they smile through their 'unlucky' fates—a condition that weakens muscles or cuts life expectancy to a brutish handful of years, a birth 'defect' or childhood trauma. No other symbol of disability is more beloved by Americans than the cute and courageous poster child—or more loathed by people with disabilities themselves" (p. 12). Pity places persons with disabilities in a totally powerless position. They are not in control of their own lives. They are childlike.

Box 3.3   Quality of Life versus End of Life

Below are several situations relating to disability and end-of-life decisions. What are your attitudes relative to each? Provide your reasons.

- A thirty-four-year-old male who has had high quadriplegia (paralysis and lack of sensation from the neck down) for five years is on a ventilator and is institutionalized in a nursing facility. He demands removal of the ventilator, which will result in his death from asphyxiation.
- A twenty-six-year-old female with severe cerebral palsy requests that a hospital provide her with medications to ease discomfort while she starves herself to death.
- A twenty-five-year-old woman in a persistent vegetative state (PVS) has been unconscious for five years. Her family requests that the nursing facility discontinue artificial hydration and nutrition, which will result in her death within several days.
- An eighteen-year-old woman who has been in a PVS for one year is dependent on a ventilator for breathing. Her family requests that the ventilator be removed, which will result in her death in a matter of hours.
- An eighty-six-year-old woman in a PVS is dependent on a ventilator for breathing. Her family demands that all measures be taken to prolong her life, while her physicians advocate removal of the ventilator, which will result in her death.
- A forty-one-year-old woman has been in a PVS for fifteen years. Her husband requests the cessation of artificial hydration and nutrition, which will result in her death within several days. Her parents strongly disagree and sue to continue artificial hydration and nutrition to keep her alive.

1. In each situation above, what do you think would be the moral choice? Why?
2. To what extent do each of these cases involve disability rights?
3. To what extent does consciousness versus unconsciousness influence your beliefs relative to disability rights in each case?
4. How do social constructions and social policies influence the situations above?

For a fuller discussion of the cases described in this exercise, we refer you to Mackelprang and Mackelprang (2005). (The final case above is illustrative of the Terry Schiavo case, which gained national attention in 2005.)

They are dependent. They are damaged goods. They are not normal. They are not capable of taking care of themselves. They are not a force to be reckoned with. No one would want to be like them (Shapiro, 1993).

This absolutely damning stereotype is constantly used by charities in order to raise funds. "The crippled child becomes a poor soul whose disability evokes pity and guilt and the spirit of giving" (Bogdan & Biklen, 1993, p. 74). This pity is the foundation of telethons; the most infamous of these is the Jerry Lewis Labor Day Telethon. Johnson (1992) points out the various complaints about this telethon by disability leaders who detest the paternalism that pervades the weekend's events. Telethons portray persons with disabilities as children even when they are adults. Disability leaders object to the images portrayed in telethons that objectify and minimize the lives and accomplishments of persons with disabilities. They are portrayed as the saintly objects of charity, forever hoping for a cure that will allow them to find meaning in life. Telethons ignore issues such as inaccessible communities and the need for environmental change, placing the sole emphasis on curing the individual rather than intervening in the environmental obstacles standing in the way of people's access to jobs, buildings, transportation, health care, and recreation. Finally, fund-raising efforts such as the Jerry Lewis telethon promote the belief that being disabled is alien and unnatural (Johnson, 1992). Lewis has acknowledged the underlying driving force of his efforts. Lewis states: "I'm telling people about a child in trouble. If it's pity, we'll get some money. I'm just giving you facts. Pity? You don't want to be pitied because you're a cripple in a wheelchair, stay in your house" (qtd. in Sweet, 2001, p. 50).

Compare the pity-based telethon approach to Spain's progressive policies concerning the blind. In Europe, the blind have received special attention dating back to the Middle Ages, when prisoners of war were intentionally blinded and returned to their homes rather than kept as prisoners or executed. This was considered an expedient and humane way of dealing with prisoners. Garvia (1996) recounts that in the nineteenth century, blind citizens in Spain organized, and that today Spain has "professional blind," those who use their blindness as a source of income. There are multiple lotteries in Spain, including the Cupón de la ONCE (Organización Nacional de Ciegos Españoles), which is staffed by more than 20,000 "registered" blind and disabled people who run the lottery (AngloInfo, 2006). ONCE meets public demand and employs blind people to do so.

Another insidious compartmentalization of persons with disabilities centers on the "sick" role. Largely because of the medical paradigm, society perceives persons with disabilities as being sick. While many persons with disabilities have health-related problems, most are not physically ill. Yet the medical establishment views and treats disability as sickness. Richard Salsgiver's experiences with medical professionals relative to his cerebral palsy illustrate this situation:

Recently, I have been experiencing some problems directly connected to aging and cerebral palsy. They are neurological in nature, and I chose to see a rehabilitation physician rather than a neurologist. In talking about my problem, he referred to my loss of nerve function as being related to a "sick" part of the nerve. Unfortunately for him, this precipitated an hour-long discussion of the difference between what is sick and what is a natural consequence of aging. I'm not sure this is how he preferred to spend his time, but when we were through, he had at least heard my perspective.

Devore and Schlesinger (1999) describe components of the sick role. Persons filling this role are not held responsible, and they are excused from being productive. For this privilege, they have certain duties. First, they must want to get well at any cost. They must follow their treatment plans and take their medicines without protest, and in a passive and pleasant manner. Second, they must be grateful for what they receive.

This compartmentalization perpetuated by the medical model results in the extensive subjugation of persons with disabilities through the reinforcement of their dependency on medical providers and on society. It assumes that persons with disabilities need not work; others will care for them and shelter them from harm. Persons with disabilities will stay at home. They will remain with their parents as long as they can. If they work, it will be at a safe and predictable job. Finally, this stigma results in the expectation that persons with disabilities should be pleasantly accepting and grateful for the meager offerings of society. Persons with disabilities must constantly strive to become "healthy" and "normal," and they must do it with a smile.

The sick role that is imposed on them prevents persons with disabilities from learning the skills necessary for economic survival and advancement. Persons with disabilities are denied the opportunity to take risks and to make mistakes. They are not encouraged to go out on their own, to break away from their parents. They are not encouraged, particularly by medical professionals, to take control of their lives.

As previously discussed, one of the most overtly hostile implications of the moral and medical models is that persons with disabilities are a threat to the fabric of society (Arokiasamy et al., 1978). According to the moral model, disabled people are aberrant or sinful and should be avoided and prevented from perpetuating their deviant natures. Because they bring forth the displeasure of God, they are a menace to be feared. The medical model views the menace in terms of reproduction and the future of humans. Disability threatens the future integrity of the human species. Therefore, persons with disabilities need to be prevented from reproducing. Persons with developmental disabilities usually fall into this category. In addition, society perceives certain people with disabilities as personally dangerous and a threat to life and limb. Persons with AIDS and persons with mental health disabilities fall into the category of a personal threat to society (Arokiasamy et al., 1978).

While all the above elements of oppression are perpetrated by society, the final element of oppression, blaming the victim, relieves society of any responsibility in the oppression of disabled people.

Blaming the Victim

Both Goldenberg (1978) and Pharr (1988) discuss the concept of blaming the victim, a process in which those in authority or positions of respect fault injured parties for externally imposed problems. Blaming the victim provides justification for discrimination, whether based on race, gender, age, sexual orientation, disability, or other characteristics. Pharr points out that this is the major mechanism for the internalization of stereotypes. Longmore (1997) calls it "individualistic claptrap usually fed to disabled people. It keeps us believing that if our lives are limited, it is because of our disabilities or lack of pluck" (p. 14).

Before the independent living movement began in the 1960s, this explanation for the individual's lack of success dominated rehabilitation treatment. DeJong (1979) discusses the rehabilitation model, in which the locus of the problem is the individual. It is the individual who makes it or does not. Much of this has to do, according to the early rehabilitation model, with the perseverance, the personal responsibility, and the individual effort of the person in rehabilitation. The professionals provide the institutions, model, and tools needed to achieve success, which is defined by the professionals and can be achieved if individuals demonstrate compliance, perseverance, and dedication. If rehabilitation fails, it is the failure of the individual to overcome his or her disability, not the failure of the process or the structure (Arokiasamy et al., 1978).

Richard Salsgiver has experienced the blaming-the-victim mentality throughout his life.

> When institutionalized as a teen, I received physical therapy three times a week, and my therapists complained constantly when I did not reach the goals they set for me that I simply wasn't trying hard enough. Therapists, physicians, and other treatment team members repeatedly conveyed this message to my parents, who then joined the chorus of voices telling me that I was not trying hard enough. I was somehow responsible for my deficiencies, and if I just tried harder, I could indeed walk—and walk normally.
>
> As an adult, I experienced blaming the victim within the medical model when working as an administrator at the chancellor's office of the California State University. As part of my duties, I regularly attended meetings of the directors of programs servicing students with disabilities on the CSU campuses. At one such meeting held in San Francisco, several program directors met for lunch. Most of them had degrees in rehabilitation counseling or human services, and only two of us at the table were persons with disabilities. The conversation turned to individual students and their lack of achievement and, except for the other director with a disability and myself, everyone joked about their students'

lack of progress. Their humor centered on their students' dependency, their unwillingness to leave home or find a job after graduation, or their lack of motivation to obtain passing grades.

When the other director with a disability and I challenged their arguments and attitude, everyone at the table became quiet. When I started to talk about the nature of oppression and disability, they discontinued eye contact. Upon finishing dessert, all the nondisabled directors got up and left, while the remaining director and I sat in stunned silence, just looking at each other and shaking our heads.

Some disabled persons accept the blaming-the-victim mentality and internalize others' explanations that they are, and will forever be, deficient. On the other end of the spectrum are those who internalize this medical model–based explanation and constantly strive to overcome their disability by performing spectacular deeds and feats. These persons are known in Disability culture as "supercrips." They may reason that no matter the expense in time or energy, they will be as normal as possible. They climb mountains to prove their normalcy. They walk at great expense rather than being one of those "handicapped" people using a wheelchair. They deny their pain so that their peers and society accept them as normal. They disavow their connection with other persons with disabilities, internalize ableist messages, and deny the existence of oppression.

Franklin D. Roosevelt was the personification of the supercrip. Paul Longmore, a historian who specializes in the history of persons with disability, talked about this phenomenon in an address before the California Disability Leadership Summit in October of 1993:

> What Franklin Roosevelt did was to strike a bargain with the American people. Franklin Roosevelt presented himself as an "overcomer," someone who never succumbed to self-pity—who never gave in to his disability—someone who was ceaselessly striving after the example of nondisabled people, someone ceaselessly trying to recover his "normality." The image he presented of overcoming became the required mode of self-presentation for people with disabilities in the three generations since Roosevelt's era. He created a new social identity of overcoming. He made an implicit bargain with the nondisabled majority in society. The terms of the bargain of overcoming go like this: society says, "We will extend provisional and partial toleration of your public presence as long as you display ceaseless, cheerful—cheerful is a very important part of this—striving toward normality."

FDR was indeed a supercrip—this was the only way he could succeed as president of the United States.

Denial of Disability

Before the emergence of the independent living movement in the 1960s, disabled persons expressed the positive components of their identity through the process of either pretending they were not disabled or redefining obvious disabled attributes in a nondisabled fashion. This process is known as denial and uses up a tremendous amount of physical and psychological energy. Up until the mid-1960s, the survival and success of persons with disabilities in the face of societal oppression depended to a large degree on denial and hiding disability components.

Wright (1983) concludes that children with physical disabilities develop psychosocially similarly to children without disabilities because of denial. Denial allows persons with disabilities to go forward in the face of the adversity of oppression that results from negative social constructs of disabilitiy. It allows many children and adults with disabilities to fill in the gaps created by the view that disability is aberrant, nonspiritual, and unnatural. Richard Salsgiver's experiences as a child illustrate.

> When I was a kid, I pretended that my crutches were not really crutches but were my horse on which I rode. I would throw my crutches to the ground and jump on the ground, pretending that I was jumping off my horse. When I was in high school, I used canes rather than crutches. I would pretend they were like the cane used by Bat Masterson, the fictional TV hero. When I was in college, I pretended my wheelchair was a bicycle. I took an attribute directly connected to my disability and turned it into a nondisability entity.

For the few persons with disabilities who "make it" in Western society historically and currently, the mechanism of denial goes beyond the individual with the disability to the world around him or her. Many successful disabled persons have the ability to convince those around them either that they are not disabled or that their disability is far less severe than it is.

To illustrate, we again turn to Franklin D. Roosevelt, the thirty-second president of the United States, who was severely disabled from polio. In order to be elected and supported as president of the United States, he was required to hide his disability from the public. Gallagher (1985) paints a vivid picture of the extent to which FDR used his powers of persuasion to create an illusion of nondisability. The public went along with the "splendid deception":

> This largely voluntary suppression of an important aspect of the President's life was an extraordinary thing. That Roosevelt pulled it off in the 1930s is in part a tribute to the close, harmonious relations he maintained with the working press and to the affection and respect accorded the President by the reporters. In a sense, however, this veil of silence about the extent of the President's handicap required the unspoken acquiescence of everyone—Roosevelt, the press, and the American people.
>
> In a very real way a great nation does not want a crippled man as its President: It does not wish to think of its leader as impaired. Roosevelt was undeniably and obviously a crippled man. Literally millions of people saw him moving down his railroad ramp, bent over like a praying mantis, or hobbling

painfully slowly on the arm of his son. Crippled or not, the nation wanted this man, with all his magnificent qualities, as its leader. So an agreement was struck: the existence of FDR's handicap would simply be denied by all. The people would pretend that their leader was not crippled, and their leader would do all that he could not to let them see that he was. The generally accepted line was that FDR had had polio and was now a bit lame; he had been paralyzed, but now he was recovered. He was a "cured cripple." (p. 96)

Richard Salsgiver experienced this individual and societal denial early in his career.

My colleagues and friends would never acknowledge my disability, and on those rare occasions when the subject came up, their comments usually centered on their estimation that I was not really "handicapped." It was as if this was the highest compliment they could give me, a person with a disability, to show their acceptance. My incorporation of a positive disability self-identity occurred after I became involved in the independent living movement when I moved to California. Over the course of several years in California, my disability identity became deeply embedded in my identity and changed my self-concept.

The change in my identity became obvious several years later when my wife, Pam, and I returned to Pennsylvania to visit relatives and friends. We stayed for awhile at the home of a friend and fellow mental health professional with whom I had worked at a partial psychiatric ward day hospital for children and adolescents before moving to California. In the course of several conversations, we discussed the many happenings in our profession, including an increased awareness of disability as a minority/civil rights issue. During one of these discussions, she said to me, "But you aren't really disabled." I replied, "But I *am* a person with a disability. It is as much a part of my identity as my family, my profession, my intelligence." I realized that for my friend and for most Americans, telling people with disabilities that they are not really disabled or handicapped is the highest of compliments.

Shapiro (1993) recounts a similar exchange at the memorial services for Timothy Cook, a disability rights fighter, when friends and colleagues got up and complimented him by saying they did not see him as disabled. "It was as if someone had tried to compliment a black man by saying, 'You're the least black person I ever met,' as false as telling a Jew, 'I never think of you as Jewish,' as clumsy as seeking to flatter a woman with 'You don't act like a woman'" (p. 3).

Even today, for the author and many other persons with disabilities, creating the illusion of nondisability is an important skill for success in the nondisabled world. By passing as nondisabled, disabled persons engage in denial and improve opportunities for acceptance. However, denial comes at great expense. Some individuals never develop the survival mechanism. For those who do, the physical and psychological effort it takes to maintain denial is costly, resulting in internalized ableism and leaving little energy for work, family, and recreation.

SUMMARY

Oppression inevitably affects the identity of persons with disabilities (Large, 1993). Some persons with disabilities internalize society's stereotypes in much the same way that some African Americans (Solomon, 1976), ethnic minorities worldwide, women, and gays and lesbians (Pharr, 1988) respond to their oppression. Internalized racism affects the identity of people of color. Internalized heterosexism affects the identity of LGBTQ individuals. Internalized ableism influences the identity of disabled persons.

People with disabilities are oppressed in American society and most other places in the world. The oppression takes on the form of containment, the feeling that they are expendable, compartmentalization, and blaming of the victim. People with disabilities are contained geographically (in institutions), psychologically, and economically. People with disabilities are treated as expendable through inaccessible health care and euthanasia. The compartmentalization of people with disability results in stereotyping leading to imprisonment at the bottom rungs of society. And people with disabilities are blamed for their oppression. All these oppressive experiences relate to the social paradigms of disability. The two main culprits remain the moral model and the medical model.

DISCUSSION QUESTIONS

1. In human services, do you think it is important to understand that persons with disabilities experience oppression?
2. How would you use issues of oppression in working with people with disabilities?
3. If the moral model of disability stems from religion, can institutionalized religion play a role in facilitating the empowerment of people with disabilities?
4. Upon graduation, you will most likely be employed in a medical-related agency. How will knowledge of the medical model inform your practice with persons with disabilities?

PERSONAL NARRATIVE: ABBY KOVALSKY

Abby Kovalsky, LCSW, is disabilities project coordinator for Jewish Family and Children Services in San Francisco, California. Abby has been very active in the independent living movement for many years. She has myasthenia grāvis, a neuromuscular disability that produces symptoms such as weakness of the voluntary muscles, including the facial muscles and muscles that affect speech and swallowing.

My disability is myasthenia gravis. I was diagnosed with MG at age sixteen. Before my disability, I did not know any children who were disabled, but I did know a few adults. One had a developmental disability. All the children in the neighborhood made fun of her, including me. But a part of me felt sorry for her. There was a store owner in the neighborhood who had an adult daughter with severe cerebral palsy. She was on the telethon every year and was kind of a celebrity. She was always dressed beautifully, with makeup and a lovely hairdo. Other than that, I don't remember much about her.

Becoming disabled in adolescence was devastating. I had never heard of myasthenia gravis and could barely pronounce it. I thought that if I got proper medical care it would go away. Because it affected my speech, facial muscles, eyes, and limbs, I was very limited in physical activity. It progressed rapidly and I spent a lot of time in the hospital. We had to move to New York from Connecticut during my senior year in high school because I needed specialized medical care. I didn't want to see my friends. I was embarrassed because I couldn't smile or speak clearly. Slowly, they stopped calling and visiting. I don't think they knew how to act around me either. Over time, I became more and more isolated.

My mother became overprotective after I became disabled. The doctor told her I couldn't be emotionally upset or I could get worse. So she walked on eggshells around me. My mother was also ashamed of my disability. I can remember being in line at the market with my mother. We knew the people who worked there because it was a neighborhood store. The man at the cash register, whom we both knew well, asked my mother what was wrong with my voice. She told him that I had a cold. Later, when I asked her why she said that, she said my condition was none of his business. I knew then how she felt about me.

My college career was interrupted by hospitalizations. When I was able to return to college, I decided to go into medical research. Everyone told me the load was too much. All my classes had laboratories; it was like taking a double load. In a sense, I was my own role model. The more people told me I shouldn't go into medical research, the more determined I was to prove them wrong. As a result, I entered a PhD program in medical microbiology and immunology.

I was in my third year of the PhD program when I decided to take a leave of absence from the program to rethink my goals. I had just completed a peer counseling course at the local center for independent living (CIL), and I was going to volunteer there. At the same time, when I left my graduate program, a job opened at the CIL for an information and referral counselor. I was hired. I was twenty-nine years old, and after thirteen years of living with MG, this was the first time I identified as a person with a disability, not a sickness. It was a major transition.

I had a real role model at the CIL—my supervisor, a licensed clinical social worker. Since that time, there has never been a doubt in my mind that I am a person with a disability. It is so much a part of who I am today. It feels liberating. I swore to myself that I would never again hide anything about my disability.

There is no generalized way in which I see others with disabilities. As people with disabilities, we are as varied as any other group of people in the community. I can tell you I see all of us as people, with whatever baggage we have.

I definitely think there is a Disability culture. For me, any group that has been so totally discriminated against for unsubstantial reasons has commonalities that are unique to that group. There is a history, a language, and a rich montage of art forms relating to disability.

My supervisor at the CIL encouraged me to apply to social work school. I did, got accepted, and formally left my PhD program for an MSW program. I was more assertive when I applied for vocational rehabilitation services in social work school: they paid half of my tuition at a private institution. Unfortunately, social work has not been as accepting as I had hoped.

When I was in social work school, I was railroaded into my placements because the field placement person decided that the only agency that would accept me was a rehabilitation hospital. She never bothered to send my packet of practicum materials to any other agencies, and I had no interviews. I was enraged. I wanted my social work education to be in the health track, but if my first-year placement was in a hospital, I wanted a different placement in my second year. Instead of having a second-year placement that met my needs, I was placed in a setting otherwise used for first-year placements because the supervisor had no problem with my disability. Again, I was not given an opportunity to interview with other agencies or determine my placement—I had little choice in the matter.

Upon graduation, after getting straight A's and having excellent references from my social worker, I had directors of hospital social work departments tell me I should go into administration. Again, there was this concern that doctors wouldn't understand me. I offered to work two weeks for free at one hospital just to prove I could do the work. I was angry. Here I was in a profession where I thought people are supposed to be caring and sensitive. Was I wrong!

From the school personnel (who had an obligation once I was accepted to the program to do all they could for me) to social workers in practice (who are some of the most prejudiced people I have met), I learned the hard way about outright discrimination. I have also experienced rude questions and comments from doctors with whom I have worked. (Interestingly, these doctors were older women.)

Social work was not the first place I experienced discrimination. For example, when I first graduated from college, I wanted to apply to a training program in laboratory technology. Yet I was told by most schools that I shouldn't even bother applying because the doctors would have a hard time understanding me. Since this was a very competitive field that paid quite well, I didn't waste my time applying. Even though educational and employment discrimination were not new to me, I guess I expected social workers to be different. That made my treatment in the social work profession especially hard to deal with.

The biggest obstacle people with disabilities face is discrimination, pure and simple. I experience discrimination and stereotyping in my everyday life. People assume that because I have a speech impairment I must also be deaf or "mentally retarded." The ADA was too little, too late for me. Perhaps I have been helped by 504 [section 504 of the Rehabilitation Act of 1973] in some ways.

The major issue around disability continues to be unabated discrimination. This one issue has serious consequences in every aspect of a disabled person's life, from employment to housing to dating to raising a family. It's the age-old dilemma, learning to tolerate people who are different. The difference between other minority groups and the disabled is that anyone can become disabled at any time. I think this touches a vulnerable place in all of us that we don't want to acknowledge. The paradox, as I see it, is that until people with disabilities are a solid part of the workforce, with earning power and voting power, it will be slow going. However, it is hard to develop earning power when we are shut out of the job market. The flip side is that, for people who are not able to work, society needs to acknowledge their value as human beings even though they are not part of the Puritan work ethic.

On a personal level, I joined a dating service a year and a half ago. All I hear from the agency is that everyone who reads my profile and then sees my photo is basically not willing to meet someone with my disability.

As we all know, we cannot legislate attitudes. What must happen is education of the masses, constant and persistent, and, in every way possible, creation of opportunities for people to have contact with people with disabilities. The agency at which I work sponsors an educational program for nondisabled children under the auspices of the program I coordinate, where speakers with disabilities go into the classroom. I spent two years looking for work. I had lots of interviews. One person had the audacity to say to me, "I had to meet you, you look so good on paper, but we don't have any openings." I knew this statement was not true, because I had answered an ad in the paper and knew the agency was looking for a person to talk about living with a disability. It is a powerful experience for these children. They ask questions and learn about advocacy, rights, and prejudice. People with disabilities become more human and less frightening to them.

People have many differences; disability is just another way people are different. I have always felt different from others in many ways, and my disability is one of those ways. However, before I developed an identity as a person with a disability, I thought it was terrible to be a person who was disabled. I never asked anyone with a disability if it was terrible; I just assumed so because that is what I heard from others.

The older I get, the more comfortable I become with the way I am, although there are still times when I am struck in a vulnerable way by something someone might say or the stares I still get. I have been discriminated against most definitely; the most traumatic area has been in employment. However, I have also been successful. What helped me to be successful was sheer determination. I do get tired sometimes of having to fight for everything, but I continue to move on.

As for my mother, she has grown. It was recently that she said to me, "I am very proud of you. You could have just spent your life as a vegetable."

SUGGESTED READINGS

Fadiman, A. (1997). *The spirit catches you and you fall down: A Hmong child, her American doctors, and the collision of two cultures.* New York: Farrar, Straus and Giroux.

Gallagher, H. G. (1985). *FDR's splendid deception.* New York: Dodd, Mead.

Racino, J. A. (1999). *Policy, program evaluation, and research and disability: Community support for all.* New York: Haworth Press.

Wright, B. (1983). *Physical disability—a psychological approach* (2nd ed.). New York: Harper & Row.

REFERENCES

Albrecht, G. (1992). *The disability business: Rehabilitation in America.* Newbury Park, CA: Sage.

Altshuler, S. A., Mackelprang, R. W., & Baker, R. L. (2008). Youth with disabilities: A standardized self-portrait of how they are faring. *Journal of Social Work in Disability and Rehabilitation, 7*(1), 1–18.

AngloInfo. (2006). *The Spanish lottery.* Retrieved October 16, 2006, from http://barcelona.angloinfo.com/countries/spain/lottery.asp

Arokiasamy, C. M., Rubin, S. E., & Roessler, R. T. (1978). Sociological aspects of disability. In S. E. Rubin & R. T. Roessler (Eds.), *Foundations of the vocational rehabilitation process* (pp. 123–155). Baltimore: University Park Press.

Asch, A. (1994). The human genome project and disability rights. *Disability Rag, 15*(1), 12–15.

Asch, A., & Fine, M. (1988). Introduction: Beyond pedestals. In M. Fine & A. Asch (Eds.), *Women with disabilities: Essays in psychology, culture, and politics* (pp. 1–37). Philadelphia: Temple University Press.

Blumberg, L. (1994). Eugenics vs. reproductive choice. *Disability, 15*(1), 3–11.

Bogdan, R., & Biklen, D. (1993). Handicapism. In M. Nagler (Ed.), *Perspectives on disability: Text and readings on disability* (2nd ed., pp. 69–76). Palo Alto, CA: Health Markets Research.

Bryant, M. D. (1993). Religion and disability: Some notes on religious attitudes and views. In M. Nagler (Ed.), *Perspectives on disability: Text and readings on disability* (2nd ed., pp. 91–95). Palo Alto, CA: Health Markets Research.

Chestnut, M. (2001, March). A reality check with Martha Beck. *O: The Oprah Magazine,* pp. 151–152.

Coulter, D. L. (1993). Beyond Baby Doe: Does infant transplantation justify euthanasia? In M. Nagler (Ed.), *Perspectives on disability: Text and readings on disability* (2nd ed., pp. 507–514). Palo Alto, CA: Health Markets Research.

DeJong, G. (1979). *The movement for independent living: Origins, ideology and implications for disability research.* East Lansing: Michigan State University, Center for International Rehabilitation.

Devlieger, P. (1995). Why disabled? The cultural understanding of physical disability in an African society. In B. Ingstad & S. R. Whyte (Eds.), *Disability and culture* (pp. 94–106). Berkeley: University of California Press.

Devore, W., & Schlesinger, E. G. (1999). *Ethnic-sensitive social work practice* (5th ed.). Pacific Grove, CA: Brooks/Cole.

Eckstein, C. M. (1996–1997). One of our children is dead. *Ability Network Magazine, 5*(2). Retrieved from http://www.ability.ns.ca/v5n2/v5n2p37.html

Fadiman, A. (1997). *The spirit catches you and you fall down: A Hmong child, her American doctors, and the collision of two cultures*. New York: Farrar, Straus and Giroux.

Farley, J. E. (1995). *Majority-minority relations*. Englewood Cliffs, NJ: Prentice Hall.

Gallagher, H. G. (1985). *FDR's splendid deception*. New York: Dodd, Mead.

Garvia, R. (1996). The professional blind in Spain. *Work, Employment and Society, 10*(3), 491–508.

Goldberg, R. (1998, June 7). Protesters arrested outside assisted suicide conference. *Detroit Free Press*. Retrieved from http://www.freep.com/news/mich/qassist7.htm

Goldenberg, I. (1978). *Oppression and social intervention: Essays on the human condition and the problems of change*. Chicago: Nelson-Hall.

Groce, N. (2005). Immigrants, disability, and rehabilitation. In J. H. Stone (Ed.), *Culture and disability: Providing culturally competent services* (pp. 1–13). Thousand Oaks, CA: Sage.

Harkins, S. (1994). No villains: The Corey Brown saga. *Disability Rag, 15*(3), 3–7.

Helander, B. (1995). Disability as incurable illness: Health, process, and personhood in southern Somalia. In B. Ingstad & S. R. Whyte (Eds.), *Disability and culture* (pp. 73–93). Berkeley: University of California Press.

Ho, M. K. (1987). *Family therapy with ethnic minorities*. Newbury Park, CA: Sage.

Ingstad, B., & Whyte, S. R. (1995). Disability and culture: An overview. In B. Ingstad & S. R. Whyte (Eds.), *Disability and culture* (pp. 3–32). Berkeley: University of California Press.

Johnson, M. (1991). Cripple—the word we love and hate. *Disability Rag, 12*(2), 27–28.

Johnson, M. (1992). "Jerry's kids": Ethics of the Jerry Lewis Labor Day Telethon. *The Nation, 255*(7), 232–234.

Jones, A. (1995). Why Tony Coelho fights for the disabled: Epilepsy kept him from Vietnam—and Jesuits. *National Catholic Reporter*, January 20. Retrieved October 4, 2008, from http://findarticles.com/p/articles/mi_m1141/is_/ai_16625598?tag= artBody;col1

Large, T. (1993). The effects of attitudes upon the blind: A reexamination. In M. Nagler (Ed.), *Perspectives on disability: Text and readings on disability* (2nd ed., pp. 165–168). Palo Alto, CA: Health Markets Research.

Liu, G. Z. (2005). *Best practices: Developing cross-cultural competence from a Chinese perspective*. In J. H. Stone (Ed.), *Culture and disability: Providing culturally competent services* (pp. 65–85). Thousand Oaks, CA: Sage.

Livneh, H. (1980). Disability and monstrosity: Further comments. *Rehabilitation Literature, 41*, 280–283.

Livneh, H. (1982). On the origins of negative attitudes toward people with disabilities. *Rehabilitation Literature, 43*, 338–347.

Livo, N. J., & Cha, D. (1991). *Folk stories of the Hmong: Peoples of Laos, Thailand, and Vietnam*. Englewood, CO: Libraries Unlimited.

Longmore, P. K. (1987). Elizabeth Bouvia, assisted suicide and social prejudice. *Issues in Law & Medicine, 3*(2), 141–168.

Longmore, P. K. (1993, October). *History of the disability rights movement and disability culture.* Address delivered to the California Disability Leadership Summit, Anaheim, CA.

Longmore, P. K. (1997). I am terminally ill, and I have been for the last forty-three years. *Ragged Edge, 18*(1), 13–15.

Mackelprang, R. W. (2005). Terry Schiavo—a response to Richard Salsgiver. *SCI Psychosocial Process, 18*(3), 187–189.

Mackelprang, R. W., & Salsgiver, R. O. *(1996). People with disabilities and social work: Historical and contemporary issues. Social Work, 41*(1), 7–14.

Mackelprang, R. W., & Salsgiver, R. O. (2003). Christopher Reeve: Not Superman, just a man. *SCI Psychosocial Process, 16*(1), 40–41.

Mackelprang, R. W., & Mackelprang, R. D. (2005). Historical and contemporary issues in end-of-life decisions: Implications for social work. *Social Work, 50*(4), 315–324.

Montgomery, C. (1998). The tactics of survival. *Ragged Edge, 19*(3), 18–20.

Morris, J. (1991). *Pride against prejudice: Transforming attitudes to disability.* Philadelphia: New Society.

Nicolaisen, I. (1995). Persons and nonpersons: Disability and personhood among the Punan Bah of Central Borneo. In B. Ingstad & S. R. Whyte (Eds.), *Disability and culture* (pp. 38–55). Berkeley: University of California Press.

Pharr, S. (1988). *Homophobia: A weapon of sexism.* Inverness, CA: Chardon Press.

Rhodes, R. (1993). Mental retardation and sexual expression: An historical perspective. In R. W. Mackelprang & D. Valentine (Eds.), *Sexuality and disabilities: A guide for human service practitioners* (pp. 1–27). Binghamton, NY: Haworth Press.

Rothman, D. (1971). *The discovery of the asylum: Social order and disorder in the new republic.* Boston: Little, Brown.

Russell, B. (1965). *A history of Western philosophy and its connection with political and social circumstances from the earliest of times to the present day.* New York: Simon & Schuster.

Salsgiver, R. O. (2005). A context for Terri Schiavo. *SCI Psychosocial Process, 18*(3), 185–186.

Salsgiver, R. O., Watson, A., Cooke, J., & Madison, L. S. (2004). Spiritual/religious access for women with disabilities. *SCI Psychosocial Process, 17*(1), 27–32.

Santana-Martin, S., & Santana, F. O. (2005). *An introduction to Mexican culture for service providers.* In J. H. Stone (Ed.), *Culture and disability: Providing culturally competent services* (pp. 161–186). Thousand Oaks, CA: Sage.

Shapiro, J. P. (1993). *No pity: People with disabilities forging a new civil rights movement.* New York: Times Books.

Skotko, B. (2005a). Mothers of children with Down syndrome reflect on their postnatal support. *Pediatrics, 115,* 64–77.

Skotko, B. (2005b). Prenatally diagnosed Down syndrome: Mothers who continued their pregnancies evaluate their health care providers. *American Journal of Obstetrics and Gynecology, 192,* 670–677.

Smart, J., & Smart, D. (1991). Acceptance of disability and the Mexican American culture. *Rehabilitation Counseling Bulletin, 34*(4), 357–367.

Solomon, B. (1976). *Black empowerment: Social work in oppressed communities.* New York: Columbia University Press.

Sweet, R. (2001). At least they got my name right. *Ragged Edge, 5,* 50–52.

Talle, A. (1995). A child is a child: Disability and equality among the Kenya Maasai. In B. Ingstad & S. R. Whyte (Eds.), *Disability and culture* (pp. 56–72). Berkeley: University of California Press.

tenBroek, J., & Matson, F. W. (1959). *Hope deferred: Public welfare and the blind.* Berkeley: University of California Press.

U.S. Preventive Services Task Force. (1996). *Guide to clinical preventive services* (2nd ed.). Washington, DC: U.S. Department of Health and Human Services, Office of Disease Prevention and Health Promotion.

Whyte, S. R. (1995). Disability between discourse and experience. In B. Ingstad & S. R. Whyte (Eds.), *Disability and culture* (pp. 265–291). Berkeley: University of California Press.

Wiggam, A. E. (1924). *The fruit of the family tree.* Indianapolis, IN: Bobbs-Merrill.

Wolfe, K. (1993). The bible and disabilities: From "healing" to the "burning bush." *Disability Rag, 14*(3), 9–10.

Wright, B. (1983). *Physical disability: A psychological approach* (2nd ed.). New York: Harper & Row.

4

Disability Culture

I have developed an identity as a Deaf person. I went from being a child in a hearing school who had "trouble hearing," felt I was different, and just couldn't seem to succeed in school, and not understanding what being deaf meant or even that I was in fact deaf, to readily identifying myself as Deaf, understanding what that means to me and others, and I embrace it comfortably.

—Martha Sheridan, Gallaudet University

STUDENT LEARNING OBJECTIVES

1. To identify how culture is developed and transmitted
2. To understand the development of a culture of Disability
3. To be able to compare and contrast Disability culture and racial/ethnic culture
4. To be able to identify elements of the cultural development and mainte-nance of devalued groups
5. To understand the national and international implications of the concept of a culture of Disability

A culture of spinal cord injury? Deaf heritage? Blindness as an element of diversity? Until the last generation, these things were unheard of. Persons with disabilities have been defined by their differences, and their differences have always been perceived as pathological. Franklin D. Roosevelt went to great measures to hide his wheelchair from the public. Why? His wheelchair was a sign of weakness, a cause for shame. Roosevelt reacted to this societal ableism by seeking to hide the fact that polio made the use of a wheelchair necessary for mobility. A man without two good legs for walking was not a whole man. Arguably, if FDR were to run for president in this era of mass television coverage, he probably would not have a chance of being elected president. Controversy raged about whether the FDR memorial in Washing-ton, D.C., should acknowledge his disability and use of a wheelchair; the wheelchair was finally included. Even Bob Dole's war injury was a topic of discussion when he ran for president of the United States. He was adept at hiding his impairment, usually by holding a pen in his injured hand.

After an automobile accident left Tim Johnston (pseudonym) with para-plegia, he felt the same way Roosevelt seems to have felt. His wheelchair was a cause of shame. An avid recreational athlete before his injury, he saw no way that he could participate in sports again. He told his wife to divorce him and find a "whole" man. He was mortified at the thought of being seen in public with others in wheelchairs. He internalized all the ableist messages he had received throughout his life and accepted his lot as "half a man," who "look[ed] like some freak." Like Roosevelt, Johnston saw his disability as a cause for shame and self-doubt. Unlike Roosevelt, however, Johnston lives in an era in which people with disabilities are beginning to take pride in their whole selves, disability and all.

CULTURE

Some writers on culture and even some experts on disability argue against the existence of a Disability culture. Batavia (2001) questions the efficacy of people using the concept of oppression from a cultural/identity standpoint to achieve political aims. DePoy and Gilson (2004), while recognizing some advantages to the concept of Disability culture, see a distinction between disability identity and cultural Disability identity. Since language and mores are basic components of traditional conceptualizions of culture, they believe the concept of Disability culture falls short in terms of developing a unified disability language and in explaining the lives of affluent people with disabil-ities. Indeed, one of the authors of this text, in his pursuit to establish a program with a foundation in Disability culture, has run into resistance from those whose teaching and research agendas are in culture. This resistance is based upon the assumption that Disability culture is a misnomer. Despite the issues raised by those who question the existence of Disability culture, overall, the view that Disability culture is a legitimate and important frame-work for intellectual discovery is growing among scholars (Jakubowicz & Meekosha, 2002). In fact, many believe that to disregard Disability culture is to weaken the aggregate importance of culture in human behavior. Ignoring the cultural components of disability limits our ability to understand social interaction from a cultural perspective.

To discover the culture of Disability, we must first understand some of the elements of culture in general. The poet T. S. Eliot (1949) discussed three important conditions for culture that influence the ways culture has been viewed for much of this century. First, he contended there must be an organic structure to foster the transmission of culture; in other words, the culture must have a way of being passed along to others. Eliot believed the family to be the primary means by which culture is transmitted, but others can perform this function as well. Second, he believed in the existence of local cultures within larger cultures. These cultures have been largely geo-graphically determined, although with modern technology, geographical boundaries are becoming less important. Finally, Eliot recognized the existence of unity and diversity within cultures. Both the diversity and the strength of commonalities within each culture led him to conclude that culture is "not merely the sum of several activities, but a way of life" (p. 40).

Eagleton (1978) suggests that culture can mean "a society's 'structure of feeling,' its lived manners, habits, morals, values, the learned atmosphere of its learnt behavior and belief." In the societal context, it can mean "a society's whole way of life in an institutional sense, the totality of interacting artistic, economic, social, political, ideological elements which composes its total lived experience" (pp. 4–5). Thompson, Ellis, and Wildavsky (1990) suggest two ways of defining culture: "One views culture as composed of values, beliefs, norms, rationalizations, symbols, ideologies, i.e., mental products. The other sees culture as referring to a total way of life of people, their interpersonal relations as well as their attitudes" (p. 1).

Storey (1993) discusses the meanings of popular culture. Popular culture can be defined as culture that is widely accepted or favored. Storey separates high culture, which comes from the upper classes, from popular culture, which comes from the people or the masses.

By combining all these perspectives, we conclude that culture is a way of thinking, feeling, and believing—a stored knowledge that guides people's lives. In part, culture is developed as a social legacy, learned when one belongs to a group. Forged by constant conscious and unconscious influences as well as social and political forces, culture affects its members from birth to death. On an individual level, feelings, reactions, and behaviors become second nature in the context of cultural experiences and identities (Epstein, 1973; Milner, 1992; Storey, 1993).

Culture influences society's expectations about how people should act. Rules that govern interpersonal and social interactions are developed within cultural contexts. Social and political structures and organizations are reflections of the cultures in which they are developed. Conversely, power structures and the dominant classes of society do not merely rule but lead society morally and intellectually (Milner, 1992; Storey, 1993).

In great measure, culture provides people with meaning in life. It is transmitted through a number of means. Families are usually the first context in which the meanings and rules of life are developed. The meanings and values of attributes such as gender, religion, sexuality, education, socioeconomic status, and disability are conveyed within families beginning at birth and continuing throughout life. Family therapists Minuchin and Fishman (1981) describe one way Puerto Rican families and communities transmit life meaning to their children as they search for that meaning. "In a playground in Central Park, a Puerto Rican mother watches her three-year-old son playing in the sand box. An older woman tells her in Spanish that her son has a very nice *cuadro* (picture or image). She says that he will grow up to become a teacher. The prediction obviously pleases the mother. . . . A child's *cuadro* floats above his head, for everybody who is knowledgeable to see and transmit. Puerto Rican parents search for a child's *cuadro,* unaware that they are contributing to its construction" (p. 73).

The Puerto Rican *cuadro* embodies a search for individual meaning and identity. Others may not call the image a *cuadro,* but their search for identity is similar. Families and communities are the immediate transmitters of meanings that are strongly influenced by their cultural evolution (Epstein, 1973). Reciprocally, over time, individuals and groups influence their cultures. For example, in traditional European American culture, the roles of men and women were sharply defined. Married men were expected to work outside the home and be the financial providers for families, while women were expected to be homemakers and the primary caregivers of children. These strictly defined *cuadros* for men and women have been evolving dramatically in recent generations to the point that roles ascribed to people based on gender have expanded significantly—for example, most women now work outside the home.

For Susan, born in 1933 in the United States to European American parents, life was mapped out clearly. Her father worked outside the home, and her mother's job was to raise children. She always assumed her life would be the same. Finding a profession or developing a career never crossed her mind. From her earliest memories, she learned from her family, friends, school, church, and community that marriage and motherhood were her destiny. Susan graduated from high school, married at age eighteen, and bore and raised six children. "I never considered doing anything else. That's what women were supposed to do." However, her daughter Rachel, born in 1956, was born as times were changing. As in her mother's era, girls' sports were not sponsored by her high school, as reflected in her high school yearbook, in which forty pages were devoted to boys' sports, and two pages to girls' recreational activities. However, Rachel saw female role models with careers outside the home. Unlike her mother, she was encouraged to take math and science courses in high school, and she also emulated her father's example as a first-generation college student. When she told her minister she wanted to be a nurse, he envisioned her volunteering her talents, a vision she rejected. During Rachel's thirty-year marriage, she has worked as a nurse and shared child-rearing responsibilities for four children with her spouse. Earning and parenting responsibilities are not as tightly defined by gender as in her mother's marriage. Culture evolved even further for Rachel's children. Rachel graduated from high school shortly after Title IX was passed, providing equal opportunities for females' sports and recreation. Her three daughters played high school sports, and one attended college on an athletic scholarship, opportunities never available to their mother or grandmother. Her son was able to take home economics courses, and her daughters could take auto mechanics courses in high school. All four children attended college, with no thought of gender differentiation. One daughter has a doctorate in the physical sciences, and her husband has relocated for her career purposes. Each of the three generations has married and had children later than the previous generation, with each subsequent generation wanting fewer children. The average education level of each generation has also risen.

Though changes in the family have occurred over the last fifty years, many elements in their lives have remained the same. Their European American heritage continues to be a source of identity. Stories of ancestors have been passed through the generations. For the most part, political beliefs have been passed from generation to generation. Individuals may differ on political issues; however, the commitment of family members to the U.S. system of government is steadfast. The religious and spiritual heritage of the family has been conveyed through several generations. They continue to have a strong work ethic, while the family's culture has evolved, with an increasing emphasis on education. Susan, Rachel, and their families are an example of evolution with constancy that has occurred in a culture over the last sixty years. Family and gender roles have evolved, while many sociopolitical values have remained relatively unchanged.

It is important to recognize that families like Susan's have had the advantage of being part of the dominant culture of North America. However, when people belong to groups that are in the minority or without power, their experiences can be very different. Their cultures are in danger of devaluation and oppression. Marxism suggests that power differentials are based on economics and production. Historically, relationships between dominant and subservient classes have included master-slave, lord-peasant, and bourgeois-proletariat relationships. Similarly, feminism has viewed culture and the causes and effects of oppression from a gender perspective, according to which women and their place in society have been devalued (Storey, 1993). Persons from racial and cultural minorities have also been subjected to attempts to destroy their cultures and pressures to assimilate into the dominant culture.

Disability culture is one of the central concerns regarding the formation and continuation of the disability community. For people with disabilities, it is an issue of public policy (Racino, 1999). What we call Disability culture in this text is synonymous with what Longres (2000) sees as a community of interest and identity. Disabled persons have formed communities based on their common experiences, which come directly from their minority group status (Fine & Asch, 1993). Because of this experience, their communities are also communities of interest. Consequently, disabled persons—that is, people who identify as disabled and embrace disability—have recognized the importance of moving the agenda of independence and equality forward through the political process. Disabled persons and their allies have become active in developing political agendas and establishing policies that recognize Disability culture and educating both disabled and nondisabled persons about Disability culture. Riddell and Watson (2003) affirm a connection between the political process of advocacy and resistance and the development of the Disability culture. Through this political process, a system of "signs, symbols, tools and beliefs," a kind of "social order," communicates, reproduces, and explores the common experience of persons with disabilities (p. 5). It is the common experience of oppression and survival of marginalization that forms the basis of the culture: people with disabilities have forged a group identity. They share a common history of oppression and a common bond of resilience. They generate art, music, literature, and other expressions of their lives and their culture, drawn from the experience of disability (Brown, 1996).

Both authors of this text have experienced the commonality of experience expressed in Disability culture many, many times. It is a joining together of persons with disabilities across the dimensions of ethnicity, gender, class, type of disability, and political perspective. Richard Salsgiver has experienced this Disability culture for most of his life:

> When I was executive director of an independent living center, I spearheaded projects facilitated by a board president who was African American, a vice president who was Latina, and a board member who played out the role of protagonist, who was a Republican white male. Within that group, there existed an unspoken understanding of the experience of being disabled. We at times disagreed on strategy but almost always agreed on end goals.
>
> When employed as an administrator for the California State University system, I met another administrator in the finance department who used crutches as the result of polio contracted at the age of seven. In the cafeteria one day, we struck up a conversation. We began to talk about our experiences growing up as persons with disabilities. It amazed me how many similar experiences he and I had. The one that stands out centers on being paraded naked as adolescents in front of physicians, both male and female, so that they could address our abnormalities. We talked about the feelings of shame and humiliation this parade created. It was an experience that happened to both of us even though we were three thousand miles apart and from different ethnic backgrounds. It was an experience few other groups of people could share.

Similarly, the common worldview of Disability culture stems directly from the experiences of disabled persons in society and their struggles to emerge from marginalization and oppression with dignity and freedom. It is a worldview antithetical to that of the dominant society but shared by individuals who have experienced oppression, including indigenous peoples, ethnic and cultural minorities, LGBTQ people, and women.

CULTURE AND OPPRESSION

Mahatma Gandhi's experiences as a young lawyer illustrate the development of identity in the presence of oppression. Raised in India as a British subject, he went to law school in London then in 1893 went to British-ruled South Africa to practice law for one year. As an Indian, he was denied rights and abused by the government. He stayed in South Africa for two decades, fighting for the rights of Indian people and other non-white people. Under Gandhi's leadership, oppressed peoples galvanized and acted collectively. They forged an identity under the most trying of circumstances. Returning to India in 1915, he used skills and strategies he had developed in South Africa to lead India to independence from colonialism.

As another example, the term *Palestinian* today has dramatically different meaning contemporarily than a century ago. Prior to the creation of an Israeli state, Palestinians were people of both Jewish and Arab heritage. However, in recent decades, the complex conflicts in the Middle East, including the limited rights of Arabs in Israel, have led to a Palestinian identity among diverse groups of people of Arab descent. The creation of the Palestinian Liberation Organization in the 1960s contributed significantly to this contemporary identity (Khalidi, 1997).

Forced deportation of Africans to the Western Hemisphere provides another example of cultural development in the face of oppression. As a result of the deplorable conditions and oppression of the slaves, people forced into slavery were unable to carry on traditions and pass down cultures intact, and subsequent generations of slaves lost much of their unique cultural identity. One of the ways slavers kept slaves subjugated was to strip them of a collective identity. Holloway (1990) observes that slaves, especially those who labored in proximity to European Americans, "were forced to give up their cultural identities to reflect their masters' control and capacity to 'civilize' the Africans" (p. 16). Families and friends were always at risk of forced separation. "Masters" forbade the observance of African traditions by slaves. Stripping slaves of individual pride and collective identity helped keep them subjugated. However, though unique African cultural identities could not be preserved undefiled, they were replaced with the beginning elements of African American culture. As Holloway points out, traditions and elements of various African cultures were incorporated in a new environment.

The history of colonization by Europeans throughout the world provides multiple examples of attempts to strip people of their culture and identity. As European Americans encroached on Native lands such as North America, Australia, and New Zealand, indigenous people were forced off their lands. The traditions that had sustained them for millennia were wrested from them and replaced by reservations, preserves, geographic limitations, and government control. For example, Berthrong (1976) states, "It was the policy of the United States government to grind the Cheyenne into cultural submission and remold them into replicas of white, Christian farmer-citizens with red skins" (p. viii). Attempts to impose a white brand of "self-sufficiency" were met by formidable challenges and with failure as Natives struggled to maintain their identities as unique peoples. Prior to colonization, widely dispersed indigenous groups, tribes, and nations had unique identities. However, colonization foisted similar policies and experiences upon them. Consequently, widely diverse groups share identity and commonalities resulting directly from their experiences with oppressive governmental actions.

Jewish tenacity in maintaining identity during the Holocaust is an example of the importance of culture and heritage. Elie Wiesel (1995), a survivor of the Holocaust, provides an example of the importance of cultural identity: "We practiced religion even in a death camp. I said my prayers every day. On Saturday I hummed Shabbat songs at work, in part, no doubt, to please my father, to show him *I was determined to remain a Jew* even in the accursed kingdom" (p. 82). Even as Jews were being humiliated, tortured, and murdered by the millions, they clung to their identity as a people. Years later in 1992, the Dalai Lama asked Wiesel "about the secret of Jewish survival, wondering how it could be applied to his own people, also exiled, its religion also threatened: 'Despite the persecution and hatred that surrounded you, you managed to keep your culture and memory alive. Show us how. . . . We Tibetans have much to learn from our Jewish brothers and sisters'" (Wiesel, 1995, pp. 226–227).

Although Jewish survivors maintained their Jewish identity, the Holocaust also changed them, individually and as a group. Upon liberation, many Jewish youths were housed and schooled together in supervised group settings. Jewish counselors were employed to help survivors readjust to life in a post-Holocaust world. Wiesel (1995) recounts his experiences as follows: "Poor counselors, did they think they could educate us? . . . The youngest among us had a fount of experiences more vast than the oldest of them. . . . Imperceptibly the roles were reversed, and we became their counselors, feigning docile submission to their authority only because ours was superior" (p. 111). These youths and other survivors had developed an identity of their own, a culture not transmitted by family but forged through common experiences. Though they were orphans, they shared a deep and abiding identity. They came from different countries and survived different camps, but they shared bonds forged and solidified from similar experiences.

Disabled people share a history of devaluation and oppression with racial and ethnic minorities such as African Americans, Native Americans, and European Jews. In Europe and the United States, social Darwinism of the late nineteenth and early twentieth centuries defined persons with disabilities as a major source of social ills. Social workers and other people in general were taught the virtues of eugenics and were encouraged to permanently segregate persons with a variety of disabilities (Devine, 1912). Extant wisdom of the times caricatured people with disabilities as sexually immoral and in need of segregation from the rest of society. Forced sterilization was common, and institutionalization was encouraged. "Feebleminded" women were especially dangerous and were thought to be highly fertile and major transmitters of venereal disease (Adams, 1971; Rhodes, 1993).

Nazi Germany produced the ultimate in discrimination against persons with disabilities. Hitler's minions trained exterminators, using persons with disabilities as subjects, before they began mass exterminations of Jews. In "hospitals" like Hartheim, "those deemed mentally, morally, or physically unfit to participate" in society were euthanized (Levy, 1993, p. 267), while their murderers kept detailed records of their executions to perfect their killing techniques. Unlike ethnic and racial groups, persons with disabilities have not had centuries of collective identity and history to aid them in rejecting stereotypes and overcoming discrimination. It is only recently that collective disability identity has been developed and fostered (Hallahan & Kauffman, 1994). This identity has been manifested in organizations like People First, Not Dead Yet, the National Council on Independent Living, and ADAPT. Like post-Holocaust Jews and indigenous peoples worldwide, disabled people are acknowledging and rejecting societal devaluation and oppression. Previously, dependence and isolation produced powerlessness and resulted in internalized ableism. Now, people with disabilities have begun to claim their identities and their power.

MINORITY STATUS AND CULTURE

The meaning of disability has been heavily influenced by society and by human service professionals. Disability has often been a cause for grieving and a sense of loss rather than joy and celebration for families (Featherstone, 1980). The focus by physicians' attention has been cure at best, improvement at worst. Until recently, children with disabilities were segregated from the community, and sometimes from their families. People with mental health disabilities were kept in institutions, often under subhuman conditions. Children with intellectual disabilities were often removed from their families and placed in large facilities. For example, one of the authors has a family member who lived his entire life in a state-run institution with several hundred beds that was labeled a "training school for the mentally retarded." His family placed him there because they were strongly advised that it was the best place for him. Had he been born forty years later, he could have grown up in his family's home and attended public schools. The facility in which he lived and died is closed, and residents have been moved to the community.

Devalued populations such as ethnic minorities and persons with disabilities are often forced to transmit culture primarily in untraditional ways. Eliot's view (1949) of family as the primary cultural transmitter is not always possible. For example, families of forced laborers and slaves have often been unable to transmit culture because of forced separations. When families of persons with disabilities adopt the negative attitudes and stereotypes of the aggregate culture, they avoid association with others with disabilities. At best, they are a neutral influence and can become deterrents to the transmission of Disability culture. Persons with disabilities living in families in which they are the only person with a disability may be forced to rely on nonfamily to convey culture. The community of disabled persons, therefore, is critical in the development and sharing of identity and life meaning. The communities are brought together based on geography; disability type; common activities; and, in recent decades, the virtual world that connects people worldwide.

Historically, isolation has been a major obstacle for persons with disabilities in developing culture. Isolated from others with disabilities, people with disabilities have been given little opportunity for shared development. Society has labeled them as hopeless and has treated them accordingly. Furthermore, the energy it has taken to survive has contributed to this isolation. Lack of access to employment, education, transportation, and housing has produced poverty and has restricted access to society. For some people with physical disabilities, the lack of attendant care to assist with basic activities of daily living has created overwhelming physical demands. Communication barriers have isolated deaf and hard-of-hearing people. People with visual disabilities have faced environmental barriers. Thus, many people with disabilities have been isolated and forced to expend so much energy on basic survival that their participation in society is limited.

Although people with disabilities have been isolated from each other, they have shared many common experiences that have allowed the rapid growth of a collective identity. Since the early 1960s, social and political activism with the goal of creating civil rights legislation has facilitated the coming together of persons with disabilities to share and develop collective identities. Over the last generation, the technology explosion and access to the virtual world have dramatically improved communication. For example, early U.S. independent living leaders visited Japan to educate their disability advocates. Today, Japanese independent living activists are further spreading this expertise by training independent living leaders throughout Asia. IDEAnet and DREDF have Web sites devoted to national and international disability law and policy. Increasingly, a pool of educated persons with disabilities is telling its stories, using literature, the arts, oral traditions, and educational institutions to raise awareness of the lives and contributions of people with disabilities. Disability studies programs in higher education are proliferating. Culture, developed in isolation, is being integrated, enriched, and further developed in groups, leading to the creation of a new and evolving heritage, and perceptions of culture as a way of life are evolving rapidly in the disability community.

The existence of local cultures within larger cultures is manifested in unique ways within minority communities. Different Native American nations, for example, have different cultures. However, they share many commonalities because of their backgrounds and their similar experiences with colonizers, missionaries, and other outsiders. Similarly, persons with different disabilities have different life experiences but shared identities as well. For example, persons with blindness experience the world differently than persons with mental health disabilities. However, they have much in common. Both live in a society that perceives them as different, deficient, and pitiable. Historically, both groups have lacked civil rights protections and have experienced discrimination in education, employment, socialization, and entertainment. These experiences have provided a common ground and culture within the larger disability community. However, each group still maintains its uniqueness.

Because of the isolation and powerlessness experienced by persons with disabilities, the nondisabled world has historically assigned labels, roles, and identities to them. Unlike racial and ethnic minorities, however, persons with disabilities have not always had families and communities to reject or insulate them from ableist identities ascribed by the dominant culture. Rather than celebrating the uniqueness and capabilities of their children who have disabilities, families, guided by the medical profession, have been susceptible to feelings of loss, grief, and shame (Ziolko, 1993) and to transmitting their negative feelings and beliefs to their children.

A burgeoning culture of Disability is filling this cultural void. This development is strongly reflected in the language of disability. Increasingly, life with a disability is being perceived as different, not deficient (Gerber, Ginsberg, & Reiff, 1992). People are not "confined" to wheelchairs; instead, they use wheelchairs for mobility. The *Disability Rag,* an early militant disability newspaper, portrays persons with disabilities as having "disability cool." As societal barriers are eradicated, the opportunities for persons with disabilities are expanding. The *cuadro* for persons with disabilities is, increasingly, being defined *by* persons with disabilities. Ed Roberts defined himself on national television when he corrected Larry King's reference to him as a victim of polio. He acknowledged his disability but refuted the victim label applied by King, a label readily accepted in an ableist society.

Disability art reflects the Disability culture. Actress Marlee Matlin won an Academy Award for her portrayal of a student at a school for deaf people in *Children of a Lesser God.* Since then, she has shown herself to be a solid actress whose disability influences but does not define her roles in such series as *Picket Fences* and *The West Wing. Sue Thomas: F.B.Eye* was a television show based on the experiences of a deaf FBI agent. Author and cartoonist John Callahan's first book, *Don't Worry, He Won't Get Far on Foot,* chronicled his life with quadriplegia and is full of cartoons and experiences with which people with mobility disabilities readily identify. Callahan (1989) scoffs at the notion that life with quadriplegia is a tragedy, and he yearns for the day when people with disabilities will be able to thrive in a society "based on incentive and encouragement. They will be free to develop their talents without guilt or fear—or just hold a good steady job" (p. 187). Since then, he has become a nationally syndicated columnist and has written other irreverent books that prominently display a disability theme. Comedian Josh Blue won the 2006 *Last Comic Standing* using jokes about his cerebral palsy as fodder for his routines.

The 1992 film *The Waterdance* portrays the cultural commonalities among persons who become disabled in the midstream of their lives. *The Waterdance* depicts the experiences of three young men in a rehabilitation center after each has experienced a spinal cord injury. It demonstrates the frustration they feel in confronting the stereotypes and oppression of American culture regarding disability. The film portrays forms of this oppression ranging from the removal of self-control to sexual and social isolation. The film shows how a white racist, an African American, and a Latino are forced to join together to remove barriers to the fulfillment of their needs. The characters, created by Neal Jimenez in his attempt to share his own experience of disability, touched the essence of the commonality of Disability culture (Stanley, 1992). The "waterdance" is the dance of the common experience of being disabled that transcends ideology, ethnicity, and class. *Beyond Victims and Villains*, a compendium of contemporary plays by disabled playwrights edited by Victoria Ann Lewis (2006), serves to further incorporate disability consciousness in modern-day dialogue.

Wade (1994) describes the essence of disability art as a reflection of the disability experience. Disability art educates the world about the disability experience, displaying both the tragedy and celebration of disability:

> Disability Art. The tragedy of Cripple played for all it's worth. But real, not the safe, comfortable tragedy of Jerry's slobber. All the things THEY pray not to be: in your face. Taking 'em to the back ward. Making sure they smell the pissy sheets we've been lying on 'cause the "nurse" ain't in the mood this week. Throwing the spotlight on the festering bedsore health care reform don't cover. Showing 'em that swastika the nice boy down the street carved into our front door with his Boy Scout knife.
>
> Disability Art. The celebration of Cripple for all it's worth. The jazz. The sass. The triumph over. The movement. The revolution. The making it, big time. Disability Cool. Disability hot. The red hot power of Different with a capital D. Flaunting it. The bodies electric. Sequins on the scars. Get ready for the close-up Mr. De Mille. The celebration of me. Deeply me. Me in all my Cripple wholeness. Coming at you from the inside out. (p. 29)

Disability art serves as the bridge between the reality of disability and mainstream society and culture (Younkin, 1989).

An important manifestation of the collective development of culture was the 1988 uprising at Gallaudet University, after which the first deaf president in the school's history was installed. For more than a century, schools for the deaf have been used as a means of educating deaf people. Historically, these schools have been run and operated by hearing professionals to help those who are deaf and hard of hearing. Such schools have isolated and kept deaf people subservient; however, they have also given them a sense of community and shared identity, thus contributing to the development of a strong Deaf culture. The Gallaudet uprising was a manifestation of this culture, as alumni, students, and faculty rejected the appointment of a hearing president, which resulted in the university choosing its first deaf president, I. King Jordan, in more than a century of its existence. This protest demonstrated Deaf cultural awareness and Deaf pride, resulting in a determination that leadership for the group should come from one of its own members.

In spite of tremendous opposition, people from diverse backgrounds have developed and clung to their cultural identities with tenacity. In so doing, they have had to surmount personal, physical, social, and societal barriers. Culture has provided them with an identity, a reason for living, and meaning in life. Disabled persons have learned from other minorities the importance of culture in developing personal identity and strength, and in social and political action as well. Majority groups may define minority groups by their differences and perceived deficiencies. However, a strong sense of identity empowers people to preserve their cultures in the face of great opposition (Hallahan & Kauffman, 1994; Spekman, Goldberg, & Herman, 1992).

DEVELOPMENT OF DISABILITY CULTURE

Disability culture requires a nontraditional way of viewing disabled people. Historically, a focus on functional limitations has predominated research and practice with persons with disabilities (Hahn, 1991). This focus assumes that the major problems facing persons with disabilities reside within the person. Hahn (1991) states, "From this viewpoint, disability resided exclusively within the individual; and emphasis was centered on a clinical assessment of a person's remaining skills. Little interest was devoted to external restrictions in the individual's social and work environment" (p. 17). This emphasis on functional limitations is often expressed in a medical model approach that defines persons with disabilities based on individual deficiencies and biology, definitions used to justify denying people their rights to full participation in society (Mackelprang & Salsgiver, 1996; Meyerson, 1990).

Traditional views of persons with disabilities relegate them to the roles of patients and clients in need of social aid and professional services. Traditional approaches also make them more vulnerable to devaluation and discrimination. Present-day policy in China mandates the abortion of fetuses with disabilities and the sterilization of women known to be at risk of having children with disabilities. Though most countries have not instituted policies such as those in China, it is important to recognize that it has been legal to discriminate against disabled people throughout most of history. In the United States, discrimination in most areas of non-federally funded public life was legal until passage of the Americans with Disabilities Act in 1990. Other countries have followed ADA with similar laws, which we discuss further in chapter 5. In addition, disability history is replete with forced sterilizations and laws prohibiting the marriage of people with disabilities.

The cultural perspective for viewing the lives of persons with disabilities requires a dramatic change of focus. Disability culture strikes against the "naming activity that erases diversity and wants homogeneity above all else" (Noble, 1993, p. 52). Life with a disability becomes something to celebrate rather than mourn. Disability is seen as a form of diversity, not deficiency. People with disabilities are viewed as individuals and citizens rather than clients and patients. The problems facing persons with disabilities are recognized as environmental rather than residing exclusively within the individual. Because people with disabilities have been denied basic rights as a group, the focus of intervention becomes one of civil rights rather than individual treatment. Access to full societal participation is recognized as allowing persons with disabilities to be part of society rather than struggle merely to survive (Hirsch, 1995; Johnson, 1996).

DISABILITY CULTURE AND LIBERATION

The U.S. independent living movement and other disability rights movements began to change the social and personal identities of persons with disabilities from one of passive victim to assertive leader. The independent living movement manifested in the political action of persons with disabilities in the 1960s and continues today. In part, its philosophical roots came out of work by social psychologists in the mid-1940s. Researchers such as Roger Baker, Lee Meyerson, and Beatrice Wright, using the theoretical framework of Kurt Lewin, forged the foundation of a new way of looking at disability. They put forth the idea that rather than a characteristic of an individual, disability, with its narrow stereotypes and limited identity, was in fact a societal construct (Fine & Asch, 1993). Another component of the philosophical foundation of the social/minority model is rooted in conservative economics. Simply stated, it is the belief in free market theory and the concept that all individuals have the right to choose their life's direction. All people should have the right to compete. None should be locked out of the marketplace (DeJong, 1979). These two perspectives were welded together to form the social/minority model of disability, which became the cornerstone of the independent living movement, which resulted in the development of a positive Disability culture.

The social/minority model of disability rests upon certain assumptions. First, disabled people comprise a minority group in the same way as ethnic minorities, women, gays and lesbians, and people who are older (Wright, 1983). Along with this minority status come all the stereotypes of ableism and internalized ableism. Second, and related to the first assumption, the concept of disability is a social construct. This social picture of disability rests upon cultural tenets about disability. These beliefs manifest themselves in the stereotypes of and discrimination against persons with disabilities (Fine & Asch, 1993; Harlan & Robert, 1998). Third, the "problem" of disability lies with the social construct of disability rather than with the individual (DeJong, 1979; Harlan & Robert, 1998). There is nothing innately wrong with the person with a disability. He or she merely represents a piece of the grand diversity that is human society. Disabled people belong in the spiritual and natural universe. Disability may play only a small part in a person's life, or it may be a major force. Fourth, when there is a problem concerning disability, we begin finding solutions by addressing the social construct and the related barriers to individual and group fulfillment (DeJong, 1979). In other words, intervention with persons with disabilities goes beyond the disabled individual to the economic, political, and social arenas. Changing the social context is the key issue concerning the problem of disability. Disability's main problem is its social definition. Fifth, disabled persons should be in control of their own lives just as nondisabled persons are. This has several implications. Persons with disabilities have a right to independence but must take on the responsibilities that are a part of independence (DeJong, 1979). They must demand their political and economic freedom and continually work for it in both the political and economic arenas. This is not only the responsibility of disabled people; it is also that of professionals who work with them, and of society as a whole. Professionals can help disabled persons by teaching them political and economic skills as well as helping them participate in the political and economic process for the empowerment of disabled people. In addition, in professional treatment, independence means the person with a disability has absolute control. The professional becomes merely a consultant. Disabled people make the decisions about what happens in their lives, particularly when they receive social and health services.

Important to this alternate perception of disability is the view of persons with disabilities as having interrelated, shared customs and traditions. When we view the origins of the problems that persons with disabilities face as coming primarily from the environment rather than from individual pathology, it becomes possible to think of a culture of Disability. Just as survivors of the Holocaust developed a culture, persons with disabilities have much in common. When Tim Johnston was first injured, he shared the dominant cultural perspective—having a disability was a cause of shame and embarrassment. However, within weeks, Tim had begun to meet others with spinal cord injuries (SCI). Over time, he found himself connecting through the Internet with SCI persons throughout the world. Like Tim, they had all gone through the shock of losing the ability to walk. They had all known the embarrassment of losing volitional control of their bladders and of having bladder accidents. They shared the common experience of having nondisabled people assume they were unable to speak for themselves because they used wheelchairs for mobility.

Even those whose SCI occurred thousands of miles apart had commonalities. Soon Tim found himself sharing the language and culture of SCI. When Tim called himself a "T-12 para" (a person with a spinal cord injury at the twelfth thoracic level), everyone in his newfound culture understood. When Tim talked about his "Quickie," his friends knew he was talking about his wheelchair. When a non–wheelchair user walked by and someone called her a "TAB," they all knew she was being called "temporarily able-bodied." Conversely, it was a sign of solidarity of their shared experience when he and his friends referred to each other as "gimp" or "crip." The use of those labels by an outsider, on the other hand, would have been considered offensive. Whether they had been injured in California; Cali, Columbia; or Copenhagen, Denmark, their experiences were similar.

Even though he acquired his disability as an adult, Tim's disability provided an opportunity for him to become part of a new culture. Though Tim had to make many adjustments to his disability, paraplegia gradually lost its negative meaning. He resumed his athletic life, participating in activities such as wheelchair basketball, adapted track and field, and waterskiing. Tim was able to eschew society's view of him and others like him.

Though born with a disability, it was in adulthood that Carolyn Jenkins (pseudonym), a friend of one of the authors, found Disability culture. The third of five children, Carolyn was born with spina bifida in 1963. Her eagerly anticipated birth turned out to be extremely traumatic for her parents. She had surgeries to close the neural tube in her thoracic spine and to place a shunt to drain fluid from her brain. The family pediatrician told Carolyn's parents she would likely not live to adulthood and that she would never be able to live independently of them. Some of her earliest memories are of numerous doctor visits. Physical touch, during her childhood and adolescence, was either painful or part of the process of caregiving. She learned to accept the way people treated her as an object rather than as a complete human being, such as when, at age fourteen, she was paraded half-naked in front of several physicians. Entering puberty and dressed only in panties, she was forced to walk across a stage so they could observe her gait.

The devotion of Carolyn's parents to her led them to treat her as their "special" child. Her family was protective of her, wanting to shield her from the cruelty of others. All of Carolyn's siblings grew up, moved out of the home, and married. Carolyn, however, never considered independence from her family or marriage as possibilities in her life.

Carolyn attended "special" classes in public school, eventually graduating from high school. She found part-time work as a secretary, using paratransit to get to work. Though capable of driving with hand controls, she was terrified of driving and had never considered acquiring a driver's license. She had experienced crushes on men but had never considered the possibility that a man might be interested in her romantically.

When she was twenty-five years old, Carolyn was still living with her parents. Because her parents were aging and she was frightened about her future, it was at this point that Carolyn entered counseling. She wanted to be independent of her family but felt unsure of herself. She was also fearful of being disloyal by leaving the family home but was afraid of burdening her parents by continuing to live with them.

In counseling, it became clear that she had the intellectual and physical capabilities to live independently. However, she felt incapable of living independent of her family. Living in an apartment on her own seemed impossible. Though her siblings grew up and went through the regular life transitions of leaving home, developing financial independence, and starting families, Carolyn's family had never considered these possibilities for her. She continued to be juvenilized. Her family had relied on the advice of the best professionals. Carolyn had internalized the ableism that defined her as dependent, fragile, and incompetent—a definition that had been conveyed by family, professionals, and society as a whole.

An integral part of counseling and growth for Carolyn was connecting her with others who had similar life experiences. The first time she met Marnie, another woman with a disability, there was an immediate connection. They developed an immediate sisterhood forged from shared circumstances. Both remembered wondering why their families never talked to them about growing up, getting married, and moving away, as they had with their siblings. Both remembered shunt revision surgeries and hospital experiences that were strikingly similar. Both mourned the fact that they had always experienced their bodies as painful and as objects of probing and invasion, not as pleasant and as a source of pleasure and competence. Both had experienced objectification by health care providers, and isolation from peers. As a result, their self-concepts and the meanings they ascribed to their disabilities were similar.

Though previously unbeknownst to each other, Carolyn and Marnie shared a cultural identity. As persons with disabilities, they shared many commonalities but were isolated from others like themselves. Unfortunately, because of their isolation, they received cultural messages about disability from persons without disabilities who ascribed negative and limiting meanings, roles, and identities to their disabilities. With few or no role models with disabilities, their disabilities were defined as negative, shameful, and a cause for mourning. Their treatment was similar to the treatment experienced by racial and ethnic minorities; however, they did not have families and communities to buffer and correct the ableist identities ascribed by the dominant culture.

As Carolyn and Marnie became involved in their local independent living center, they found others who took pride in their disabilities. They met the director of the independent living center, a woman with quadriplegia who lived independently with the aid of attendants. They were impressed by a blind independent living specialist who was a strong disability advocate. They saw a group of people with intellectual disabilities who were moving from an institution to supported apartments. Others with mental health disabilities were active in advocating for themselves. Though their disabilities were varied, they shared bonds forged from a determination to overcome devaluation. In numbers, they rejected society's views of them as powerless and invalid.

As Carolyn and Marnie got to know each other and as they began to network with other people with disabilities, a transformation occurred. As Carolyn stated, "I got so mad when Marnie told me about what people had done to her. She was smart, attractive, and a lot of fun. All those people were so wrong to tell her [that she was incompetent]. It was wrong that she couldn't go to school with the other kids." As Carolyn saw the prejudice and discrimination directed against Marnie, something happened to her. "Gradually, I began to realize all those things they did to Marnie they did to me too! And it was just as wrong. I got mad." Carolyn began to reject the limitations and stereotypes she had passively accepted for years. Carolyn began to realize that instead of psychotherapy to correct her personal deficiencies, she needed skill development and independent living counseling to help her gain confidence and competence.

ADVOCACY AND CULTURAL DEVELOPMENT

Political activism has resulted in environmental change, and it has reinforced the sense of unity and pride among persons with disabilities as they forge an identity as disabled people. Every culture has stories from which its myths are garnered. Every culture has its heroes and icons, and Disability culture is no exception. The 1988 Gallaudet uprising announced to the country that Deaf people are a force to be heard. In 1980, Patrisha Wright, a woman with a visual disability, set up shop in Washington, D.C., representing the Disability Rights Education and Defense Fund to advocate the civil rights of persons with disabilities. Mentored by Judy Heumann, a prominent leader in the disability movement, Wright had repeatedly seen the discrimination and patronization that people with disabilities experience. Wright's work was instrumental in facilitating passage of the ADA (Shapiro, 1993).

With leaders like Bob Kafka, members of the militant group ADAPT (which began as American Disabled for Accessible Public Transit and now stands for American Disabled for Attendant Programs Today) have fought for the rights of people with disabilities, especially for accessible transportation. ADAPT has led protests throughout the country for persons with disabilities, using tactics such as bus stoppages and sit-ins. In 1986, one of the authors engaged in a protest against a local transit authority whose board repeatedly denied accessible transportation services to persons with disabilities while offering a "free-fare" zone geared at affluent businesspeople. Several local members of ADAPT pleaded with the board to make basic transportation available to people with disabilities for doctor's visits, work, and entertainment. When that did not work, several members descended on the free-fare zone to take advantage of the free bus rides. Members of ADAPT with severe physical disabilities were helped to transfer from their wheelchairs to the first step of the bus, where they slowly wriggled up the stairs on their backs to the bus floor for their free rides. In the meantime, other protesters ran with their wheelchairs to the next bus stop, where the riders would disembark. In this way, members of ADAPT brought attention to the discrimination they faced daily. At the same time, their sense of empowerment and unity was a source of great pride. While the transit authority board, comprised exclusively of nondisabled people, expected them to be thankful for the minimal, expensive service they received, they knew they were citizens who were being denied access because they were different. They had no reason to feel thankful, and much reason to feel outraged.

Persons with disabilities in the United States are indebted to disability rights leaders and advocates like Judy Heumann, Ed Roberts, Patrisha Wright, I. King Jordan, Justin Dart, and Evan Kemp Jr. Disabled persons in other countries also have leaders, such as England's Tom Shakespeare as well as the UK Disabled People's Council. These pioneers have helped usher in a new era in which persons with disabilities are afforded human rights that nondisabled persons take for granted. They also serve as role models for young and newly disabled persons, who have protections and opportunities unimagined a generation ago. These leaders and others at national, regional, state, and local levels are creating and developing a new international disability culture (Shapiro, 1993).

In addition, culture is being developed through other means (Holcomb, 1996). Places like Gallaudet University are breeding grounds for deaf and hard-of-hearing people to nurture their culture. Places like summer camps for youths with disabilities have allowed people to share hopes, desires, experiences, and fears they cannot share with people without disabilities— who would not understand them anyway. Performers like Marlee Matlin and Chris Burke, who has Down syndrome, provide examples that invalidate traditional views of persons with disabilities. Movies such as *Gaby: A True Story, Passion Fish, The Waterdance, Coming Home, Children of a Lesser God,* and *39 Pounds of Love* portray people with disabilities as loving, competent, and vibrant human beings, in contrast to movies that portray them as evil or incompetent, such as *A Fish Called Wanda* and *It's a Wonderful Life* (see box 4.1). People like John Callahan and Josh Blue provide disability humor. Academic organizations such as the Society for Disability Studies are affording scholars and educators opportunities to develop and transmit knowledge about disabilities. Some colleges and universities are developing disability curricula and creating disability studies programs.

Box 4.1 Mass Media and Disability

View a film such as *Million Dollar Baby* or *Whose Life Is It Anyway?* in which the lives of individuals with disabilities are portrayed as worse than death. Then watch a film such as *The Waterdance* or *Murderball.* How does each of these portray the lives of disabled persons? What messages do audiences bring away with them? How do they reinforce or weaken common perceptions and stereotypes of disability?

This generation is ushering in a new disability era. Increasingly, people with disabilities are defining their lives rather than accepting pathology-laden roles and labels placed on them by the dominant society. People who are born with and acquire disabilities have role models who are forging new vistas of civil rights and societal participation. Out of adversity, a Disability culture is being created, as are many disability-specific subcultures. Increasingly, disability is becoming defined as different, not bad; persons with disabilities are thriving, not just surviving. New generations of persons with disabilities can continue to build a rich heritage and to transmit positive Disability culture, thereby becoming a social and political force in society.

SUMMARY

Culture is a way of thinking, feeling, and believing—a stored knowledge that guides people's lives. In part, culture is a social legacy, learned as a result of a person's membership in a group. Forged by constant conscious and unconscious influences as well as social and political forces, culture affects its members from birth to death. On an individual level, feelings, reactions, and behaviors become second nature in the context of these cultural experiences.

When people belong to groups that are in the minority or without power, their experiences can be negative, and their cultures in danger of devaluation and oppression. Persons with disabilities have been defined by their differences, and their differences have always been perceived as pathological. Persons with disabilities share a history of devaluation and oppression with racial and ethnic minorities such as African Americans, Native Americans, and European Jews.

Unlike ethnic and racial groups, persons with disabilities do not have centuries of collective identity and history to aid them in rejecting stereotypes and overcoming discrimination. Perceptions of culture as a way of life are evolving rapidly in the disability community. Because of isolation and powerlessness, persons with disabilities have been assigned labels, roles, and identities by the nondisabled world. An emerging culture of disability is beginning to change the pejorative construction of disability of the past. It will be a slow process. This development is strongly reflected in the language of disability. Increasingly, the media displays life with a disability as less of a tragedy and more of an integrated process. Throughout history, minorities have struggled to maintain their cultural roots. They have used culture to overcome oppression and adversity. People with disabilities are learning from other minorities the importance of cultural framework in order to achieve political and economic goals leading to personal independence.

Human service practitioners must be knowledgeable of the language and history that make up this culture. They must be aware of the resources of this culture and be able to help the person with a disability establish links with this culture.

DISCUSSION QUESTIONS

1. What is culture? What is the culture of Disability?
2. What are some of the ways culture is conveyed?
3. What are some similarities and differences between ethnic culture and Disability culture?
4. Many persons with disabilities have led lives isolated from others with similar disabilities. How do their combined experiences contribute to Disability culture?
5. What are some ways to promote and enrich Disability culture?
6. Why is knowledge of Disability culture important to practitioners?

SUGGESTED READINGS

Brown, S. E. (1996). Deviants, invalids, and anthropologists: Cross-cultural perspectives on conditions of disability in one academic discipline. *Disability and Rehabilitation, 18*(5), 273–275.

Callahan, J. (1989). *Don't worry, he won't get far on foot: The autobiography of a dangerous man.* New York: William Morrow.

Hahn, H. (1991). Alternate views of empowerment: Social services and civil rights. *Journal of Rehabilitation, 57,* 17–19.

Hallahan, D. P., & Kauffman, J. M. (1994). Toward a culture of disability in the aftermath of Dino and Dunn. *Journal of Special Education, 27*(4), 496–508.

Harlan, S. L., & Robert, P. M. (1998). The social construction of disability in organizations. *Work and Occupations, 25*(4), 397–437.

Holcomb, T. K. (1996). Development of deaf bicultural identity. *American Annals of the Deaf, 142*(2), 89–93.

Noble, M. (1993). *Down is up for Aaron Eagle: A mother's spiritual journey with Down syndrome.* San Francisco: Harper.

Riddell, S., & Watson, N. (Eds.). (2003). *Disability, culture and identity.* London: Pearson Hall.

Stanley, J. (1992, May 10). Paralyzed writer directs own story. *Los Angeles Chronicle (Datebook)*, p. 35.

Storey, J. (1993). *An introductory guide to cultural theory and popular culture.* Athens: University of Georgia Press.

REFERENCES

Adams, M. (1971). *Mental retardation and its social dimensions.* New York: Columbia University Press.

Batavia, A. I. (2001). The new paternalism: Evaluating the idea of disabled persons as oppressed minority. *Journal of Disability Policy Studies, 12*(2), 107–113.

Berthrong, D. J. (1976). *The Cheyenne and Arapaho ordeal.* Norman: University of Oklahoma Press.

Brown, S. E. (1996). Deviants, invalids, and anthropologists: Cross-cultural perspectives on conditions of disability in one academic discipline. *Disability and Rehabilitation, 18*(5), 273–275.

Callahan, J. (1989). *Don't worry, he won't get far on foot: The autobiography of a dangerous man.* New York: William Morrow.

DeJong, G. (1979). *The movement for independent living: Origins, ideology and implications for disability research.* East Lansing: Michigan State University, Center for International Rehabilitation.

DePoy, E., & Gilson, S. F. (2004). Rethinking disability: Principles for professional and social change. Belmont, CA: Thompson/Brooks/Cole.

Devine, E. (1912). *The family and social work.* New York: Survey Associates.

Eagleton, T. (1978). The common idea of culture. In P. Davison, R. Meyersohn, & E. Shils (Eds.), *Literary taste, culture and mass communication: Vol. 1. Culture and mass culture* (pp. 3–25). Cambridge: Chadwyck-Healey.

Eliot, T. S. (1949). *Notes towards a definition of culture.* New York: Harcourt Brace.

Epstein, S. (1973). The self-concept revisited. *American Psychologist, 28,* 404–416.

Featherstone, H. (1980). *A difference in the family.* New York: Basic Books.

Fine, M., & Asch, A. (1993). Disability beyond stigma: Social interaction, discrimination, and activism. In M. Nagler (Ed.), *Perspectives on disability: Text and readings on disability* (2nd ed., pp. 61–74). Palo Alto, CA: Health Markets Research.

Gerber, P. J., Ginsberg, R., & Reiff, H. B. (1992). Identifying alterable patterns in employment success for highly successful adults with learning disabilities. *Journal of Learning Disabilities, 25,* 475–187.

Hahn, H. (1991). Alternate views of empowerment: Social services and civil rights. *Journal of Rehabilitation, 57,* 17–19.

Hallahan, D. P., & Kauffman, J. M. (1994). Toward a culture of disability in the aftermath of Dino and Dunn. *Journal of Special Education, 27*(4), 496–508.

Harlan, S. L., & Robert, P. M. (1998). The social construction of disability in organizations. *Work and Occupations, 25*(4), 397–437.

Hirsch, K. (1995). Culture and disability: The role of oral history. *Oral History Review, 22*(1), 1–27.

Holcomb, T. K. (1996). Development of deaf biocultural identity. *American Annals of the Deaf, 142*(2), 89–93.

Holloway, J. E. (1990). The origins of African-American culture. In J. E. Holloway (Ed.), *Africanisms in American culture* (pp. 1–18). Bloomington: Indiana University Press.

Jakubowicz, A., & Meekosha, H. (2002). Bodies in motion: Critical issues between disability studies and multicultural studies. *Journal of Intercultural Studies, 23*(3), 237–252. Retrieved February 15, 2007, from Expanded Academic ASAP via Thomson Gale.

Johnson, J. D. (1996). Critical missing ingredients: The expertise and valued roles of people with disabilities. *NAMI Advocate, 19*(5), 10.

Khalidi, R. (1997). *Palestinian identity: The construction of modern national consciousness.* New York: Columbia University Press.

Levy, A. (1993). *The Wiesenthal file.* Grand Rapids, MI: William B. Eerdmans.

Lewis, V. A. (2006). *Beyond victims and villains: Contemporary plays by disabled playwrights.* New York: Theatre Communications Group.

Longres, J. (2000). *Human behavior in the social environment* (3rd ed.). Itasca, IL: F. E. Peacock.

Mackelprang, R. W., & Salsgiver, R. O. (1996). Persons with disabilities and social work: Historical and contemporary issues. *Social Work, 41*(1), 7–14.

Meyerson, L. (1990). The social psychology of physical disability: 1948 and 1988. In M. Nagler (Ed.), *Perspectives on disability: Text and readings on disability* (pp. 13–23). Palo Alto, CA: Health Markets Research.

Milner, A. (1992). *Contemporary cultural theory: An introduction.* St. Leonards, NSW, Australia: Allen & Unwin.

Minuchin, S., & Fishman, H. C. (1981). *Family therapy techniques.* Cambridge, MA: Harvard University Press.

Noble, M. (1993). *Down is up for Aaron Eagle: A mother's spiritual journey with Down syndrome.* San Francisco: Harper.

Racino, A. R. (1999). *Policy, program evaluation, and research in disability: Community support for all.* Binghamton, NY: Haworth Press.

Rhodes, R. (1993). Mental retardation and sexual expression: An historical perspective. In R. W. Mackelprang & D. Valentine (Eds.), *Sexuality and disabilities: A guide for human service practitioners* (pp. 1–27). Binghamton, NY: Haworth Press.

Riddell, S., & Watson, N. (2003). Disability, culture and identity: Introduction. In S. Riddell & N. Watson (Eds.), *Disability, culture and identity* (pp. 1–18). London: Pearson Hall.

Shapiro, J. P. (1993). *No pity: People with disabilities forging a new civil rights movement.* New York: Times Books.

Spekman, N. J., Goldberg, R. J., & Herman, K. L. (1992). Learning disabled children grow up: A search for factors related to success in the young adult years. *Learning Disabilities Research & Practice, 7*(3), 161–170.

Stanley, J. (1992, May 10). Paralyzed writer directs own story. *Los Angeles Chronicle (Datebook)*, p. 35.

Storey, J. (1993). *An introductory guide to cultural theory and popular culture.* Athens: University of Georgia Press.

Thompson, M., Ellis, R., & Wildavsky, A. (1990). *Cultural theory.* Boulder, CO: Westview Press.

Wade, C. M. (1994). Creating a disability aesthetic in the arts. *Disability Rag, 15*(6), 29–31.

Wiesel, E. (1995). *All rivers run to the sea: Memoirs.* New York: Alfred A. Knopf.

Wright, B. (1983). *Physical disability—a psychological approach* (2nd ed.). New York: Harper & Row.

Younkin, L. (1989). Crips on parade. *Disability Rag, 10*(3), 30–33.

Ziolko, M. E. (1993). Counseling parents of children with disabilities: A review of the literature and implications for practice. In M. Nagler (Ed.), *Perspectives on disability: Text and readings on disability* (2nd ed., pp. 185–193). Palo Alto, CA: Health Markets Research.

5

Disability Laws, Policies, and Civil Rights

STUDENT LEARNING OBJECTIVES

1. To understand the historical foundations of the laws, policies, and civil rights processes regarding disabled people in the Western world
2. To recognize the evolving perceptions and treatment of people with disabilities in societies worldwide
3. To be able to identify both disability-specific and broad-spectrum approaches to disability rights
4. To understand key pieces of legislation that affect the lives of persons with disabilities in the West
5. To be able to compare and contrast multiple disability rights laws in different countries
6. To understand the role of the United Nations and the international community in evolving disability policy and approaches to disability

The twenty-first century has brought an evolving place for disability in societies worldwide. The moral model, which has existed from the beginning of recorded history, and the medical model, which has been prevalent in recent centuries, are beginning to be challenged. Alternate models have long existed; however, new laws and policies being implemented worldwide demonstrate increasingly wide acceptance of disabled people as part of a diverse world community.

In this chapter, we discuss historical and contemporary disability laws and policies. For millennia, moral model–based laws and policies focused on the confinement, exclusion, and societal protection of people with disabilities. More humane policies have attended to social welfare needs of treatment, protection, and care, albeit by keeping disabled people dependent. In recent decades, social model– and civil rights–based policies have been implemented that promote the participation and rights of disabled people based on two general approaches to disability rights. One approach is broad-spectrum laws that promote participation and rights of people in general, including those with disabilities. For example, the 1982 Canadian Charter on Rights and Freedoms as well as the 1996 South African constitution address civil rights broadly, with disability as one component. The second approach is laws that are specifically designed for disabled people and groups. Japan's 1993 Disabled Persons' Fundamental Law and Australia's 1992 Disability Discrimination Act are examples of laws that specifically target disability rights.

It is important to understand that the view of disability as a unifying concept is a relatively recent phenomenon. Quetelet's concept of the normal man, discussed in chapter 1, provides a framework according to which people with atypical physical, mental, and intellectual characteristics fall outside the range of normal, leading society to view them collectively as abnormal and pathological. This conceptualization made explicit previously unarticulated assumptions and homogenized the treatment of diverse disability groups that had previously been devalued in similar ways but were treated based on their specific disability.

Our discussion of disability law begins with a review of the Middle Ages through the nineteenth century. Then we cover laws and policies throughout the twentieth and into the twenty-first centuries. This is followed by an examination of disability laws and policies of the countries that have addressed disability as a human rights issue over the last generation, beginning with the U.S. Americans with Disabilities Act, which is considered the model for subsequent laws. In the final section of the chapter, we examine definitions of disability in selected countries and examine the role of the United Nations in shaping disability policy.

DISABILITY LAWS AND POLICIES THROUGHOUT HISTORY

Disability Law and Policy: The Middle Ages through the Eighteenth Century

From the eleventh to the fourteenth century, people's lives were primarily determined by their immediate locales. In feudal England, families were tied to the land on which they lived, which was owned by the local feudal lord. Home and workplace were one and the same. One's community was limited to small social and geographical circles. Individuals and families were the subjects of local lords, who exerted political and economic control, with the church also exerting a strong influence. Labor was not a marketable commodity (that is, one was not compensated for one's labor with hourly wages); the products of working the land were (Gleeson, 1999). According to Lefebvre's (1991) concept of social space, the three dimensions of private, intermediate, and public spaces were intimately connected. Private places such as the home were located in intermediate social spaces such as the land on which people worked and the workshops in which artisans labored. Even those who were forced to beg or seek alms or who were cared for by local monasteries, churches, or synagogues did so within tight geographical spaces.

Throughout the Middle Ages in Europe, treatment of disabled folks was handled within families or in local communities by poorhouses operated by churches and feudal hierarchies (Metzler, 2006). Some disabled people, such as those with birth trauma that resulted in what we today call cerebral palsy, had crosses shaved on the back of their heads or were tied to pews in churches, where the populace was expected to do their charitable duty by providing them support. Lepers were a special class in both Muslim and European Christian communities. Both religious perspectives separated lepers from the general populace; this stigma dated back to ancient scriptural texts. In Europe, lepers were forced to live outside cities and towns or were institutionalized. In the thirteenth century, under Louis XIII, there were an estimated 2,000 "lazar" houses (leper houses named after the biblical Lazarus) and an estimated 19,000 leper colonies in Christian Europe. As the incidence of leprosy declined in the fourteenth century, probably due to the end of the Crusades and the isolation of persons infected with leprosy, leper colonies and institutions started declining, to the great joy of the populace (Foucault, 2006). However, Foucault recounts that in the sixteenth century, people with a different perceived scourge, venereal diseases, started sharing space with the lepers who remained. Foucault states: "Lepers were far from overjoyed at having to share their spaces with these newcomers to the world of horror" (p. 7). According to Foucault, venereal diseases were considered so abhorrent that for a time, even the lepers rejected those infected.

As the Middle Ages drew to an end, those with intellectual and mental health disabilities were labeled fools, idiots, and simpletons and were ostracized and driven from the public. As early as the fourteenth century, it was common practice in Europe to drive the insane from towns, leaving them to run wild in the hills, often in the hopes that traveling traders might help them relocate. Foucault discusses the Ship of Fools, the towns' practice of turning their insane over to riverboat captains to rid themselves of those they considered mad. Often, these people would disembark in cities where they were forced to live as beggars, roamed the countryside, or were confined to asylums. As is common today, society's marginalia were sometimes forced to live as transients.

For most of the Middle Ages and the Renaissance, disability laws and policies were based on the moral model. However, between the 1400s and 1700s, constructions of the moral model of disability evolved from religiously to secularly based explanations. Through most of the first half of the millennium, the church dominated perceptions and treatment of disabled folks. The church taught that humility was a virtue and the possession of worldly goods should not be a priority. The plight of people with disabilities was explained through spiritual lenses; for example, the church taught that disability existed to help those who were more fortunate be grateful for their blessings, or that poor people and persons with disabilities provided those with wealth an opportunity to work toward their salvation by donating alms. The mentally ill were thought to possess some sort of knowledge akin to religious experience and revealed the limits of the world to those who were not mentally ill (Khalfa, 2006). As the Renaissance progressed, reason and rational thought increased in importance, as contrasted to religious explanations of the world. As Khalfa (2006) states, "From a Christian point of view, human reason is madness compared to the reason of God, but divine reason appears as madness to human reason" (p. xvi). Rational philosophers such as René Descartes (1596–1650) considered the mad to be an aberration and the antithesis of reasonable society. The emphasis on logical thought, combined with the Reformation, resulted in the diminution of the church's influence in defining the meaning and determining the treatment of disability, and the increased control of secular governments. Increased secular influence, with its emphasis on capital development, resulted in greater measures to control and confine those considered unreasoned and deviant, who were considered a drain on society.

With urbanization and industrialization, increasing emphasis was placed on social control. For example during the sixteenth century, in London, the asylum Bedlam became notorious for its deplorable conditions. The 1500s were a time of what Foucault refers to as the Great Confinement in Europe. All groups of poor individuals and vagrants were treated the same, whether disabled or not. In Nuremburg, Germany, taxes were collected to fund lodging for so-called madmen in prison. In 1575 England, under Queen Elizabeth I, an act was passed that mandated that each county have an institution for the punishment of vagabonds and relief of the poor in which disabled persons would be confined. In 1656 Paris, by royal decree, the first *hôpital général* was created as an instrument of order to keep the undesired away from the public. By 1676, every city in France was ordered to have one of these hospitals. However, they were not devoted to treatment, but to confinement and punishment. Once inmates were committed, the institution had absolute power over their release. Hospital administrators were appointed for life and were equipped with tools such as gallows, iron collars, and dungeons (Foucault, 2006).

The Elizabethan Poor Laws of 1601 in England instituted policies for caring for the poor, including disabled individuals, who were considered the worthy poor. The Poor Laws remained essentially intact in England until 1834 and were the foundation for subsequent European and American social policies for centuries (Trattner, 1999). As Gleeson (1999) states, they "introduced a strict sense of dependency based upon the physical inability to labour, and established a system of compulsory local taxation [parish rates] to support the relief of the 'impotent.' Thus, physically impaired people became established—in law at least—as social dependants, whose proper place in the new market order was based on the economic margins reserved for those unable to sell their labour" (p. 103).

The Poor Laws created secular policies that separated disabled poor folks from the unworthy poor. They classified disabled people as helpless, and they provided money or food for subsistence. Disabled persons benefited from policies that classified them as needing help. Concomitantly, however, they disadvantaged disabled people because they were expected *not* to work, their governmental supports were substandard, and they were subject to stringent social controls. Thus, though these laws were more humane than previous laws, people with disabilities were relegated to dependence on society and to limited means.

In the 1700s in both Europe and the United States, disabled people were primarily considered inferior to the nondisabled, and this inferiority compelled the wealthy and religious to provide for them out of a sense of duty and in accordance with the law. In 1750, the English colony of Connecticut determined that families had primary responsibility for "idiots, impotent, distracted, and idle persons." In the absence of family, the colony assumed responsibility. Those disabled from war were a notable exception in that their disabilities were beyond their control and veterans held a place of appreciation.

Nineteenth-Century Disability Law and Policy

The rise of the Industrial Revolution and capitalism in the nineteenth century corresponded with increased urbanization and markedly amplified the distance between private, community, and public spaces. Religious care for poor and disabled individuals was increasingly perceived as encouraging dependence and laziness. The growth of capitalism and industrialization placed the workplace squarely outside the immediate home and in the larger community as wages were earned in the factories. Family caregiving roles, traditionally handled by women, now became a form of nonwork, an uncompensated arena of labor. The newly wealthy controlled the economic conditions of workers. Snyder and Mitchell (2006) observe that charity was used to ensure that the rich would attain salvation by caring for those less fortunate. It also provided subsistence for people such as disabled persons, who are negatively affected by the inequalities inherent in capitalism. Private charity was provided through businesses, religious organizations, and civic groups. Public charity, or welfare, was paid for through taxation. Charity became an insidious and effective tool of social control, as recipients were dependent on the largesse of contributions and taxes paid by the wealthy. Social unrest or civil disobedience brought the immediate threat of diminution or complete removal of the meager resources that trickled down from the economic elite. Poor and disabled people were further controlled by the threat that resources would be withheld unless they followed strict moral and behavioral codes imposed by charitable organizations and subscribed to the political ideologies of the ruling elite. Significantly, those who were physically unable to work were deemed more worthy than people with mental disabilities, and resources were distributed accordingly. Many of these social forces that rose to prominence in the nineteenth century continued throughout the twentieth century and still exist today.

The nineteenth century was a time of a growing middle class, who were also morally obligated to donate to the poor and disabled through donated time, charitable contributions, and taxation. Snyder and Mitchell (2006) contend that the proliferation of organized charities precipitated an ironic social phenomenon by which some in the middle class became dependent on disabled people: "With the development of organized social charities in the nineteenth century, the management of 'social dependents' became legitimated as an occupation and provided stable professional careers for middle-class professionals" (p. 56).

In part, the nineteenth century witnessed the invention, expansion, and legitimization of a number of helping professions, including medicine, nursing, social work, and psychology. Ostensibly, these occupations were created to help the sick and disabled and others in need. However, they have also maintained social control through the doctor-patient, professional-client, and service provider–service recipient hierarchies. Disabled individuals are seen as dependent on professionals, charitable organizations, and governments for their maintenance. They must depend on professionals for permission to use society's services and benefits. For example, physicians give prescriptions and orders, not suggestions or advice. Psychologists and social workers diagnose clients and determine who receives access to societal resources. Unacknowledged is the fact that these very professionals are dependent on their patients and clients for their own livelihoods. Without disabled folks, the poor, and the sick, health and human services professionals would be unnecessary.

We suggest that, in most cases, the need for charities is positively correlated with social inequalities, and that the greater the discrepancies in the distribution of societal resources, the greater the need for welfare and charity is. Furthermore, charity and welfare for disabled persons perpetuate a myth that people with disabilities are parasitic, constantly feeding off those who have. An alternate view is that the structures and systems that create the need for charity depend on disabled folks and others traditionally labeled dependent as much as the latter does on the former. The systems that provide charity and welfare are closely tied to the systems that maintain social and economic inequalities. Furthermore, without charity and social welfare, the hierarchies, social inequalities, and power differences inherent in these societies would be exposed, creating societal unrest. Thus, charity and welfare are tools the elite can use to discourage revolt and revolution.

Partially in response to the social and political unrest due to social and economic inequalities, Germany instituted unique disability policies in the second half of the nineteenth century. In 1883, under Otto von Bismark, Germany became the first country to institute health insurance for workers with employer-employee cost sharing. This was followed in 1884 by a workers' compensation law for disabled workers, the costs of which were borne exclusively by employers. Then, in 1889, Germany instituted an old age and disability social security pension funded by workers. At a time when the average German life expectancy was forty-five years, the eligibility age was set at seventy years then was lowered to sixty-five years in 1916 (SocialSecurityOnline, nd). It was supported by mandatory employer and employee contributions. France instituted a similar law in 1898, the Protection of Victims of Work Accidents Act (IDEAnet, 2003a). The laws of the late 1800s rewarded the contributions of elderly and disabled workers, defining benefits as a social responsibility rather than a charitable handout, a fundamental departure from previous policies that denigrated the poor and recipients of charity. In other words, recipients deserved these benefits as payment for their contributions to society.

Statutes such as the Bismark laws were highly progressive for their time and provided a model for employment-based income maintenance, retirement, and medical insurance programs in other countries. However, as Liedtke (2006) states, they also laid a foundation for an eventual trap that has limited societal participation for disabled persons. Though they were originally designed to aid people who are disabled or no longer *capable* of working in paid employment, they have led to an expectation that people should not work when they reach a certain age or if they have certain characteristics that are labeled disabilities. When German social security was instituted, the age of eligibility was twenty-five years beyond life expectancies of the time. Contemporarily, people are routinely living twenty-five years beyond expected, and sometimes mandatory, retirement ages.

Twentieth-Century Disability Laws and Policies

As we discuss disability law over the last century, we examine the development of these policies to provide a glimpse of the evolution of societal attitudes throughout the twentieth century. We also provide examples of laws and policies from multiple countries. While we discussed ableist, and often draconian, disability policies in chapter 1, we focus here on laws that have promoted the inclusion of disabled persons. Disability laws during the last half of the twentieth century tended to provide progressively greater coverage. First, they were initiated to provide benefits and protections to those disabled by war, then broadened to cover people with work-related disabilities, and then eventually broadened again to cover all disabled persons. This reveals the irony that wars have been one of the most important motivations to benefit all disabled persons, primarily, it seems, because war veterans are considered to be among the most worthy.

In the United States, there were several key legislative initiatives that led to expanded societal participation of disabled individuals during the twentieth century. Below, we discuss some of the most important, including the National Defense Act of 1916, the National Rehabilitation Act of 1920, the Social Security Act of 1935, Social Security Disability Insurance, Supplemental Security Income, the Rehabilitation Act of 1973, the All Handicapped Children Act of 1975 and its various updates and amendments, and the Americans with Disabilities Act of 1990.

Employment and Education

The beginnings of any concerted effort in dealing with services directed toward persons with disabilities in the United States can be found in the National Defense Act of 1916. The focus of the service components of this act centered on the training of soldiers disabled in World War I so that they could compete for jobs in civilian life. Four years later, the concept of vocational rehabilitation expanded from a focus on soldiers to the public in general in the form of the National Rehabilitation Act of 1920. Funds were provided for job training, job counseling, job adjustment, job placement, and accommodations such as prosthetics. The National Rehabilitation Act of 1920 created a cost-sharing program between the states and the federal government. The federal government picked up half the costs of rehabilitation in return for the development of a state plan, an annual report on costs and services, the creation of a comprehensive state program, and assurances that the federal funds would not be used for buildings and equipment (Albrecht, 1992).

Similar policies were passed in France in the first two decades of the twentieth century, such as an occupational retraining act, a 1916 law giving war "invalids" priority in public-sector jobs, and laws that instituted a disability pension that required private-sector employers to employ war invalids (Cooper, 2000). In Germany, disability activism was strong, particularly among the blind and deaf. For example, the Reich Association of the Blind, formed in 1912, eventually had 14,000 members. Organizations also formed for the Deaf and physically disabled (Poore, 2006). These organizations helped expand rights that were originally afforded veterans to all disabled persons. Unfortunately, when the Nazis took power, these organizations, and many of their members, were doomed.

The Rehabilitation Act of 1973

The second half of the twentieth century saw expanded laws relative to the education and employment of adults. The Rehabilitation Act of 1973 was the culmination of many years of struggle on the part of a variety of political forces, including persons with disabilities involved in the early independent living movement. The Rehabilitation Act of 1973 included several significant components that mandated services and civil rights for persons with disabilities involved in federally funded programs. The act established the Rehabilitation Services Administration within the Department of Health and Services. It established the policy that the most severely disabled persons should receive priority in rehabilitation services. This emphasis was in direct opposition to the historic approach to rehabilitation called "creaming," accepting the least disabled person for rehabilitation services in order to quickly close the case (DiNitto & Cummins, 2006). The Rehabilitation Act of 1973 established the rule that all consumers receiving rehabilitation services must have an individualized written rehabilitation program to ensure they have input in their services. The act also created the Architectural and Transportation Barriers Compliance Board to facilitate the elimination of architectural barriers in public places to persons with disabilities. The act funded a national center for the deaf-blind and increased funding to rehabilitation research. The 1978 amendments to the Rehabilitation Act of 1973 established the National Institute of Handicapped Research, now called the National Institute on Disability and Rehabilitation Research, and established funding for independent living centers and for employer incentives to train and hire persons with disabilities (Albrecht, 1992).

Section 503 of the Rehabilitation Act of 1973 required entities contracting with the federal government in excess of $2,500 (recently updated to contracts of $150,000 for firms of 150 or more employees) to establish affirmative action plans for persons with disabilities. Section 503 requires employers to initiate affirmative action for all employment openings, including those in administration. Affirmative action applies to promotion and upgrading as well as layoff and termination. Affirmative action programs must include outreach practices to agencies and organizations that are likely to have access to qualified persons with disabilities. The employer must periodically review job qualifications to determine if they adequately reflect the essential functions of the job and do not systematically screen out persons with disabilities. Employers need to consider job applicants who are persons with disabilities for other positions in the company for which they may qualify. Employers must develop internal practices and procedures to ensure management's cooperation in affirmative action programs for persons with disabilities (Department of Labor, 1992).

Section 504 of the Rehabilitation Act of 1973 guaranteed that employers contracting with the federal government could not discriminate against persons with disabilities. Section 504 was different from social services–type legislation in that it defined devices used by disabled people, such as wheelchairs, as different modes of functioning in regular society and defined them as permanent legitimate tools necessary for some to navigate society rather than special benefits (Longmore, 2003).

Health Care and Income Maintenance Laws and Policies

The Social Security Act of 1935, the product of a long and arduous battle by Franklin Delano Roosevelt, has become the cornerstone of social welfare related to disability. The act provided permanent public assistance to the elderly, persons who were blind, and children with disabilities (Albrecht, 1992). In 1956, Congress enacted the Social Security Disability Insurance (SSDI). Based upon an individual's prior payments to Social Security, SSDI expanded coverage to all persons with disabilities. SSDI defined physical and mental disability in terms of the inability to hold any employment at any geographic location in the country (Berkowitz, 1987). There are three general categories of persons with disabilities who qualify for benefits under SSDI: (1) insured workers who become disabled for a year or more and who are under sixty-five years of age; (2) widows, widowers, and divorced wives between the ages of fifty and fifty-nine who are disabled and who also meet the widows' or widowers' benefits criteria; and (3) the disabled sons and daughters of an entitled worker (Albrecht, 1992). When Social Security was enacted in 1935, the average life expectancy in the United States was just under sixty-five. Two decades later, the law was expanded to cover disabled workers under sixty-five years. At the same time, life expectancies were increasing. The Social Security Administration and Social Security Disability Insurance provided important benefits for retired and disabled workers, providing them financial independence heretofore unavailable. However, they have evolved into policies that discourage disabled people from working at the risk of losing the very benefits they need to survive. As we mentioned previously, similar laws had been instituted decades earlier in countries like France and Germany.

In 1974, Congress implemented Supplemental Security Income (SSI), which provides an income floor for persons with disabilities and the elderly. SSI, which replaced state-run programs, is paid from the general revenues of the federal government. Some states supplement this minimum income from state funds. Generally, to qualify for SSI, an individual must have little or no income or resources and must be considered medically disabled. In addition, to become eligible for SSI, people must be unemployed or, if employed, their earnings must be less than the limits set each year by the Social Security Administration. These limits are called "substantial gainful activity" (Social Security Administration, 1994). Eligibility for SSI is determined by the state, and payments are administered by the federal Social Security Administration. SSI eligibility is especially important because most SSI recipients qualify for Medicaid coverage and services.

Persons with disabilities who receive either Social Security Disability Insurance benefits or Supplemental Security Income benefits qualify for the Plan for Achieving Self Support (PASS). A PASS allows persons with disabilities to return to work by setting aside moneys earned to achieve a specific vocational goal within a certain amount of time so they maintain medical benefits through SSDI and SSI. The primary goal of the PASS program is to help persons with disabilities move to employment. Recent changes in the Social Security Administration's policy on PASS appear to be discouraging this innovative program (Ervin, 1997).

In addition to the implementation of income maintenance programs, laws have been passed in the United States to provide health care benefits for elderly and disabled persons. Medicaid, made a part of the Social Security Act in 1965, provides health care for people who are aged and disabled and who are also poor. Persons with disabilities who qualify for SSI automatically qualify for Medicaid, which provides physician and hospital services, including inpatient and outpatient hospital care, and laboratory and X-ray services. Medical services are reimbursed by the government. Persons with disabilities with substantial work histories and Social Security tax payments may qualify for Medicare. Medicare, also enacted in 1965, is a hospital and medical insurance plan for the retired. Hospital insurance is compulsory, and additional medical insurance is voluntary. Benefits under the hospital insurance plan include hospital services, limited skilled nursing home care, and home health care services. The supplemental medical insurance provides coverage for physician services and outpatient hospital care (DiNitto & Cummins, 2006). In 2006, Medicare Part D, which provides coverage for prescription drugs, was implemented.

The United States is unique in its health policies. While it spends far more per capita than any other country on health care, it is one of the only industrialized countries that does not have universal health coverage. The other, South Africa, is engaged in plans to implement universal health coverage, as is Mexico, which has an economy that struggles mightily in comparison to the United States. England became the first country to implement universal health coverage in 1948, with other British Commonwealth as well as other European countries following thereafter. Canada passed enabling legislation for universal health coverage in 1964. The Japanese have universal health coverage, purchased through employers or governmental entities. U.S. health policies negatively affect disabled persons in important ways. First, because disabled people often have publicly funded insurance such as Medicaid, which is available only to the poor, they are in constant danger of having benefits cut to assuage the concerns of the middle and upper classes, which bear the primary costs. Second, disabled people who work are severely penalized through the loss of health care coverage. For some who have significant medical costs, the expense of working becomes prohibitive. Although the United States has the most sophisticated and technologically advanced health care in the world, health policies, including unequal resource distribution, have led to decreased life expectancies, increased infant mortality, and other morbidities for disabled persons and others (Altenstetter, 2003; Deber, 2003; Kennedy, 2003; Rodwin, 2003).

The All Handicapped Children Act of 1975 and the Individuals with Disabilities Education Act (2004)

The All Handicapped Children Act of 1975 is one of the few pieces of legislation known to professionals in human services and education by its original number, Pub. L. No. 94–142. The All Handicapped Children Act of 1975 went through several levels of evolution and was renamed the Individuals with Disabilities Education Act (IDEA) in 1990, and most recently the Individuals with Disabilities Education Improvement Act, which Congress last modified in 2004, with the changes effective in 2006. Individuals from birth up through the age of twenty-one years are covered under this historic act. IDEA stipulates that "free appropriate public education" be provided at public expense to all children, including children with disabilities from age three through twenty-one years. The education of children with disabilities should be provided in the most open and "normal" environment possible (the least restrictive environment). When children need to be diagnosed, be evaluated, and receive prescriptions, the diagnosis, evaluation, and prescription should not produce stigmatization and discrimination. Parents and the child need to be primary players in any remedial or pedagogical plan established for the child's education (Albrecht, 1992; Altshuler, 2007).

The original legislation provided for the establishment of an Individual Education Program (IEP). IDEA maintains the IEP as the central process in the education of a child with a disability. These plans should delineate the current level of education of the child, the goals and objectives of the child's educational process, specific services needed and when they need to be provided, and the method by which the plan's implementation will be evaluated. The educational environment in which the child is to be educated is established in the IEP. The IEP process addresses whether or not a child with a disability is placed in a regular classroom or special education. Regular classroom placement is determined by the degree to which the student with a disability will benefit from being educated with nondisabled students. It must be ensured that the child's behaviors and needs do not disrupt other students' learning or make it impossible to meet the educational needs of the student with the disability ("Inclusion," 1995).

The interactive component of IDEA, and the central position of the child and parent, is emphasized in the IEP process (Altshuler, 2007). The child, the parents, other individuals at the parents' request, the student's teacher, a school district representative, and other individuals at the school district's request must be involved in the creation of the IEP. If the school, student, or parent is considering placing the student with a disability in a regular class- room, the teacher of the classroom in which the student seeks placement should be part of the process ("Inclusion," 1995).

Part C (previously Part H) of IDEA mandates that participating states provide early intervention services to children with developmental disabili- ties from birth to their third birthday. In addition, Part C covers children and youths to age twenty-one. State participation is not mandatory, but strong financial incentives for state participation are offered by the federal govern- ment. The objective of Part C is to provide early intervention in the context of the child's environment with maximum family involvement in the total care of the child with a disability. Crucial to this objective is the individual- ized family service plan (IFSP). The IFSP is developed in a similar manner to the IEP. The child's parents and family play a crucial role. The IFSP team may include an advocate or person outside the family at the parents' request. Other team members should include a service coordinator, the evaluations and assessment professional, and the service provider. Since the focus of the IFSP is both the child and the family, the IFSP may include services to the family that will facilitate growth of the child with a disability. As the child with a disability moves closer to the age of three, a plan of transition to Part B of IDEA or other preschool services should be included in the IFSP. Each participating state should have an agency in place to administer Part C, utiliz- ing an advisory council (Bernstein, Steitner-Eaton, & Ellis, 1995).

It is important for disabled youths and their loved ones to understand some of the unique qualities of IDEA as a disability law. First, it covers dis- abled youths through age twenty-one or until high school graduation, whichever comes first. Second, it mandates public support of substantial ser- vices, placing financial and service responsibility on states and schools. Third, it mandates substantial involvement of both disabled individuals and their families. Fourth, IDEA is *entitling* legislation: not only are people *eligi- ble* for services, but schools and states are *responsible* for providing services. Once people turn twenty-two years old or graduate from high school, they are no longer entitled to IDEA services; however, they continue to be eligible for protection against discrimination under other laws such as the Americans with Disabilities Act. In addition, family members are no longer privy to information without the consent of the disabled individual. It is especially important for individuals and families to be aware that services such as test- ing and counseling that were previously mandated and paid for by public entities are now the responsibility of disabled individuals (Altshuler, 2007). For example, a $1,000 psychological aptitude test paid for by a primary or secondary school becomes the financial responsibility of the individual once the individual graduates or reaches twenty-two years of age, whichever comes first.

DISABILITY RIGHTS AS CIVIL RIGHTS

Disability rights is a new concept that developed in the last half of the twentieth century. In the United States, the disability rights movement arose from the civil rights movement in the 1960s and the women's rights movements of the 1970s. Other industrialized countries went through similar experiences. Even so, eligibility for protections from disability laws is based on impairments of normal functioning. The *International Classification of Impairments, Disabilities, and Handicaps,* produced by the World Health Organization (1980), provided an international model for understanding illness and disorders using three criteria: (1) impairment, (2) disability, and (3) handicap. *Impairment* was defined as an abnormality in psychological, physiological, or anatomical body structure, appearance, or organ or system function. Examples of impairments include blindness, deafness, paralysis, intellectual limitation, and depressed mood. *Disability* was defined as a functional restriction or limitation arising as a consequence of impairment with regard to individual activity and functional performance. This includes difficulty seeing or speaking, eating, or moving around. *Handicap* involves the individual disadvantages that limit "normal" role functions (such as employment, housing, and transportation) and that result from disability and impairment. Handicaps account for social influences that disadvantage people with impairments (United Nations, 1990).

In the United States, the Americans with Disabilities Act defines people with disabilities as those who (1) have impairments that limit life activities, (2) have a history of such impairment, or (3) are perceived to have such an impairment. The Australian Disability Discrimination Act of 1992 defines disability in relation to a person as:

(a) total or partial loss of the person's bodily or mental functions; or

(b) total or partial loss of a part of the body; or

(c) the presence in the body of organisms causing disease or illness; or

(d) the presence in the body of organisms capable of causing disease or illness; or

(e) the malfunction, malformation or disfigurement of a part of the person's body; or

(f) a disorder or malfunction that results in the person learning differently from a person without the disorder or malfunction; or

(g) a disorder, illness or disease that affects a person's thought processes, perception of reality, emotions or judgment or that results in disturbed behavior; and includes a disability that:

(h) presently exists; or

(i) previously existed but no longer exists; or

(j) may exist in the future; or

(k) is imputed to a person.

These definitions are all based on medical model criteria. We suggest an alternate definition. We acknowledge that disabled people have atypical characteristics or functioning, that is, functioning that falls outside the margins of Quetelet's "normal" curve. These atypicalities produce social and societal responses that often disadvantage and can result in the oppression of disabled persons both individually and as a class. However, even though we disagree with the internal pathology–based definitions of disability, we still applaud the impact of recent disability civil rights laws and policies. In this section, we begin with an in-depth discussion of the ADA, then summarize laws from several countries.

THE AMERICANS WITH DISABILITIES ACT OF 1990

The Americans with Disabilities Act of 1990 was a civil rights landmark for persons with disabilities. With the ADA, Congress acknowledged that 43 million Americans with disabilities had been subjected to serious and pervasive discrimination. Congress also acknowledged that unlike other populations who have experienced discrimination, persons with disabilities have had no recourse within the law to deal with this discrimination. Thus, the ADA was enacted to prevent further discrimination and to promote the rights of persons with disabilities.

The ADA is considered one of the most comprehensive pieces of civil rights legislation in the history of the United States and, at the time it was passed, in the world. The ADA has five parts. Title I addresses issues of discrimination in the employment of persons with disabilities. It deals with the definition of disability and outlines reasonable accommodations in the workplace, what is considered undue hardship in not providing accommodations, and essential functions of the job. Title II applies the ADA to public entities, including public transportation. Like Section 504 of the 1973 Rehabilitation Act, the ADA sets no funding limitations; all government activity is covered. Government agencies were required by the ADA to develop transition plans that assess physical barriers in the public entity's facilities and create a detailed plan to make the facilities accessible. Government agencies were required by the ADA to complete a self-evaluation analyzing all services, policies, and practices to determine whether or not they comply with the ADA. Then a plan was to be formulated for bringing those things that did not comply with the ADA into compliance. Title III brings the Civil Rights Act of 1964 and the Rehabilitation Act of 1973 into the private sector for persons with disabilities. Basically, it makes discrimination against persons with disabilities in public accommodations and in commercial facilities illegal. If services are provided, services must be made available to persons with disabilities. Title IV mandates the establishment of telecommunications relay services. Title V contains several miscellaneous provisions and exclusions, including alternate access to phone services (Jarrow, 1992). We will address Titles I through III.

The Americans with Disabilities Act defines disability based upon the definitions established under the Rehabilitation Act of 1973. Disability means "(1) a physical or mental impairment that substantially limits one or more of the major life activities of such individual; (2) a record of such an impairment; (3) being regarded as having such an impairment" (Equal Employment Opportunity Commission & U.S. Department of Justice, 1991, p. I-25). A significant impact of this definition is that it encompasses the individual who is considered disabled out of prejudice or bias. Individuals who are stereotyped as persons with disabilities can be defined as disabled under the ADA. They are legally entitled to reasonable accommodation. The ADA defines physical or mental impairment as "(1) Any physiological disorder or condition, cosmetic disfigurement, or anatomical loss affecting one or more of the following body systems: neurological, musculoskeletal, special sense organs, respiratory (including speech organs), cardiovascular, reproductive, digestive, genito-urinary, hemic and lymphatic, skin, and endocrine; or (2) Any mental or psychological disorder, such as mental retardation, organic brain syndrome, emotional or mental illness, and specific learning disabilities" (Equal Employment Opportunity Commission & U.S. Department of Justice, 1991, p. I-26).

And finally, major life activities are defined by the ADA as "caring for oneself, performing manual tasks, walking, seeing, hearing, speaking, breathing, learning, and working" (Equal Employment Opportunity Commission & U.S. Department of Justice, 1991, I-27). Although the definitions appear at first glance to be fairly clear cut, there are many conditions that fall into gray areas. such as obesity and infertility. Each of these requires individual legal cases to determine if, in fact, the condition can be defined as a disability under the ADA and thus requires reasonable accommodation on the part of the employer.

Title I of the ADA defines reasonable accommodation. Reasonable accommodation is a modification or adjustment to a job, the work environment, or the way things usually are done that enables a qualified individual with a disability to enjoy an equal employment opportunity. An employer cannot deny an employment opportunity to a qualified applicant or employee because of the accommodating process. The obligation to provide a reasonable accommodation applies to all aspects of employment; it is ongoing and may arise anytime that a person's disability or job changes. Potential employees with disabilities must be accommodated in the job application process to enable qualified applicants to have an equal opportunity to be considered for the job. Reasonable accommodation must be provided to enable an applicant or a current employee to perform the essential functions of a job. An employee with a disability must be accommodated not only in terms of the tasks of the job but also in the benefits and privileges of employment like training, social events, and health programs (Equal Employment Opportunity Commission & U.S. Department of Justice, 1991).

The following are examples of reasonable accommodation. In recruitment, an employer sends notices of jobs to various organizations where persons with disabilities are likely to be found, such as independent living centers. In the application process, the employer provides assistance in filling out an application form or provides the application in a form (e.g., Braille) that is accessible to a person with a visual disability or a person who lacks manual dexterity (Johnson, 1992). In the actual job performance, an employee with a disability may be reassigned to a job with essential functions that he or she can perform, or jobs may be restructured so that the nonessential functions are redistributed. Most of the time, reasonable accommodation means obtaining assistive equipment or devices; providing qualified readers and interpreters; modifying examinations, training materials, or policies; reassigning a job; permitting use of accrued paid leave or unpaid leave for necessary treatment; providing reserved parking for a person with a mobility impairment; or allowing an employee to provide equipment or devices that an employer is not required to provide. In benefits, the employer ensures that the office picnics or other social activity events are held in an accessible place (Equal Employment Opportunity Commission & U.S. Department of Justice, 1991).

Title I of the ADA defines the concept of essential function. Essential functions of a position are the basic tasks that a person must be able to perform in order to fulfill the purpose of the position. They have to do with the purpose and intended results of a position rather than with how the job is typically performed. Essential functions do not include marginal functions (Equal Employment Opportunity Commission & U.S. Department of Justice, 1991) and do include functions that must be performed by the person who holds the position. For example, if a person is hired to enter data into a computer, an essential function of that job is data entry. It is not the ability to type or even to see. If a person is hired to teach math, the essential function of that job is to transmit knowledge to students. It is not the ability to stand in front of a class; it is not the ability to write on the chalkboard. If a person is hired to unload a truck, the essential function is moving the material inside the truck to a designated place. The essential job function is not lifting x number of pounds. Essential functions may include a wide span of functions when there are a limited number of other employees available to perform the necessary job tasks. For example, it may be an essential function for a file clerk in a very small and busy office to answer the telephone, greet people entering the office, and process incoming and outgoing mail.

And finally, essential functions are highly specialized functions of a job or position. For example, a company may want to expand its market into Mexico. For a new sales position, in addition to sales experience, it may require a person to communicate in Spanish. Another example is a university that wants to hire a professor to teach industrial social work. An essential function of this position is having knowledge of employee assistance programs. In these examples, the essential job functions of speaking Spanish and knowledge of EAP programs have to do with the purpose and intended results of the positions.

Title I of the ADA also deals with the concept of undue hardship. Undue hardship means significant difficulty or expense on the part of the employer in order to accommodate the disabled person. This is determined generally through a comparison of the cost of an accommodation to the overall fiscal resources of the employment organization, and the total number of employees hired by the company. The Equal Employment Opportunity Commission, in looking at comparative resources in determining whether or not an employer is compliant with the ADA, seeks data that substantiate that an employer has sought outside resources for reasonable accommodation (Equal Employment Opportunity Commission & U.S. Department of Justice, 1991). Finally, it is an undue hardship for an employer when an accommodation would negatively affect the basic nature and operation of the business.

Title II applies the ADA to public entities, including those that supply public transportation. All government activity is covered, whether or not the public entity has a contractual agreement with the federal government. The ADA mandates the following: (1) Agencies must make information on the ADA, including the rights of persons with disabilities, available to applicants, employees, and consumers of the agency's services. (2) At least one employee must be designated to coordinate efforts to comply with the ADA and carry out the responsibilities under the ADA. (3) Agencies must have procedures for dealing with complaints that are published and available. (4) Government agencies are required by the ADA to complete a transition plan and self-evaluation. The self-evaluation is a self-analysis of all services, policies, and practices to determine whether or not they comply with the ADA. (5) A transition plan must assess physical barriers in the public entity's facilities and detail the plan to make the facilities accessible (Jarrow, 1992).

Title III of the ADA provides basic civil rights to persons with disabilities in the private public-service sector. Persons with disabilities have the right to equal enjoyment of goods, services, facilities, advantages, and accommodations of any place of public accommodation. This also applies to services and establishments that are leased by commercial enterprises. Public accommodations cannot circumvent the law by providing goods or services that are different or separate from those offered to the general population unless they equalize accommodations; for example, special restrooms may be separate from regular restrooms. Goods and services must be offered in the most integrated setting appropriate to the needs of the individual. Service providers like liability and health insurance companies cannot offer policies that discriminate against persons with disabilities. Commercial facilities may not refuse to serve individuals who associate with people known to have disabilities (Equal Employment Opportunity Commission & U.S. Department of Justice, 1991).

DISABILITY LAWS IN MULTIPLE COUNTRIES

The ADA was a landmark in disability law in that it framed disability as a civil rights issue. Previous to passage of the ADA, the United States and other countries offered rights to disabled persons in a variety of forms. For example, in the United States, discrimination was forbidden in governmental activities, but not in commercial concerns. As early as 1975, France passed a disability law providing for the integration of disabled persons in work, education, and social life. In 1982, Canada amended its Charter of Rights and Freedoms, making nondiscrimination on the basis of disability a constitutional mandate. Statutorily, the 1985 Canadian Human Rights Act prohibited disability discrimination (Department of Justice Canada, 1976–1977). In 1990, shortly before the United States passed the ADA, France implemented a statute that criminalized disability discrimination in the workplace (Burgdorf, 1998).

Multiple countries have passed laws acknowledging and protecting disability rights. We will now investigate disability civil rights laws in multiple countries throughout the world. Countries have taken two general approaches to disability laws. The first approach is disability-specific legislation. Alternatively, countries have passed general civil rights laws that include disability.

In our analysis, we summarize laws and policies from selected countries as tracked by DREDF and by IDEAnet. The Disability Rights Education and Defense Fund (DREDF), founded in 1979 and directed by disabled persons, is a leading U.S. disability advocacy and policy development organization. "The mission of the Disability Rights Education and Defense Fund is to advance the civil and human rights of people with disabilities through legal advocacy, training, education, and public policy and legislative development" (DREDF, n.d.1). DREDF has begun tracking international disability law and policy. The International Disability Educational Alliance Network (IDEAnet) is a global network of individuals and institutions working together on issues of importance to people with disabilities.

Australia: Disability Discrimination Act of 1992

Australia was one of the first countries to pass a disability civil rights law subsequent to the passage of the ADA in the United States. The 1992 Australian Disability Discrimination Act has much in common with the ADA; however, it is broader in scope. For example, unlike the ADA, the Australian Disability Discrimination Act's antidiscrimination provisions apply to private clubs. Main provisions of the act are outlined below.

(a) [The goal of the act is] to eliminate, as far as possible, discrimination against persons on the ground of disability in the areas of:
    (i) work, accommodation, education, access to premises, clubs and sport; and

(ii) the provision of goods, facilities, services and land; and

(iii) existing laws; and

(iv) the administration of Commonwealth laws and programs; and

(b) to ensure, as far as practicable, that persons with disabilities have the same rights to equality before the law as the rest of the community; and

(c) to promote recognition and acceptance within the community of the principle that persons with disabilities have the same fundamental rights as the rest of the community. (Australian Attorney General's Department, 1992)

Harassment is forbidden, and people who make complaints relative to violation of the act are protected from retaliation. Consequences of violation of the Australian Disability Discrimination Act include incarceration and monetary penalties.

Chile: 1994 Law No. 19.284

Law No. 19.284 acknowledges that persons with disabilities should enjoy full societal integration and the same rights the constitution affords all people. The law obligates the state to provide disability prevention and rehabilitation. It establishes that prevention and rehabilitation of disabilities are the obligation of the state, and that upholding the rights of persons with disabilities is the duty of society and of their families. It provides for public disability access in education, media, buildings, and transportation. The law is to be enforced through "local police judges," to whom disabled people who experience discrimination go for remedy. This local enforcement can result in wide variability in application of the law. In addition, sanctions for discrimination are monetary and not delineated in the law. Disability accommodation is not identified as a requirement. IDEAnet (2004) considers this more of a social welfare rather than an antidiscrimination law.

China: 1990 Law of the People's Republic of China on the Protection of Disabled Persons

The Chinese law covers people with a broad range of "abnormalities," including speech, hearing, visual, physical, and mental disorders and mental retardation. It provides preferential treatment for veterans injured while protecting the interests of the people. This law guarantees the right of disabled persons to education and protects their right to employment. Prevention is emphasized in the law. One interesting element of the Chinese law is its emphasis on social control. The law states, "Disabled persons must abide by laws, carry out their due obligations, observe public order and respect social morality. Disabled persons should display an optimistic, and enterprising spirit, have a sense of self-respect, self-confidence, self-strength and self-reliance, and make contributions to the socialist construction" (DREDF, n.d.2) Disabled people are expected to be appreciative, and public dissatisfaction with their situation is not acceptable. However, this is not unique to people with disabilities in China. Peterson (2007) has noted that the Chinese government's emphasis on the collective is generalized to disabled people. The collective has a duty to disabled people, yet people with disabilities are expected to have positive attitudes, and it is not acceptable to make disability rights a political issue.

Hong Kong: 1995 Disability Discrimination Ordinance, Chapter 487

In the final years before unification with mainland China, Hong Kong passed two antidiscrimination ordinances: one dealing with women, and the other with disabled persons. The Disability Discrimination Ordinance led to the creation of the Equal Opportunities Commission to oversee their implementation. The Disability Discrimination Ordinance prohibits discrimination in a wide range of activities and areas, including education, employment, government activities, and public access (Equal Opportunities Commission, 1997). It has been hailed as one of the most far-reaching disability laws in Asia. Peterson (2005) outlines strengths of the law while critiquing the implications of enforcement. As implemented, the focus is on "conciliation" rather than advocacy, and the primary function of the Equal Opportunities Commission in disputes has been to maintain a neutral stance in private conciliation efforts. Disabled complainants and advocates have experienced frustration that the onus of enforcement is placed on the individual and must include conciliation. Some have advocated a more immediate legal approach that provides for prompt redress and rectification of violations.

Argentina: 1981 Comprehensive System of Protection for Persons with Handicaps Act (Law 22431)

Since Argentina passed this law for persons with disabilities, it has lived through civil unrest, revolution, revolt, and military rule. Governmental changes and stability since 2003 have provided optimism for disabled persons in Argentina. Law 22431, passed in 1981, has provided a foundation for multiple subsequent laws dealing with protections in employment, education, and community access. Argentina has traditionally turned responsibility for specific laws and implementation over to local jurisdictions; therefore, the rights of disabled persons have varied throughout the country (IDEAnet, 2007). In 1997 Argentina created the National Disability Council, which is "comprised of officials from the provinces and from the Municipality of Buenos Aires, who have a high level of authority within their respective jurisdictions, and representatives of non-governmental organizations (and) is responsible for preserving the role of the provinces and the municipality of Buenos Aires in the orchestration of national policies for complete prevention-rehabilitation and comparison of opportunity for persons with disabilities" (Comisión Nacional Asesora para la Integración de Personas Discapacitadas, n.d.). Argentine law has a wide scope, but enforcement is uneven.

Bolivia: 1995 Law No. 1678 of Persons with Disabilities

The Bolivian law includes provisions for including disabled persons in employment, education, health, and social security. It led to the creation of the National Committee on the Disabled Person, which has the responsibility to implement policies and protect the rights of people with disabilities. The committee employs a social model approach to disability, but general societal acceptance and provision of the resources to implement provisions of the law continue to be problematic (Japan International Cooperation Agency, 2002).

Canada: 1982 Canada Act and the Canadian Charter of Rights and Freedoms

Canada's approach to disability rights is general rather than specific in focus. Title 15(1) of the Canada Act states, "Every individual is equal before and under the law and has the right to the equal protection and equal benefit of the law without discrimination and, in particular, without discrimination based on race, national or ethnic origin, colour, religion, sex, age or mental or physical disability" (Department of Justice Canada, 1982). Prior to this act, the Canadian government passed the Canadian Human Rights Act of 1976–1977, which prohibited discrimination based on disability and set up a human rights commission (Department of Justice Canada, 1976–1977). Nondiscrimination legislation was a precursor to the equal rights legislation implemented five years later. The Human Rights Act has been updated several times, with the latest iteration in 2002. The Canadian Employment Equity Act prohibits discrimination in employment: "The purpose of this Act is to achieve equality in the workplace so that no person shall be denied employment opportunities or benefits for reasons unrelated to ability and, in the fulfillment of that goal, to correct the conditions of disadvantage in employment experienced by women, aboriginal peoples, persons with disabilities and members of visible minorities by giving effect to the principle that employment equity means more than treating persons in the same way but also requires special measures and the accommodation of differences" (DREDF, 1995). This law goes beyond ensuring equal rights by requiring special accommodation. Violations of these laws are civil rather than criminal infractions, generally with monetary liability. Unlike the laws of the

United States and some other countries that approach discrimination and civil rights categorically (e.g., based on gender, disability, race, and ethnicity), Canada's legislative approach treats traditionally disadvantaged groups universally; that is, without singling out specific populations. Mayerson and Yee (2001) suggest Canada's approach to civil rights may be superior to that of the United States, citing the Supreme Court of Canada case *Eldridge v. British Columbia,* in which the Supreme Court acknowledged that laws requiring equal treatment, such as the equal protection clause in the U.S. Constitution, can perpetuate discrimination in cases when *equal* treatment would disadvantage disabled persons.

United Kingdom: 1995 Disability Discrimination Act

The primary disability rights legislation in the United Kingdom is the Disability Discrimination Act (DDA). Similar to the ADA, the DDA has provisions relating to employment, public transportation, public accommodations and services, education, and telecommunications. The United Kingdom instituted the first disability legislation in 1944. This piece of legislation relied on voluntary compliance in disability discrimination until the 1995 DDA. IDEAnet (2003f) states, "The DDA contains a variety of measures aimed at preventing discrimination toward disabled persons and ensuring equal rights to employment; access to facilities, goods, and services; and in purchasing or renting property. It also established the National Disability Council whose purpose is to advise the Secretary of State on the operation of the legislation and matters of discrimination and ways to reduce and eliminate it." The 1995 DDA provided general disability rights but was seen as a disappointment by disability advocates, who had lobbied for full civil rights but got significant but limited protections. To further strengthen disability rights, the royal government passed the Disability Rights Commission Act (Office of Public Sector Information, 1999), which created the Disability Rights Commission, a governmental body to promote equalization, prevent discrimination, and advise the government relative to disability law and policy. This commission is afforded investigatory authority to rectify discrimination that has occurred. In 2005, the DDA was updated and amended to broaden protections relative to transportation, renting, and private clubs (Disability Rights Commission, 2007; Office of Public Sector Information, 1995). The 2005 DDA makes it unlawful for operators of transport vehicles to discriminate against disabled people. It makes it easier for disabled people to rent property and for tenants to make disability-related adaptations. Private clubs with twenty-five or more members are enjoined from excluding disabled persons on the basis of their disability. It also ensures that discrimination law covers all the activities of the public sector and requires public bodies to promote equality of opportunity for disabled people. Finally, it extends protection to cover people who have HIV/AIDS, cancer, and multiple sclerosis from the moment they are diagnosed.

France: 1975 Law 75–534

The 1975 Law 75–534 was revolutionary for its time. Whereas in the United States, the Rehabilitation Act pertained to entities receiving government funding or support, Law 75–534 made the integration of disabled people in education, the workplace, and social life a national obligation. It made public and private sector groups and organizations responsible for achieving this goal. Since 1975, France has passed multiple laws further strengthening disability rights. In 1987, Law 87–517 strengthened the obligations of employers with twenty or more employees, requiring 6 percent of the workforce to be people with disabilities. Law 89–486 provided for educational reforms for disabled youths, and Laws 91–663 and 2005–102 included measures strengthening access to housing, the workplace, and public buildings. Law 2001–1066 protects disabled persons from discrimination based on health or disability. The Conseil national consultatif des personnes handicapées is comprised of people from multiple private and governmental organizations who participate in policy making and governmental advising relative to disability (IDEAnet, 2003a). However, in spite of progressive laws, disabled people in France still face discrimination and exclusion, particularly in the workplace (Jolivet, 2004, 2005).

Japan: 1993 Disabled Persons' Fundamental Law

Shortly after World War II, Japan instituted welfare-oriented laws. Following the United Nations International Decade of Disabled Persons from 1983 to 1992, Japan moved toward policies of full inclusion of disabled persons, passing the Disabled Persons' Fundamental Law in 1993. In addition, Japan modified other laws and regulations to include disability rights, and finally, in 2004 the law was modified to include antidiscrimination provisions (Umeda, 2005). The Disabled Persons' Fundamental Law classifies disabilities into three distinct categories—physical, intellectual, and mental—a system that has been criticized by Japan's disability advocates as too limited in scope. Defining disability categorically by diagnosis rather than by the impact it has on people's lives significantly increases the likelihood that people who do not meet medical diagnostic criteria will be excluded from civil rights protections. Other disability laws in Japan typically address one of the three categories of disability, not disability in general, thus perpetuating this concern (IDEAnet, 2005b).

It is important to note that Japanese disability rights advocates have been leaders in the Asian disability rights movement. In 1981, U.S. disability rights advocates, including Judy Heumann and Ed Roberts, visited Japan in conjunction with the International Year of Disabled Persons, and in 1986 the first Japanese center for independent living opened. In 1999, Japanese disability activists established an international disability training program for Asian and Pacific countries. Trainees come to Japan then return to their countries to open centers for independent living. As a result of these activities, centers for independent living have opened in countries such as Mongolia, Thailand, Korea, Pakistan, Nepal, and Taiwan (Hayashi & Okahira, 2007; Peterson, 2007).

India: Persons with Disabilities Act (Equal Opportunities, Protection of Rights and Full Participation) of 1995

The 1995 Persons with Disabilities Act was a landmark law for India's disabled population (DREDF, 2000c). The act was passed in response to the 1993–2002 Asian and Pacific Decade of Disabled Persons and other United Nations actions. It spells out the state's responsibility to people with disabilities and also contains provisions relative to the prevention of impairments. Although the Persons with Disabilities Act outlines civil rights, it has a distinctly medical model focus. In order to be eligible, individuals must be certified to have at least 40 percent impairment by medical professionals in one of seven disability categories: blindness, low vision, leprosy (cured), hearing impairment, locomotor disability, intellectual disability, and mental health disability (IDEAnet, 2005a). Thus, people with other disabilities are left out, including people with epilepsy, genetic disorders, and cognitive and learning disabilities (Ghosh, 2006). The definition of disability was further expanded by the National Trust for the Welfare of Persons with Autism, Cerebral Palsy, Mental Retardation and Multiple Disabilities Act of 1999, which expanded disability categories to include autism, mental retardation, cerebral palsy, multiple disabilities, and severe disabilities (more than 80 percent disabled, as certified by a physician). Implementation of the Persons with Disabilities Act in India has been hampered by a number of social and economic conditions, including overpopulation, extensive poverty, gender-based discrimination, domestic strife, international disputes, and the devastating effects of the 2004 tsunami that hit the South Pacific (Ghosh & Bose, 2006; IDEAnet, 2005a; Srivastava, 2006; Sundaresan, 2006).

Jordan: 1993 Law for the Welfare of Disabled Persons

Jordan's Law for the Welfare of Disabled Persons defines disability as an impairment of senses or a physical, psychological, or mental ability that limits an individual from fulfilling normal daily requirements similar to those of able-bodied persons. The law states it is based on Arab Islamic values, as well as international human rights laws and declarations. Under the law, disabled persons have rights including integration into the general life of society, education and employment commensurate with their capabilities, health care, transportation, and freedom of movement and decision making, The Law for the Welfare of Disabled Persons established the National Council for the Affairs of Disabled Persons, which includes disabled individuals who advise the government on disability policy and practices (DREDF, 2000b). It is noteworthy that Jordan's law is based on both secular and religious values.

Israel: Equal Rights for People with Disabilities Law (Law 5758–1998, 305) of 1998

Law 5758–1998, 305, the Equal Rights for People with Disabilities Law of 1998, sets as its basic principles: "The rights of people with disabilities and the commitment of Israeli society to such rights, are based on the recognition of the principal of equality and the value of human beings created in the Divine Image" (DREDF, 1998b). Its purposes include full societal inclusion and affirmative corrective action. The Israeli law is similar to the ADA and contains provisions relating to employment, education, public accommodations by private entities, and barrier removal. It provides for injunctive relief, as well as civil and criminal penalties for violations of the law (IDEAnet, 2003c). Similar to Jordan's law, the foundation of the Israeli law is based on both secular and religious values.

Russian Federation: 1995 Social Protection of People with Disabilities Law No. 181

The 1995 Federal Law No. 181, the Social Protection of People with Disabilities, is the primary disability rights law in Russia. It has provisions related to information resources, education, and reductions of restrictions related to travel and transportation, housing, and employment. The law sets societal responsibilities such as hiring quotas of not less than 3 percent. It does not recognize enforceable individual rights to integration. The societal responsibility emphasis would be commendable if societal structures met their legal statutory responsibilities; however, enforcement has not fully implemented, and enforcement is minimal (IDEAnet, 2003e). The lack of individual protections makes it difficult for disabled persons to obtain personal redress for violations of the law.

Netherlands: 2002 Bill on Equal Treatment of People with a Handicap or Chronic Illness

The law in the Netherlands, unanimously passed by the Dutch parliament, covers people with disabilities and chronic illness in employment, education, and transportation. It is similar in concept to the ADA, but significantly less comprehensive. It does not cover areas such as public access, housing, and communication. Prior to this law, the Netherlands treated disabled persons as objects of public welfare; this law treats disabled persons as subjects deserving of civil rights (IDEAnet, 2003d). It is noteworthy that the Ministry of Health, Welfare, and Sport places responsibility for independence on disabled persons: "The Ministry of Health, Welfare and Sport encourages people with disabilities to be as independent as possible. They must be able to use the same facilities as anyone else. Special measures are needed only when this is not possible. In the past, people with disabilities were often regarded as medically unfit. Services and aids were provided on that basis. The current policy is not to shut them away in institutions, but to give them a place in the community" (Ministry of Health, Welfare, and Sport, 2007).

It is important to note that the Netherlands has health and social programs that are available to all citizens. Universally accessible health care and explicit disability rights are especially important in the Netherlands, which has practiced euthanasia for decades and in 2002 enacted the Termination of Life on Request and Assisted Suicide Act, which formally legalized both assisted suicide and euthanasia. Without these protections, pressures to limit health care and encourage termination of disabled lives could be especially great. Even with extant policies, disability rights advocates believe the Dutch euthanasia law makes disabled persons especially vulnerable (Mackelprang & Mackelprang, 2005).

Germany: Forty-sixth Constitutional Amendment of 1998

The forty-sixth amendment to Germany's constitution is a major provision for disabled persons. Article III states, "No one may be disadvantaged or favored because of his sex, his parentage, his race, his language, his homeland and origin, his faith, or his religious or political opinions. No one may be disadvantaged because of his handicap" (DREDF, 2000a). Prior to this amendment, Germany's primary disability law was the 1986 Severely Handicapped Persons Act, which provided employment protections. The 1998 amendment framed disability as a civil rights issue, whereas Germany's approaches have traditionally had a social welfare framework. It promotes full societal participation for multiple groups. In addition, it provides additional protection for disabled persons by implying that disabled persons may be "favored" under the law. IDEAnet (2003b) observes that three disability laws have been passed subsequent to the forty-sixth amendment. They are the Act Combating Unemployment among the Severely Disabled, which provides employment and working conditions protections; Title 9 of the Social Code, which consolidates and strengthens rehabilitation and employment regulations; and the Disability Equalization Act, which addresses societal participation and requires private and public entities to remove barriers that deter the inclusion of disabled persons. Germany's recent history has particular relevance to the evolutions of its laws and policies. Its current governmental structure is relatively new, given the post–World War II dismantling of the Nazi regime. In addition in 1990, Germany was reunified from two distinctly different governments. Thus, laws and policies, including its constitution, are developing at a faster rate than those of some other governments.

Ghana: 1992 Constitution of the Republic of Ghana

Like many African governments, Ghana only recently emerged from colonial rule, establishing its current government in 1992. The constitution of Ghana contains specific provisions relative to disability civil rights protections in Chapter 5, which contains language regarding the protection of the rights of all persons, with special mention of specific groups. It states, "All persons shall be equal before the law" (5:17:2), and that a "person shall not be discriminated against on grounds of gender, race, colour, ethnic origin, religion, creed or social or economic status" (Chapter 5:17:3). In addition, Chapter 5, Section 29, provides specific protections for disabled persons regarding social, creative, and recreational activities; living conditions; employment; and public access as well as protection from discriminatory, abusive, or degrading treatment (Ghana Review International, 2002). In addition to the provisions of the constitution, Ghana's parliament enacted the Disabled Persons Act of 1993, which established the National Council on Disabled Persons. This council, which is composed of high government officials, is charged with such activities as monitoring and implementing disability policies and programs, advising the government, and preventing discrimination and exploitation. Ghana's laws contain provisions that include such language as "As far as practicable," which can be interpreted as lessening the social responsibility to ensure full inclusion.

South Africa: 1996 Constitution

South Africa's new constitution, adopted in 1996 at the end of apartheid, is unusual in its acknowledgment of a history of discrimination. Its preamble states,

> We, the people of South Africa, Recognise the injustices of our past;
> Honour those who suffered for justice and freedom in our land;
> Respect those who have worked to build and develop our country; and
> Believe that South Africa belongs to all who live in it, united in our diversity.
> (South Africa, 1996)

The bill of rights prohibits discrimination against people based on race, gender, sex, pregnancy, marital status, ethnic or social origin, color, sexual orientation, age, disability, religion, conscience, belief, culture, language, and birth. Thus, disabled people are one of several groups now protected under South African law. In 1998, South Africa passed the Employment Equity Bill, which includes antidiscrimination provisions for the same groups as those enumerated in the constitution. It offers further affirmative action provisions for three "designated groups": black people, women, and people with disabilities (DREDF, 1998a).

CONTEMPORARY INTERNATIONAL APPROACHES TO DISABILITY

In addition to laws in individual countries, the United Nations and other international organizations have increasingly emphasized disability rights in the final decades of the twentieth century and into this century. The 1981 United Nations International Year of Disabled Persons (IYDP) was a benchmark for framing disability rights as a human rights issue. The United Nations outlines the purposes of the IYDP, which was adopted by UN General Assembly Resolution 31/123.

> The theme of IYDP was "full participation and equality," defined as the right of persons with disabilities to take part fully in the life and development of their societies, enjoy living conditions equal to those of other citizens, and have an equal share in improved conditions resulting from socio-economic development.
>
> Other objectives of the Year included: increasing public awareness; understanding and acceptance of persons who are disabled; and encouraging persons with disabilities to form organizations through which they can express their views and promote action to improve their situation.
>
> A major lesson of the Year was that the image of persons with disabilities depends to an important extent on social attitudes; these were a major barrier to the realization of the goal of full participation and equality in society by persons with disabilities. (United Nations Enable, 2004)

Prior to IYDP the rights of disabled persons were addressed by general protections of many nations, but not mentioned specifically. For example, a primary purpose of the Council of Europe, established in 1949, was the protection of human rights of *all* people. Founder nations recognized the atrocities perpetuated by the Nazis not only against Jews but against disabled people and others. To prevent this from ever happening again, the Council of Europe adopted the 1950 Convention for the Protection of Human Rights and Fundamental Freedoms, which provides safeguards such as international redress for violations of rights (Council of Europe, 1950). However, IYDP was a landmark event for specifically identifying disabled people as deserving of civil rights.

Subsequent to IYDP, the UN Decade of Disabled Persons was implemented from 1983 to 1992, and other regions of the world have followed suit. The Asian and Pacific Decade of Disabled Persons was implemented from 1993 to 2002, with the African Decade of Disabled Persons of 2000–2009 and Arab Decade of Disabled Persons of 2003–2112 marking the first decade of the twenty-first century.

The rights of disabled persons have increasingly been recognized by multiple countries and international bodies due, in part, to the efforts and demands of disabled persons and disability rights proponents. Gradually, the complexity of disability in societal contexts has gained recognition. Disability is no longer defined as synonymous with illness or disease. The evolution of the meaning of disability in the World Health Organization illustrates this shift.

In 1980 the World Health Organization published the *International Classification of Impairments, Disabilities, and Handicaps* (*ICIDH*), which provided a unifying framework for classifying disease and disability. The *ICIDH* has been modified over the years, with the tenth revision of the *International Classification of Diseases* (*ICD*) completed in 1994. The *ICD* is a manual devoted to the diagnosis and classification of health conditions. It is medical and diagnostic, taking into consideration internally based pathologies. However, in the early 1990s, the World Health Organization began a multinational and multiprofessional effort to investigate functioning, impairment, and disability beyond internally based pathologies.

National governments also initiated efforts to look at disability in a comprehensive manner. Consider the model of disability developed by the Australian Institute of Health in figure 5.1. The Australian model removed sickness and disease from disability and recognized the impact of resources and inputs on the health and well-being of people, including disabled people.

The New Zealand government places disability in a societal context. The strategy developed by the New Zealand Ministry of Health, Office of Disability Issues (2001) seeks to create an inclusive society: "Disability is not something individuals have. What individuals have are impairments. They may be physical, sensory, neurological, psychiatric, intellectual or other impairments. Disability is the process which happens when one group of people create barriers by designing a world only for their way of living, taking no account of the impairments other people have" (p. 7). The New Zealand policies define disability as residing outside the individual. They make disability a creation of nondisabled society that produces barriers and imposes limitations on people with impairments.

In the early 1990s, the World Health Organization began a multinational and multiprofessional process that culminated in the development of the *International Classification of Functioning, Disability and Health,* or *ICF* (World Health Organization, 2001). The *ICF*'s framers intended it to be relevant across cultures, age groups, and genders (Centers for Disease Control and Prevention, 2006). The *ICF* is considered a companion to the tenth revision of the *International Classification of Diseases,* which contains information on diagnosis and health condition, but not on functional status, as

FIGURE 5.1 Australian Institute of Health and Welfare's Conceptual Framework for Health

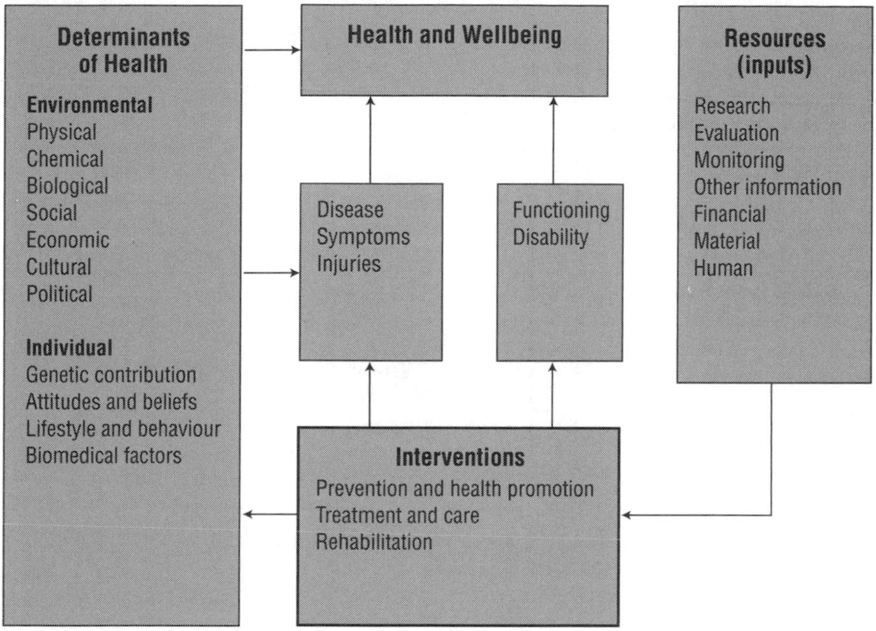

Source: Australian Institute of Health and Welfare. (2000). *Australia's health 2000: Conceptual framework for health.* Canberra, Australia: Author.

illustrated in figure 5.2. As the figure shows, disability and disease are separate domains in a category of reference classifications that are intended to be used worldwide and cover main parameters of health systems. The adjacent derived classifications are based on the reference classifications, provide additional detail, and are tailored at national and multinational levels. Related classifications "are those that partially refer to the reference classifications, or that are associated with the reference classification at the specific levels of structure only" (World Health Organization, 2004, p. 5).

Like the *ICIDH,* the *ICF* is concerned with internal determinants of disability. However, it also represents a step forward by concerning itself with the environmental contexts of disability. The activities and participation section deals with both internal and external factors and their intersection. The environmental factors section is particularly unique in its emphasis on the social and societal influences on disability and functioning. While the *ICF* retains a focus on individual pathology, its emphasis on social and societal influences on disability and functioning shifts the responsibility for enhancing life quality to the external world.

Other international organizations have framed disability in a social context. For example, the European Union–affiliated European Disability Forum

FIGURE 5.2 World Health Organization Family of International Classifications

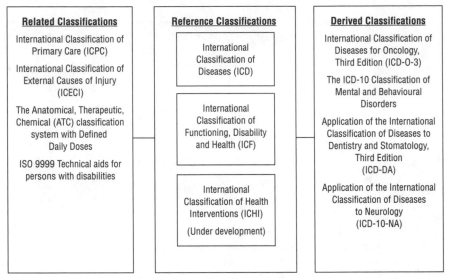

Source: World Health Organization. (2004). *Family of international classifications: Definitions, scope, and purpose.* Geneva, Switzerland: Author.

(2005), which is comprised of more than fifty organizations, including the National Federations of Disabled People of twenty-seven European countries, advocates a human rights approach to disability, including the implementation of nondiscriminatory language. The World Bank (2006) now acknowledges the importance of including disabled people in investment and economic development: "An individual with limited mobility could be at a great disadvantage in an agricultural subsistence farming society yet if that same person lived in a society with advanced services, supports and technology, he/she might encounter only few challenges. . . . To alleviate poverty, economic policies must embrace the entire population, including vulnerable groups like those with disabilities. Without integrating the disabled population, economic development efforts can not [sic] be effective since disabled people face a higher risk of poverty and poor people experience a much heightened rate of disabilities" (p. 1).

Actions of the UN have continued to evolve subsequent to the International Year and Decade of Disabled Persons. Over the last generation, the UN has been at the forefront of challenging traditional treatment of disabled people. In response to a proposal by the government of Mexico, on December 19, 2001, UN General Assembly Resolution 56/168 established the Ad Hoc Committee on a Comprehensive and Integral International Convention on the Protection and Promotion of the Rights and Dignity of Persons with Disabilities, whose purpose was "to consider proposals for a comprehensive and integral international convention to promote and protect the rights and dignity of persons with disabilities, based on the holistic approach in the work done in the fields of social development, human rights and non-discrimination and taking into account the recommendations of the Commission on Human Rights and the Commission for Social Development" (United Nations, 2007a).

In December 2006 the committee issued its final report calling for the rights of disabled persons, stating,

> The purpose of the present Convention is to promote, protect and ensure the full and equal enjoyment of all human rights and fundamental freedoms by all persons with disabilities, and to promote respect for their inherent dignity.
>
> Persons with disabilities include those who have long-term physical, mental, intellectual or sensory impairments which in interaction with various barriers may hinder their full and effective participation in society on an equal basis with others. (United Nations, 2006)

The preamble to the committee's final report places disability directly in the context of human rights, stating that "disability is an evolving concept and that disability results from the interaction between persons with impairments and attitudinal and environmental barriers that hinders their full and effective participation in society on an equal basis with others" (United Nations, 2006).

In March 2007 the Convention on the Rights of Persons with Disabilities and its Optional Protocol were adopted, with signatories from eighty-two countries, the highest number in the history of UN Convention opening days. The United Nations (2007b) calls the protocol

> the first comprehensive human rights treaty of the 21st century. . . . It marks a "paradigm shift" in attitudes and approaches to persons with disabilities . . . [and is] intended as a human rights instrument with an explicit, social development dimension. It adopts a broad categorization of persons with disabilities and reaffirms that all persons with all types of disabilities must enjoy all human rights and fundamental freedoms. It clarifies and qualifies how all categories of rights apply to persons with disabilities and identifies areas where adaptations have to be made for persons with disabilities to effectively exercise their rights and areas where their rights have been violated, and where protection of rights must be reinforced.

The Convention contains fifty disability-related protocols, including:

- The recognition that women are subject to multiple discriminations
- Assurance of equality and the best interests of children
- Assurance that disabled people have full and equal access to all areas of society
- Assurance of the right to life
- Assurance of equal recognition before the law

- Assurance of access to justice
- The right to liberty and security
- The right to freedom from cruel, inhuman, or degrading treatment (a particularly important provision in light of the Holocaust)
- The right to independent living and community inclusion
- The right to freedom of expression and opinion, and access to information

Other protections involve health, education, mobility, habilitation and rehabilitation, employment, leisure, and living conditions.

The actions of the United Nations, the European Union, regional organizations, and national governments dramatically depart from disability laws and policies of past decades and centuries. Throughout the history of the world, disabled persons have been forbidden from marrying and having children, have been forced into institutions, and have been denied liberty, freedom, and even life. We applaud recent disability laws and policies; however, disabled people are still at great risk for poverty and violation of their civil rights. Laws and policies are necessary, but not sufficient to improve the lives of disabled persons. The challenge for this generation and future generations will be to persist in continuing to change attitudes toward and actions regarding disabled persons.

SUMMARY

Through much of history, laws and policies have reflected the moral model approach to disability. Disabled persons have been considered inferior, threats to others, and have been ostracized from society. These attitudes are reflected in the laws and policies in multiple countries and cultures. Recent centuries have seen an increased emphasis on rational thought and reasoning, with a concomitant rise of medical model–based explanations of disability. The medical model brought with it the hope of treatment and cure; however, it also kept disabled persons dependent on and subservient to professionals, charities, and social service systems. Social welfare laws and charitable organizations have provided public and private benefits and services and have forced disabled persons to depend on the largesse of others. At their worst, laws and policies have restricted the rights of disabled persons to participate in society. At their best, laws and policies have provided social welfare for disabled persons.

In recent decades, laws and policies regarding disability and persons with disabilities have been evolving. Increasingly, disability is being defined from a social model perspective that emphasizes the civil rights of disabled persons. The IYDP signaled the beginning of evolving international approaches to disability. Subsequent to IYDP, multinational organizations and national governments have passed laws and implemented policies intended to include disabled persons in the fabric of society. Two challenges remain. First, the twenty-first century should be a time in which disability rights laws continue to expand and develop. Second, and just as important, disability civil rights policies need full implementation. Though many laws and initiatives have been passed and declarations made, disabled people throughout the world still experience discrimination, poverty, and lack of access to societal resources. Though important, and maybe even necessary, it is not sufficient to pass laws and initiatives; the civil rights of disabled persons must be achieved.

Judeo-Christian thought of the early Middle Ages viewed disability as a result of sin. The Enlightenment in Europe established the idea that persons with disabilities could be perfected, made "normal." America adopted these perspectives up until the independent living movement of the 1960s. This civil rights movement for persons with disabilities championed the view that lack of access in society results from architectural and attitudinal barriers rather than the dysfunction of the individual person with a disability. Much of the legislation that affects persons with disabilities is the result of the political work of persons with disabilities themselves. It is extremely important for practitioners working with persons with disabilities to be aware of these laws.

DISCUSSION QUESTIONS

1. How was disability perceived during the Middle Ages through the eighteenth century?
2. Discuss the role of religious institutions in explaining and defining the roles of disability in the Middle Ages through the eighteenth century. How does this compare and contrast to explanations and roles in contemporary religious thought?
3. How have industrialization and capitalism influenced the place of disability in society?
4. How have wars and conflicts influenced the development of laws affecting disabled persons?
5. Compare and contrast laws that provide services to people with disabilities with civil rights laws for disabled people.
6. How has the *ICF* represented a change from the *ICIDH* in its approach to explaining disability and the place of disabled persons in society?
7. What are the advantages and limitations of laws that address civil rights based on individual characteristics such as race, gender, and disability?
8. What are the advantages and limitations of laws that address civil rights universally without singling out specific groups?

SUGGESTED READINGS

Americans with Disabilities Act of 1990. Pub. L. No. 101–336. (1990).

Australian Attorney General's Department. (1992). *Australian disability discrimination act of 1992*. Canberra, Australia: Author.

Cooper, J. (2000). *Law, rights, and disability*. London: Jessica Kingsley.

DREDF. (n.d.). *About DREDF*. Retrieved August 21, 2008, from http://www.dredf.org/about.shtml

European Disability Forum. (2005). *Annual report: 2004–2005*. Brussels, Belgium: Author.

Foucault, M. (2006). *History of madness* (J. Murphy & J. Khalfa, trans.). London: Routledge.

IDEAnet. (2003). *France*. Retrieved from http://www.ideanet.org

New Zealand Ministry of Health, Office of Disability Issues. (2001). *The New Zealand disability strategy*. Wellington, NZ: Author.

United Nations. (2007). *Convention on the rights of persons with disabilities and optional protocol*. Retrieved May 19, 2007, from http://www.un.org/esa/socdev/enable/conventioninfo.htm

World Health Organization. (2004). *Family of international classifications: Definition, scope and purpose*. Geneva, Switzerland: Author.

REFERENCES

Albrecht, G. (1992). *The disability business: Rehabilitation in America*. Newbury Park, CA: Sage.

Altenstetter, C. (2003). Insights from health care in Germany. *American Journal of Public Health, 93*(1), 38–44.

Altshuler, S. J. (2007). Everything you never wanted to know about special education . . . and were afraid to ask (I.D.E.A.). *Journal of Social Work in Disability and Rehabilitation, 6*(1/2), 23–34.

Americans with Disabilities Act of 1990. Pub. L. No. 101–336. (1990).

Australian Attorney General's Department. (1992). *Australian disability discrimination act of 1992*. Canberra, Australia: Author.

Berkowitz, E. D. (1987). *Disabled policy: America's programs for the handicapped*. London: Cambridge University Press.

Bernstein, H. K., Steitner-Eaton, B., & Ellis, M. (1995). Individuals with Disabilities Education Act: Early intervention by family physicians. *American Family Physician, 52*(1), 71–76.

Burgdorf, R. L. (1998). Disability rights in the USA and abroad. *Civil Rights Journal*. Retrieved May 23, 2007, from http://findarticles.com/p/articles/mi_m0HSP/is_1_3/ai_66678527

Centers for Disease Control and Prevention. (2006). *International classification of functioning, disability and health (ICF)*. Retrieved January 2, 2007, from http://www.cdc.gov/nchs/about/otheract/icd9/icfhome.htm

Comisión Nacional Asesora para la Integración de Personas Discapacitadas. (n.d.). *National disability council*. Retrieved from http://www.cndisc.gov.ar/

Council of Europe. (1950). Convention for the protection of human rights and fundamental freedoms. Retrieved June 26, 2007, from http://conventions.coe.int/Treaty/Commun/QueVoulezVous.asp?NT = 005&CM = 8&DF = 6/27/2007&CL = ENG

Cooper, J. (2000). *Law, rights, and disability*. London: Jessica Kingsley.

Deber, R. B. (2003). Health care reform: Lessons from Canada. American Journal of Public Health, *93*(1), 20–24.

Department of Justice Canada. (1982). *Canadian charter of rights and freedoms*. Retrieved June 14, 2007, from http://laws.justice.gc.ca/en/charter/index.html

Department of Justice Canada. (1976–1977). *Canadian human rights act*. Retrieved June 14, 2007, from http://laws.justice.gc.ca/en/ShowFullDoc/cs/H-6///en

Department of Labor. (1992). 41 CFR Part 60–741: Affirmative action and nondiscrimination obligations of contractors and subcontractors regarding individuals with disabilities, proposed rule. *Federal Register, 57*(204), 48084–48122.

DiNitto, D. M., & Cummins, L. K. (2006). *Social welfare: Politics and public policy* (6th ed.). Needham Heights, MA: Allyn and Bacon.

Disability Rights Commission. (2007). *Disability rights commission of the United Kingdom*. Retrieved June 15, 2007, from http://www.drc.org.uk

DREDF. (n.d.1). *About DREDF*. Retrieved August 21, 2008, from http://www.dredf.org/about.shtml

DREDF. (n.d.2). *Law of the People's Republic of China on the protection of disabled persons*. Retrieved from http://www.dredf.org/international/china.html

DREDF. (1995). *Canadian department of justice*. Retrieved June 14, 2007, from http://www.dredf.org/international/cdaemploy.html

DREDF. (1998a). *Employment equity bill (B 60–98)*. Retrieved June 25, 2007, from http://www.dredf.org/international/safrbill60.html

DREDF. (1998b). *Equal rights for Israel for people with disabilities law, 5758—1998*. Retrieved June 23, 2007, from http://www.dredf.org/international/israel.html

DREDF. (2000a). *Germany*. Retrieved June 25, 2007, from http://www.dredf.org/international/germany1.html

DREDF. (2000b). *Laws for the welfare of disabled persons*. Retrieved June 23, 2007, from http://www.dredf.org/international/jordan.html

DREDF. (2000c). *Persons with disabilities (equal opportunities, protection of rights and full participation) act of 1995*. Retrieved June 23, 2007, from http://www.dredf.org/international/india.html

Equal Employment Opportunity Commission & U.S. Department of Justice. (1991). *Americans with Disabilities Act handbook*. Washington, DC: U.S. Government Printing Office.

Equal Opportunities Commission. (1997). *Disability discrimination ordinance*. Retrieved June 14, 2007, from http://www.eoc.org.hk/EOC/GraphicsFolder/ddo.aspx

Ervin, M. (1997). Social Security passes the buck. *One Step Ahead, 1*(5), 1–9.

European Disability Forum. (2005). *Annual report: 2004–2005*. Brussels, Belgium: Author.

Foucault, M. (2006). *History of madness* (J. Murphy & J. Khalfa, trans.). London: Routledge.

Ghana Review International. (2002). *Constitution of the Republic of Ghana*. Retrieved June 25, 2007, from http://www.ghanareview.com/Gconst.html

Ghosh, N. (2006). Disability policy and action in India: A critical review. *International Journal of Disability Studies, 2*(2), 11–26.

Ghosh, N., & Bose, P. (2006). Employment, disability and gender discrimination. *International Journal of Disability Studies, 2*(2), 4–10.

Gleeson, B. (1999). *Geographies of disability*. London: Routledge.

Hayashi, R., & Okahira, M. (2007). *The independent living movement in Asia: Solidarity from Japan*. Paper presented at the Society for Disability Studies, Seattle, WA.

Inclusion: What does the law require? (1995). *NEA Today, 13*(7).

IDEAnet. (2003a). *France*. Retrieved June 11, 2007, from http://www.ideanet.org/content.cfm?id = 5B5D75&searchIT = 1

IDEAnet. (2003b). *Germany*. Retrieved June 23, 2007, from http://www.ideanet.org/content.cfm?id = 5B5D72&searchIT = 1

IDEAnet. (2003c). *Israel*. Retrieved June 14, 2007, from http://www.ideanet.org/content.cfm?id = 5B5C76&searchIT = 1#rights

IDEAnet. (2003d). *Netherlands*. Retrieved June 23, 2007, from http://www.ideanet.org/content.cfm?id = 5B5E75&searchIT = 1

IDEAnet. (2003e). *Russian Federation*. Retrieved June 23, 2007, from http://www.ideanet.org/content.cfm?id = 5B5F76&searchIT = 1

IDEAnet. (2003f). *United Kingdom*. Retrieved June 14, 2007, from http://www.ideanet.org/content.cfm?id = 5B5F72&searchIT = 1

IDEAnet. (2004). *Chile*. Retrieved June 23, 2007, from http://www.ideanet.org/content.cfm?id = 535F&searchIT = 1

IDEAnet. (2005a). *India*. Retrieved June 22, 2007, from http://www.ideanet.org/content.cfm?id = 585871&searchIT = 1

IDEAnet. (2005b). *Japan*. Retrieved June 20, 2007, from http://www.ideanet.org/content.cfm?id = 58587E&searchIT = 1

IDEAnet. (2007). *International disability rights monitor: Argentina 2004*. Retrieved June 14, 2007, from http://www.ideanet.org/content.cfm?id = 525B

Japan International Cooperation Agency. (2002). *Country profile on disabilities: Republic of Bolivia*. Retrieved June 14, 2007, from http://www.jica.go.jp/english/global/dis/pdf/bol_eng.pdf

Jarrow, J. E. (1992). *Title by title: The ADA's impact on postsecondary education*. Columbus, OH: Association on Higher Education and Disability.

Johnson, M. (Ed.). (1992). *People with disabilities explain it all for you: Your guide to the public accommodations requirements of the Americans with Disabilities Act*. Louisville, KY: Advocate Press.

Jolivet, A. (2004). *Disability legislation to be reformed*. Retrieved June 15, 2007, from http://www.eurofound.europa.eu/eiro/2004/03/feature/fr0403106f.html

Jolivet, A. (2005). *Discontent over amendments to disability bill*. Retrieved June 15, 2007, from http://www.eurofound.europa.eu/eiro/2004/12/feature/fr0412104f.html

Kennedy, E. M. (2003). Quality, affordable health care for all Americans. *American Journal of Public Health, 93*(1), 14.

Khalfa, J. (2006). Introduction. In M. Foucault, *History of madness* (pp. xiii–xxv). London: Routledge.

Lefebvre, H. (1991). *The production of space*. Oxford: Blackwell.

Liedtke, P. M. (2006). *From Bismarck's pension trap to the new silver workers of tomorrow: Reflections on the German pension problem*. Retrieved March 30, 2007, from http://eng.newwelfare.org/?p=104

Longmore, P. K. (2003). *Why I burned my book and other essays on disability*. Philadelphia: Temple University Press.

Mackelprang, R. W., & Altshuler, S. (2004). A youth perspective on life with a disability. *Journal of Social Work in Disability and Rehabilitation, 3*(3), 39–52.

Mayerson, A. B., & Yee, S. (2001). The ADA and models of equality. *Ohio State Law Journal, 62*, 535–554. Retrieved June 14, 2007, from http://www.dredf.org/publications/adachalange.html

Metzler, I. (2006). *Disability in medieval Europe: Thinking about physical impairment during the High Middle Ages, c. 1100–1400*. New York: Routledge.

Ministry of Health, Welfare, and Sport. (2007). *Disabled people*. The Hague, Netherlands: Author.

New Zealand Ministry of Health, Office of Disability Issues. (2001). *The New Zealand disability strategy*. Wellington, NZ: Author.

Office of Public Sector Information. (1995). *Disability discrimination act 1995 (c. 50)*. Retrieved June 15, 2007, from http://www.opsi.gov.uk/acts/acts1995/1995050.htm

Office of Public Sector Information. (1999). *Disability rights commission act 1999*. Retrieved June 15, 2007, from http://www.opsi.gov.uk/acts/acts1999/19990017.htm#1

Peterson, C. J. (2005). A progressive law with weak enforcement? An empirical study of Hong Kong's disability law. *Disability Studies Quarterly, 25*(4), 21.

Peterson, C. J. (2007). *Disability law and policy in Asia: Will the international treaty promote disability progress?* Paper presented at the Society for Disability Studies, Seattle, WA.

Poore, C. (2006). Recovering disability rights in Weimar Germany. *Radical History Review, 94*, 38–58.

Rehabilitation Act of 1973. Pub. L. No. 93–112. (1973).

Rodwin, V. G. (2003). The health care system under French national health insurance: Lessons for health reform in the United States. *American Journal of Public Health, 93*(1), 31–37.

Snyder, S., & Mitchell, D. (2006). *Cultural locations of disability*. Chicago: University of Chicago.

Social Security Administration. (1994). *Red book on work incentives: A summary guide to social security and supplemental security income work incentives for people with disabilities*. Washington, DC: Department of Health and Human Services.

SocialSecurityOnline. (n.d.). *The German precedent*. Retrieved October 14, 2008, from http://www.ssa.gov/history/age65.html.

South Africa. (1996). *Constitution of South Africa*. Johannesburg: Author.

Srivastava, V. (2006). Disabling barriers to employment for women with disabilities. *International Journal of Disability Studies, 2*(2), 38–49.

Sundaresan, N. (2006). Employment rights of women with disabilities in India. *International Journal of Disability Studies, 2*(2), 27–37.

Trattner, W. I. (1999). *From poor law to welfare state: A history of social welfare in America* (6th ed.). New York: Free Press.

Umeda, S. (2005). Country report: Japan. In *International disability rights: An overview and comparative analysis of international and national initiatives to promote and protect the rights of persons with disabilities* (pp. 102–118). Washington, DC: Law Library of Congress.

United Nations. (1990). *Disability statistics compendium*. New York: Author.

United Nations. (2006). *Final report of the Ad Hoc Committee on a Comprehensive and Integral International Convention on the Protection and Promotion of the Rights and Dignity of Persons with Disabilities*. Retrieved January 3, 2007, from http://www.un.org/esa/socdev/enable/rights/ahcfinalrepe.htm

United Nations. (2007a). *Ad hoc committee on a comprehensive and integral international convention on the protection and promotion of the rights and dignity of persons with disabilities*. Retrieved May 19, 2007, from http://www.un.org/esa/socdev/enable/rights/adhoccom.htm

United Nations. (2007b). *Convention on the rights of persons with disabilities and optional protocol*. Retrieved May 19, 2007, from http://www.un.org/esa/socdev/enable/conventioninfo.htm

United Nations Enable. (2004). *The international year of disabled persons 1981*. Geneva, Switzerland: Author. Retrieved June 26, 2007, from http://www.un.org/esa/socdev/enable/disiydp.htm

World Bank. (2006). *Disability—frequently asked questions*. Retrieved December 30, 2006, from http://web.worldbank.org

World Health Organization. (1980). *International classification of impairments, disabilities, and handicaps*. Geneva, Switzerland: Author.

World Health Organization. (2001). *International classification of functioning, disability and health*. Geneva, Switzerland: Author.

World Health Organization. (2004). *Family of international classifications: Definition, scope and purpose*. Geneva, Switzerland: Author.

Part II

Disability Groupings

As we have discussed, one of the guiding tenets of the independent living movement centers on the belief that although there are differences between disability types and among people with disabilities, the life experiences of disabled folks have many commonalities and have contributed to a culture of Disability. People with a variety of disabilities share common experiences. Our view contrasts sharply with the medical model, which seeks to categorize and classify disability for the sake of treatment and study and to determine people's qualifications for benefits. Grouping then becomes a mechanism of understanding commonalities; yet to date, no one has come up with a universally accepted system of grouping disabilities. In part, this occurs because the goals of groupings differ. Groupings to determine eligibility to see a health care provider or for a government entitlement produce dramatically different results from those that influence one's social activities.

We approach disability from the perspective that if one perceives oneself as having a disability, then that individual is indeed a person with a disability. This approach is consistent with an ethnographic perspective on cultural classification that relies on group self-identification and avoids the pitfalls of stereotyping individuals. Self-declaration is also consistent with the tenets of the independent living movement. We believe it is important to understand that, because of ableism and discrimination, disabled folk have remained silent about their disabilities. Increased acceptance of disability as a social construct mitigates the need for persons with disabilities to hide or deny their disabilities and helps them embrace their full identities, disability and all.

In chapters 6 through 12, we attempt to satisfy the need to bring understanding to the differences that make up the tapestry of disability without stereotyping people or groups. Not all people will agree with our groupings, nor should they. In fact, the groupings currently used came about after much discussion, debate, and compromise. We offer the groupings as a beginning point of discussion and debate, which ultimately will result in increased understanding and knowledge, and we encourage others to add to the discussion.

Because of the diversity of disability types and because of space limitations, we have made no attempt to be comprehensive in our coverage of the range of disabilities. Conversely, we discuss some classifications of disabilities more than once. Our goal is to provide samples of the wide variety of disabilities in human existence with the expectation that readers will generalize the information to disabilities not covered. In fact, we believe that discussions of disability, like all discussions of diversity, are best conducted through finding themes, commonalities, and contrasts within and between groups rather than providing information about each group in its unique silo.

Chapter 6 addresses mobility-related disabilities. We include a discussion of several mobility disabilities that are congenital. Typically, people with these disabilities live with them throughout their lives. We also discuss mobility disabilities that are acquired later in life and to which people must adjust after living without disability.

Chapter 7 looks at the diverse world of deaf and hard-of-hearing people. The disability movement owes much to Deaf culture, which has been visible and highly developed for years. It is interesting to note that members of Deaf culture became pioneers in the disability movement by eschewing "people-first" language (e.g., "person with a disability") for "Deaf-first" language. Both the first and current editions of this book address the issue of disability-first versus person-first language, which has become an area of exploration and a source of controversy among disability advocates in recent years. However, we have also enhanced our emphasis on hard-of-hearing people and people who become deaf later in life. Though those involved in Deaf culture are a small minority, we continue to emphasize Deaf culture because of its historical contributions to the disability arena.

Chapter 8 explores persons with visual disabilities and blindness. We focus on their capabilities and discuss common misperceptions about their limitations.

Chapter 9 discusses persons with developmental disabilities, including intellectual disabilities, Down syndrome, autism, and seizure disorders. Grouping disabilities for this chapter was most difficult and controversial. Since disabilities acquired before adulthood are generally considered developmental disabilities, most disabilities found in the text could have been included in this chapter. We selected only a few. Another area of difficulty involves terminology—specifically, the use of language relative to people who traditionally have been referred to as having "mental retardation." This term has been commonly accepted in governmental and professional circles but rejected by self-advocacy groups such as People First. In recent years, the term *developmental disabilities* has been used; however, this classification mixes age and trait characteristics. Because of the pejorative and offensive connotations of the term *mental retardation,* and to differentiate it from other pre-adult disabilities, we use the term *intellectual disabilities*. We welcome further exploration of this issue.

Chapter 10 addresses mental health disabilities. In the first edition, we labeled a similar chapter "Persons with Psychiatric Disabilities"; however, we became concerned that approaching this group of disabilities from the perspective of a medical specialty (psychiatry) would be antithetical to our intent. We have revised this chapter to address mental health and mental health disabilities from a social rather than a medical model. We again provide readers with information on disabilities involving mood, thought, and anxiety and have added information on disabilities involving attention. However, we approach this content from the perspective of lived experiences and social contexts rather than diagnostic categories and labels.

Chapter 11 examines cognitive disabilities, including learning disability, attention-deficit/hyperactivity disorder, and traumatic brain injury. Again, we were able to include only a small sample of disabilities that might be considered cognitive. We also recognize that the label *cognitive disabilities* is controversial and could be applied to a variety of other disabilities. Some question the existence or the prevalence of some cognitive disabilities, especially ADD and ADHD. Some may find it strange that we have included this content in both chapters 10 and 11; however, disabilities of attention are prime examples of the difficulties of classifying disabilities in specific silos. In this situation, we took the "easy" way out by addressing them twice.

Chapter 12 is a new chapter that addresses health-related disabilities. As our last edition went to press, we recognized the gap in material relative to disabilities arising from health conditions. Traditionally, people with health-related disabilities have been classified as "sick" rather than being considered disabled. Yet the sequelae of their conditions result in widespread disabilities worldwide. This chapter addresses a small sampling of health-related disabilities including infectious illness, HIV/AIDS, cancers, autoimmune conditions, and cardiovascular conditions. We invite readers to consider how applying the social model to people with these disabilities allows us to redefine them as capable people with productive lives rather than as patients.

6

Mobility Disabilities

The doctor never told me I would never walk again. I remember
that on about my fifth day in the hospital, I said, "So what's the
deal here, doctor?" He said, "Let me put it this way, Karen: you
and I will both be able to go to McDonald's someday, but it will
take you a little bit longer than it will me because you'll either be
in a wheelchair or on crutches." Still, I had this totally positive
attitude at that time, thinking, "I'm going to walk again!" And each
time I would come out with this positive attitude, my doctors or
my therapist would say, "Well, that's a really nice attitude,
but. . . ." Eventually I got it, like everybody else who's been
through this.

—Karen Pendleton, former Disney Mouseketeer

STUDENT LEARNING OBJECTIVES

1. To understand the many varieties of disabilities related to mobility
2. To develop a very basic knowledge of the major mobility disabilities
   likely to be experienced by clients and consumers
3. To understand the similarities and differences between those who acquire
   mobility disabilities at or near birth and those who acquire mobility disabilities later in life

Mobility disability can be defined in any number of ways. For this chapter,
we define physical disability related to mobility based upon our social/
minority perspective on disability and its interplay with the variety of worlds
that are a part of contemporary society. According to the social/minority
perspective, persons with a mobility disability are those whose physical differences require them to achieve physical activities in a variety of alternate
ways. For example, persons with cerebral palsy *may* be considered to have
a mobility disability because they can achieve personal mobility differently
than persons without cerebral palsy. Persons with arm amputations *may*
consider themselves mobility disabled because, although they typically can

move themselves from one place to another, their upper-extremity mobility is affected. We say "may" because, from an ethnographic perspective, people have the right to choose the group they identify with most. Ultimately, disability, no matter what kind, has a foundation in social construction (Wright, 1988).

As a matter of convenience, we have divided mobility disability into two categories: physical characteristics affecting mobility acquired before, during, or immediately after birth, known as congenital disabilities, and physical characteristics affecting mobility acquired later in life, usually during or after childhood. Congenital disabilities include cerebral palsy, spina bifida, congenital osteogenesis, anthrogryposis, dwarfism, and congenital amputations. Some of these are included under other categories of disabilities. Physical disabilities affecting mobility acquired later in life include traumatic brain injury, stroke, amputations, muscular dystrophy, rheumatoid arthritis, multiple sclerosis, myasthenia gravis, spinal cord injury, and poliomyelitis. Conditions such as traumatic brain injury can also fall under other disability categories, such as cognitive or emotional disabilities; we deal with traumatic brain injury under cognitive disabilities. Some of these disabilities, such as muscular dystrophy, have a genetic etiology, but their physical characteristics generally do not manifest until months or years after birth. We have attempted in the following pages to define some of the more common types of physical disability affecting mobility that are encountered by human service practitioners who work with persons with disabilities.

CONGENITAL DISABILITIES

Cerebral Palsy

Cerebral palsy is one of the better-known congenital conditions resulting in mobility disability. One of the most common childhood physical disabilities, it affects 2 to 2.5 children per 100,000 in the United States. In the United States, 764,000 children and adults have cerebral palsy. Physicians diagnose about 8,000 babies and infants, plus 1,200 to 1,500 preschool-age children, with cerebral palsy every year in the United States (Krigger, 2006). Cerebral palsy is a condition that can be caused by injury to the brain at birth or during fetal development before birth. The injury may result from bleeding into the brain, lack of oxygen at or near birth, or an infection that is shared by the mother and the developing fetus. Infants who are born prematurely are especially susceptible to cerebral palsy. Cerebral palsy also may be considered an acquired disability if the cause occurs postnatally. Head injuries, infections such as meningitis, and other forms of brain damage occurring in the first months or years of life are the main causes of acquired cerebral palsy (Beers, 2003).

Cerebral palsy usually results from changes to the areas of the brain that govern motor control. The changes in the brain usually affect voluntary muscle systems. Resulting differences in muscular control vary, depending on the location and degree of the changes in the brain. Spasticity (tense, contracting muscles), athetosis (constant uncontrolled motion of limbs, head, and eyes), ataxia (poor muscle control, balance, and coordination), tremors, and rigidity can result in increased or decreased muscle tone, muscle contractions, hyperactive reflexes, slow involuntary muscle movement, and jerky movements. These neuromuscular differences can result in changes in bone structure. The muscle and bone changes result in different and unique methods of mobility and movement. Sometimes in addition to changes in muscular control, cerebral palsy results in changes in mental processes and perception as well (Krigger, 2006).

Spina Bifida

Another common childhood disability, spina bifida is a condition that results from the neural tube not closing completely during the first four weeks of fetal development. Approximately 1 out of every 1,000 infants in the United States is born with spina bifida. With spina bifida, the vertebrae and usually the spinal cord of the fetus do not develop in the usual manner. In more severe types, there is an opening in the spinal column. Neurological changes may occur because of spina bifida. The neurological changes that result from spina bifida can cause paralysis and loss of sensation in most parts of the body located below the defect in the spine. These may include the legs, feet, bladder, and bowel. The neurological changes affect a wide range of muscles, organs, and body functions. Approximately 90 percent of infants born with spina bifida survive into adulthood; generally spina bifida does not adversely affect intelligence, and the majority of individuals with spina bifida are able to take part in activities of daily living and engage in recreational sports (Barker, Saulino, & Caristo, 2002).

Spina bifida is usually classified into three types. *Myelomeningocele* results when the spinal cord and its protective covering, the meninges, protrude from the opening in the spine. Myelomeningocele is usually accompanied by hydrocephalus, where the circulation of the cerebrospinal fluid is blocked in one of the cavities of the brain. If not treated, the cavity becomes enlarged because fluid cannot drain appropriately. Brain pressure, head enlargement, and intellectual disabilities can result. *Spina bifida meningocele* is characterized by typical spinal cord development, but the meninges protrude from the opening in the column. *Spina bifida occulta* occurs when vertebral development is incomplete but the meninges are closed around the spinal cord. In this form, there are usually no differences in neurological development compared to other children (Mitchell, Adzick, Melchionne, Pasquariello, Sutton, & Whitehead, 2004).

Children with spina bifida demonstrate several unique characteristics. Some alternative mobility techniques are usually required. These may include the use of braces, crutches, and wheelchairs. Usually, some alternative bowel and bladder elimination methods are necessary. These may include special diets for bowel control and intermittent catheterization for urination. Finally, because of the use of the wheelchair and a lack of physical exercise opportunities, children with spina bifida have a tendency to be obese (Barker et al., 2002; Rollins, 2003).

Congenital Osteogenesis Imperfecta

Congenital osteogenesis imperfecta is relatively rare. Osteogenesis imperfecta is a genetic disorder that occurs in approximately 1 in 10,000 births (Marlowe, Pepin, & Byers, 2002). More popularly known as the "brittle bone disease," osteogenesis imperfecta is characterized by unusually weak bones that break or fracture with minor stress or trauma. This condition has four levels of severity. The congenital form, type 2, is the most severe; other forms range from mild to severe.

Osteogenesis imperfecta results in a change in the protein matrix of collagen fibers of bones. This change reduces the amount of calcium and phosphorus, which weakens bone structure. Physical characteristics include shortened and bowed bones resulting in bone fractures, increased elasticity of joint tissue, changed skin coloration, and changes in eye coloration (blue tinge of the eyeball). Osteogenesis imperfecta can require people to use crutches and/or wheelchairs. Sometimes surgery is necessary to strengthen bones through the insertion of steel rods placed lengthwise through the bone shaft (Plotkin & Pattekar, 2006; Rauch & Glorieux, 2004).

Arthrogryposis

Arthrogryposis, named from the Greek *arthro* (joint) and *gryposis* (crooked), is a condition in which the structure of the joints of the limbs does not develop typically, resulting in effects on the person's range of motion. In many cases, the shoulders are bent inward and internally rotated. Persons with arthrogryposis usually have extended elbows and bent wrists and fingers. The hips may form outside their sockets and are usually slightly bent. Many persons with arthrogryposis have extended knees, heels bent inward from the midline of the leg, and feet bent inward at the ankle (known as club foot). Muscles of persons with arthrogryposis have not fully developed in the typical manner (this is called hypoplasia), and their limbs tend to be tubular in shape and featureless. Fatty connective tissue is present over the side of fixed joints.

The causes of arthrogryposis are unknown. Most types are not inherited. Arthrogryposis may be primarily a neurological disorder; it may also be a muscle condition. About 1 in 3,000 infants is born in the United States with arthrogryposis; both males and females are affected (Chen, 2006).

Depending on the severity, persons with arthrogryposis may need to use crutches and/or wheelchairs for mobility. Sometimes braces are used to facilitate mobility. Other manifestations linked to the condition include changes in heart and lung function and in the strength of facial muscles (Chen, 2006; Henningsen & Smith, 2005).

Dwarfism

The Little People of America (2006a) defines dwarfism as a medical or genetic condition that causes a male or female adult to attain a height of four feet ten or shorter. In some cases, the height can be a little higher. The most frequently diagnosed cause of dwarfism or short stature is achondroplasia. Other genetic conditions that result in short stature include spondylo-epi-physeal dysplasia and diastrophic dysplasia.

Achondroplasia is the most common form of dwarfism and has an incidence of approximately 1 in 7,500 births. Infants born with achondroplasia typically have an arched skull to accommodate an enlarged brain, which is generally a characteristic of this condition. This results in a very broad forehead. The child may also develop hydrocephalus. Infants with achondroplasia typically have a low nasal bridge. Arms and legs are usually very short, and the trunk of the body appears long in comparison. The hands of children with this condition are generally short and broad. The index and middle finger are typically close together, as are the ring finger and the pinkie, giving the hand a unique appearance. Changes to the spine may result in an outward curvature of the upper back, and the legs may be bowed. Most adult males with achondroplasia are under four feet six, whereas females are typically three inches shorter than males. Children with achondroplasia may also have an atypical rib cage, including curvature of the ribs. Achondroplasia does not affect cognitive and mental abilities. The life expectancy of infants over the age of twelve months is normal (Grewal, 2004; Trotter & Hall, 2005).

Spondylo-epiphyseal dysplasia is a rare form of dwarfism. There are approximately 3.4 persons with spondylo-epiphyseal dysplasia per million of the general population. One in 100,000 live births is a person with spondylo-epiphyseal dysplasia. Characteristics of spondylo-epiphyseal dysplasia include flat facial features, myopia (nearsightedness) or retinal detachment, short-trunk dwarfism, and barrel chestedness. Also, the knees often tend to be atypical, pointing either outward or inward, which changes the walking pattern. Hands and feet appear typical. Mental and intellectual capabilities are not altered by spondylo-epiphyseal dysplasia. Adults can reach heights of two feet nine to four feet two. In some cases, the characteristics of the condition may lead to further changes in physical characteristics. For instance, retinal detachment may result in blindness. Compression of the spinal cord may result in changes in neuromuscular function (Parikh & Crawford, 2003).

Diastrophic dysplasia is a very rare form of dwarfism caused by an autosomal recessive gene mutation. One in every 500,000 in the United States, 1 in 100,000 worldwide, and about 1 in 30,000 people in Finland are born with diastrophic dysplasia. Short stature and progressive curvature of the spine are major features of diastrophic dysplasia. The pelvic bones as well as the head of the thigh bone and the tailbone may also be atypical. Fingers are short, the small bones in the hand tend to grow together, and the thumb is extended. With changes in bone structure in the hips and feet, changes in mobility may occur. Cyst-like swellings on the outer ear that develop during early infancy may later develop into cauliflower-like shapes. Generally, a quarter of individuals with diastrophic dysplasia have a cleft palate. Intelligence is generally not affected (Genetics Home Reference, 2007; Parikh, Batra, & Do, 2007).

Individuals who experience dwarfism generally prefer not to be referred to as dwarfs, but as little people. In 1957, a group of little people got together in Reno, Nevada, under the leadership of Billy Barty, a widely acclaimed actor, to form the organization Little People of America. Originally developed to provide support to little people in dealing with the challenges of dwarfism, it expanded its role to include not only personal and family support but also advocacy. Through organizations such as Little People of America, little people are coming together socially and politically to challenge stereotypes, provide mutual support, and educate not only themselves but all Americans (Little People of America, 2006b).

ACQUIRED MOBILITY-RELATED DISABILITIES

Amputation

Amputation generally is seen as an acquired mobility disability, but infants born without a limb or with a significantly changed limb are also considered a part of this group. Numbers attained by the U.S. Census remain obscure. An exhaustive empirical study completed in 2002 provides a better estimate. Dillingham, Pezzin, and MacKenzie (2002) found by looking at discharge rates in the United States between 1988 and 1996 that a total of 1,199,111 hospital discharges involved limb loss or limb deficiency, an average of 133,235 limb-loss-related discharges per year. Rates of limb loss varied, depending on the cause. Amputations due to vascular conditions resulted in the vast majority (82 percent) of limb-loss discharges. Trauma-related amputations were 5.86 per 100,000 persons in 1996. In 1996, limb loss due to malignancy was 0.35 per 100,000. Finally, the incidence of congenital deficiencies resulted in only 0.8 percent of all limb-loss-related discharges—

25.64 per 100,000 live births in 1996. With violence and war so prevalent throughout major world regions, amputations and other serious violence-related injuries are increasingly commonplace. People who experience war- and terror-related limb loss must deal with the emotional sequelae related to the violent causes of their amputations.

Two types of congenital conditions are associated with an absence of limbs at birth. In the first type, a middle segment of a limb is missing, but the parts proximal and distal to the body are intact. For example, the hand or the foot may be directly connected to the shoulder or the hip, respectively, without the middle structures. The second type more closely resembles acquired or surgical amputation, where there are no structures beyond the missing part.

In many cases, persons with lower-extremity amputations use some method of alternative mobility, usually a prosthetic device. Prosthetic devices today are designed to accommodate the mobility function altered by the amputation. Devices are designed in relation to the size, type, and area of limb change. Computer technology and alternative high-tech material are key components in contemporary design of prosthetic devices (Beers, 2003).

Stroke

Stroke is also known as a cerebrovascular accident. It occurs when blood vessels in a specific part of the brain rupture (hemorrhagic stroke) or become blocked (ischemic stroke). When oxygen fails to reach a specific part of the brain, the brain cells begin to die. In a hemorrhagic stroke, blood collects in brain tissue and blocks the normal transfer of oxygen and other blood elements. Hemorrhagic strokes are usually the result of burst aneurysms (weakened spots in the blood vessels) or of hypertension, which causes constant pressure on arterial walls, eventually leading them to leak or burst (Beers, 2003).

In the United States, between 600,000 and 750,000 individuals experience a stroke each year. Of these, 160,000 die. It is estimated that by 2050, 1.5 million Americans per year will have a stroke. Although males are slightly more likely to have a stroke, more than 60 percent of the deaths due to stroke occur in women. Certain subpopulations within the general population tend to be at high risk for strokes. These include persons with long-term alcohol or drug abuse; persons with arteriosclerosis, diabetes, or high blood pressure; and people who smoke, particularly women who smoke and use birth control pills. People who have had strokes are at a greater risk of having a stroke again (Beers, 2003; Macko, Ivey, & Forrester, 2005).

Stroke can significantly affect areas of the brain that control vital functions. These functions can include a wide range of physical, cognitive, and emotional components in human existence. Stroke can affect motor ability and control, sensation and perception, communication, psychological state and emotion, and consciousness. The most common type of stroke occurs from blockage of a middle cerebral artery, which usually causes partial or total paralysis on one side of the body. Generally, when the stroke occurs in the left middle cerebral artery (which affects the right side of the body), changes occur with speech and language. Individuals who have experienced a stroke generally approach problems and new situations differently than prior to the stroke, usually with caution. Their organizational skills are usually changed. Generally, when the stroke occurs in the right middle cerebral artery (which affects the left side of the body), individuals experience changes to their spatial perception. Their ability to judge distance, size, position, rate of movement, form, and relationship of parts is diminished. They tend to neglect their left side and show impulsiveness. When strokes occur in the left middle cerebral artery, individuals are likely to experience right paralysis and sensory loss and a loss of receptive and/or expressive communication ability (e.g., aphasia), may be more cautious, and may have an inability to engage in previously learned physical tasks (apraxia) (Beers, 2003; Macko et al., 2005).

Muscular Dystrophy

The term *muscular dystrophy* covers over forty separate neuromuscular conditions, which have in common the progressive and irreversible change of the structure and strength of muscle tissue. Some of these conditions are known as *dystrophies,* which occur when the muscles change in mass and strength from within. Others are *atrophies,* where conditions in the nervous system result in the loss of the ability to use muscles.

Duchenne muscular dystrophy is the most common and most severe form of the condition. Duchenne muscular dystrophy is a sex-linked genetic condition that nearly always occurs in young males. Duchenne's is a rare condition occurring in about 1 in 3,300 male births that results in progressive muscle weakness. Current thought in terms of etiology centers on a convergence of environmental factors and inherited propensities. Early symptoms usually begin between the ages of two and five years. Muscle change is initially limited to the shoulder and pelvic areas. An enlargement of the calf muscles in the legs is the result of the infiltration of fat and connective tissue into the muscles. Within several years, Duchenne muscular dystrophy affects the muscles of the chest and arms. With further progression of the condition, all the major muscles are affected (Beers, 2003; Emery, 2002).

The early symptoms of Duchenne muscular dystrophy may include changes in mobility and an increased need for mobility-accommodating devices. By age three to five years, generalized muscle weakness has progressed. A stabilization may occur between five and seven years, with some increase in muscle strength. Weakness progresses rapidly after age eight or nine, resulting in the need for some form of permanent accommodation for mobility, such as leg braces, a walker, or a wheelchair. By adolescence, extensive accommodation in the form of a manual or electric wheelchair is usually necessary. In the late stages of Duchenne muscular dystrophy, muscles become shorter and there is a significant loss of muscle tissue. This may result in the inability to move the major joints of the body such that they become fixed in place (fixed contractures). There may be increased changes to the spine, resulting in its curvature (known as scoliosis). Lung capacity may decrease. As the condition progresses, more accommodations may be necessary, including special controls for driving and operating vehicles, lifts, and modification to the home. Death often occurs by young adulthood. Other forms of muscular dystrophy are not nearly so severe (Beers, 2003; Emery, 2002). For example, distal muscular dystrophy is an autosomal dominant, non-life-threatening form of muscular dystrophy with onset during a person's forties to sixties, which manifests as progressive weakness in the lower legs, forearms, and hands.

Rheumatoid Arthritis

Approximately 1 percent of the adult populations of Europe and North America have rheumatoid arthritis (RA). Three-quarters of the people having RA are women. Caribbean peoples have lower rates, while some Native American groups have higher rates of RA. RA usually begins in middle age but can start at any age (King, 2006). Between 30,000 and 50,000 children in the United States have juvenile rheumatoid arthritis (Myer, Brunner, Nelson, Paterno, Ford, & Hewett, 2005). Norway has a very high rate of juvenile rheumatoid arthritis, with a prevalence of approximately 148 per 100,000 people, as opposed to about 90 per 100,000 in the United States. Juvenile rheumatoid arthritis is less common in African populations than among Europeans. Girls are twice as likely as boys to contract the condition (Hekmatnia, McHugh, Basiratnia, & Offiah, 2007).

RA is an autoimmune condition, which means that the immune system attacks parts of the body, especially the joints, because it recognizes them as foreign to the body. RA causes inflammation of the joints, but it can sometimes affect multiple body systems, including the muscles, lungs, skin, blood vessels, nerves, and eyes. In addition to joint inflammation, symptoms may include fatigue and weight loss (Beers, 2003).

RA manifests differently in each individual. Most people with RA experience fatigue, soreness, stiffness, and aching early in the course of the condition. For many, joint stiffness is worse in the mornings and after long periods of physical inactivity. Usually, several joints gradually become painful, swollen, and tender. The joints in the hands and feet are usually the first to be affected and are commonly affected bilaterally. Other characteristics of RA include loss of appetite and weight loss, a slight temperature, inflammation of the eyes, and painful breathing (Black, Tyler, & Kabat, 2006). Generally, one or more joints are affected in about half of those with RA. RA, especially the juvenile form, usually progresses in severity with time (King, 2006). Special mobility accommodations may be needed, such as canes, crutches, and walkers. Depending on the degree of change in the joint, the use of a wheelchair may facilitate mobility.

Multiple Sclerosis

Multiple sclerosis (MS) is a common disease of the central nervous system, particularly among young adults. It affects about 6 people in 10,000 in white populations, with about half the rate for non-whites. It is rarely found in people of Asian descent. For almost two-thirds of these individuals, onset occurs between the ages of twenty and forty; it is twice as common in women as men. MS has an interesting environmental characteristic. It is rare in tropical climates and is very common in persons of Western European descent who live in temperate zones above 40° north and below 40° south (Blumenthal, 2006; Lazoff, 2005; Tierney, McPhee, & Papadakis, 2006).

MS is characterized by the inflammation and the eventual deterioration of the myelin sheath, a fatty material that covers and insulates the nerves. Myelin functions similarly to the plastic covering on electric wiring. Changes in the myelin cause disruption in the ability of the nerves to conduct electrical impulses to and from the brain. This disruption results in the various characteristics of MS (Beers, 2003). Exact causes of MS are unclear, but evidence suggests it may be an autoimmune condition that is precipitated by various causes, including genetic predisposition and environmental factors such as climate and viruses. Genetic susceptibility is suggested by the fact that a slightly higher risk of MS exists in families in which it has already occurred (Tierney et al., 2006).

MS is a variable condition; the resulting characteristics depend on which areas of the central nervous system have been affected. There is no typical MS, no established pattern of development. Everyone with MS has a different set of resulting characteristics that can shift from time to time and change in severity and duration. Generally, persons with MS experience changes in vision, coordination, muscular strength, speech and communication, sexual functioning, bowel and bladder control, and cognitive functioning. One of the most common changes brought about by MS is fatigue, which can occur unpredictably and without relationship to physical activity. Persons with MS generally have a low tolerance to heat.

MS is usually progressive, with periods of symptom exacerbation and remission. Over several years, the progression of MS symptoms may require accommodation. Many persons with MS require accommodation for mobility, including the use of crutches and eventually the use of a wheelchair. Home adaptations to accommodate wheelchair use may be necessary. Sexual function changes require various types of accommodation. Changes in bowel and bladder control may require alternative methods in the form of external or internal catheters and bowel management programs (Beers, 2003; Blumenthal, 2006; Lazoff, 2005; Tierney et al., 2006).

Myasthenia Gravis

Myasthenia gravis (MG) is a chronic neuromuscular condition characterized by weakness and rapid fatigue of the voluntary muscles (those muscles controlled by will). MG may involve either a single muscle or a group of muscles. Muscle groups generally most affected control speech, chewing, swallowing, and eye movement. Muscles that control the arms and legs are sometimes affected. In some persons with MG, the weakness is limited to eye and eyelid muscles, resulting in double vision and sometimes drooping eyelids. Rest and relaxation are extremely important to help people with MG regain strength and endurance (Tierney et al., 2006).

MG can occur in people of any age and either sex, but its prevalence is highest in young women ages twenty to thirty-five and in men and women over sixty years of age. The frequency and recognition of MG is increasing. The increase in incidents occurs in individuals over the age of sixty. Between .25 and 2 people per 100,000 are affected by MG each year (Vincent, Palace, & Hilton-Jones, 2001).

Muscle weakness makes the activities of daily living difficult for people with MG. Some experience difficulty chewing and swallowing. Some have respiratory weakness. The weakness in the muscles used for breathing may result in shortness of breath and the inability to take deep breaths. Usually, persons under sixty years of age with MG do not require mobility accommodation. Most individuals with MG are treated with a combination of several drugs such as pyridostigmine and prednisone (Beers, 2003).

Spinal Cord Injury

There are no worldwide estimates of the incidence or prevalence of spinal cord injury (SCI) due to the lack of information in Asia, Latin America, and Africa. Wyndaele and Wyndaele (2006) conducted a multicountry meta-analysis of available research relative to the incidence and prevalence of SCI, primarily in industrially developed countries. They found that most countries report an incidence of between 15 to 30 per million SCIs per year. Approximately two-thirds of people with SCI have paraplegia, and a third have tetraplegia. Over three-quarters are male and the majority of injuries occur in adolescence and early adulthood. Life expectancies have increased in recent decades, especially for individuals with tetraplegia.

More than a quarter million people with SCI live in the United States, where there is an annual incidence of more than 10,000. Most SCIs results from trauma. The leading traumatic cause of SCI is automobile accidents.

Forty-four percent of all SCIs come from this cause. Other causes of SCI include violence, falls, and sports. Sports only account for 8 percent of all SCIs. Interestingly, 60 percent of sports-related SCIs are the result of diving accidents. After the age of forty-five, falls overtake automobile accidents as the number one cause of SCI. The average age at the time that SCI occurs is thirty-three, but the most frequent age of injury is nineteen (Cleveland Clinic Health Information Center, 2003).

SCI can cause partial or complete paralysis and sensory loss, depending on the severity of the injury (Tierney et al., 2006). SCI in the back results in lower body paralysis, called paraplegia, whereas arm and leg paralysis (tetraplegia) occur in SCI in the neck. The location of the injury determines the function affected. Generally, four parts of the spine are considered when one is dealing with SCI: the cervical spine, the thoracic spine, the lumbar spine, and the sacrum. The higher the injury, the more functions are affected; the more extensive the damage to the cord, the greater the neurological loss. At every level, SCI affects bowel, bladder, and sexual functioning. When the spinal cord is severed or damaged so severely that no messages can be transmitted past the damage, the SCI is complete (Cleveland Clinic Health Information Center, 2003). The discussion below assumes a complete injury to the spinal cord.

The cervical spine consists of the first seven vertebrae and eight spinal cord segments. With SCIs at C1 (first cervical segment of the spinal cord) to C3, nerves that control breathing are damaged, and a permanent ventilator or other breathing aid is required to sustain life. The C4 region affects the neck and diaphragm. Injury to this area of the spinal cord generally results in paralysis from the neck down. Head control, arm and leg movement, and bowel and bladder control are all affected. Respiratory functioning is compromised, but mechanical ventilation is usually not necessary. Mobility accommodation in the form of an electric wheelchair controlled by the mouth or chin is usually required. Home modifications and attendant care for all activities of daily living are generally necessary for independent living.

A C5 injury affects some shoulder muscles. Injury at this level usually means that head control is unaffected. The individual has some use of the arms. Persons with a C5 injury can push a wheelchair with modified rims, but usually an electric wheelchair produces better mobility. Persons with a C5 injury usually require mechanical wheelchair lifts to enter motor vehicles and can sometimes drive using modified steering and hand controls to operate gas and brake pedals.

Persons with C6 tetraplegia generally have function of the major muscles of the shoulders and wrists. They can generally control their arms and wrists and are able to weakly grasp objects. Persons with a C6 injury can usually transfer from the wheelchair without assistance. They can utilize a manual wheelchair with a great deal of precision and may be able to transfer into cars without a lift and drive with hand controls and no modified steer-ing. A person with C7 or C8 tetraplegia may have slightly weakened muscles in the shoulders and arms and still retain some finger and hand function. They are capable of self-sufficiency in activities of daily living, utilizing a wheelchair, and managing bowel and bladder functions.

Persons with T1 (first thoracic segment) paraplegia have complete hand and finger function, which allows them to engage in activities requiring fine motor skills, such as piano playing and handcrafts. People with injuries to the mid-thoracic area (T6–8) have better balance because back and chest muscles are innervated. In the absence of other problems, complete inde-pendence is ensured when the environment is accommodating. People with T12 paraplegia have full use of back and abdominal muscles. Some hip func-tion is present. Long leg braces combined with crutches allow people to walk short distances; however, community mobility still requires the use of a manual wheelchair. People with injuries to the L1–5 (lumbar) segments of the spinal cord have increased function in their legs as the level of injury descends. Community mobility may be possible for people with low lumbar injuries; however, mobility is still primarily accomplished by wheelchair. Lower leg, knee, and foot stability are affected in people with injuries to the S1–5 (sacral) segments of the spinal cord. People with paraplegia at these levels may ambulate with short leg braces, although wheelchairs are usually used for long distances to conserve energy. Bowel, bladder, and genital functioning are also affected at the sacral segments of the spinal cord; there-fore, anyone with a SCI is susceptible to alteration of function in these areas (Beers, 2003; Cleveland Clinic Health Information Center, 2003; Fries, 2005).

Persons with a SCI are prone to a number of secondary health problems. Decubitus ulcers, or pressure sores, are a primary concern of persons with SCI. These usually come about at pressure points where bones tend to pro-trude, as in the buttocks, pelvis, and ankles. They are caused by reduced blood flow and lack of sensation; they can become infected and heal very slowly (Tierney et al., 2006). Persons with a SCI must consciously relieve pressure by moving themselves or having an attendant move them at regular time intervals. Extra padding for the buttocks may be necessary, particularly in the wheelchair (Fries, 2005).

Persons with SCI are also susceptible to urinary tract infections. Urinary tract infections occur when urine is retained in the bladder and becomes infected with microorganisms. People are also susceptible to urinary tract infections when they use an internal catheter over a long period of time. For persons with SCI, urinary tract infections can be quite serious and can ulti-mately affect the kidneys. Newer antibiotics are very useful for fighting off urinary tract infections, but bacteria can become resistant to antibiotics (Beers, 2003).

Poliomyelitis

Polio is caused by a viral infection of motor neurons in the spinal cord. Since the introduction of vaccines in the early 1950s, poliomyelitis has virtually been eradicated from the Western Hemisphere; however, in the late 1990s it was the leading cause of disability in some countries such as Afghanistan. In terms of the worldwide population, between 1988 and 2001, the number of cases has dropped by 99 percent. The only countries reporting more than a hundred cases between 2000 and 2001 were India, Nigeria, and Pakistan (Tierney et al., 2006). In 2006, only 2002 cases were reported worldwide, half of which were from Nigeria (Centers for Disease Control and Prevention, 2007). The near eradication of polio can be attributed to worldwide vaccination efforts. Nevertheless, about 1.6 million persons in the United States are living with the effects of poliomyelitis contracted before the development of vaccines (Kramasz, 2005). Tens of millions live with the effects of polio worldwide. Polio causes paralysis, which may be slight or severe, depending on the number and location of motor neurons affected. Paralysis may be temporary or permanent.

A recent phenomenon called post-poliomyelitis syndrome or post-polio syndrome has occurred among persons who developed polio in the past. A fourth to a third of those who contract polio develop new symptoms of weakness, pain, and fatigue many years after recovering from the acute paralytic event. Some persons who contracted polio thirty or forty years ago are experiencing increased difficulty walking, climbing stairs, dressing, bathing, and swallowing. Persons with post-polio syndrome experience weakness and muscle atrophy in previously affected or unaffected muscles. Post-polio syndrome is not infectious but may be related to the premature aging of overworked motor neurons.

Medical researchers are not certain about the cause of post-polio syndrome. Many believe that its symptoms result to a large degree from the unusual stress placed on surviving nerve cells. With initial infection, some motor neurons are damaged or destroyed, resulting in nonfunctioning muscles or muscles with limited functioning. Usually, other motor neurons survive the polio attack and establish new nerve connections to the muscle cells. These motor neurons take over the function of the destroyed nerve cells. This process often enables a person to regain at least some use of the affected muscles. But years later, the overburdened nerve cells may begin to fail, resulting in new muscle weakness (Kramasz, 2005).

COMMON ISSUES

Prejudice, Stereotyping, and Discrimination

Whether a mobility-related disability is acquired before or at birth or sometime afterward, persons with mobility disabilities experience prejudice, stereotyping, and discrimination. The stereotypes and prejudices about persons with mobility disabilities are numerous and varied. Hahn (1988), citing the work of Livneh, points out that persons who have disabilities that affect their mobility are considered ugly. Particularly in a culture that defines beauty in a narrow and restricted sense, persons with mobility disabilities are seen as particularly offensive aesthetically, and they create an apprehension of difference—a kind of xenophobia of nonaesthetics. In addition, because of the cultural inculcation of certain mores from the Judeo-Christian heritage, Western society has developed an "existential anxiety" toward persons with mobility disabilities (Hahn, 1988, p. 39). Similarly, other cultures and societies have developed similar attitudes as a result of views of disability as being out of order with nature or with the natural order of the world. This feeds the perception that if an individual acquires a mobility disability, life ends. This view, along with the stereotype that persons with mobility disabilities are sick, promotes the idea that persons with mobility disabilities should be and are universally dependent.

Other assumptions or prejudices feed the discrimination experienced by persons with disabilities. Fine and Asch (1993) list five assumptions applied by researchers, practitioners, and people in general to persons with disabilities, including those with mobility disabilities. First, people generally assume that disability is rooted in biological dysfunction and that biological dysfunction is the primary driving force in their lives; they are "confined" by and "victims" of their disabilities. For example, Johnny, who has spina bifida, cannot do well in school because of his spina bifida. Sam has trouble making friends because he is "confined" to a wheelchair. Sandra, who seeks counseling for her depression, is depressed because she was a "victim" of polio at the age of six and has used crutches ever since. Second, people generally assume that mobility-related disability is the cause of the problems that people face. The human-built world is never viewed as the cause of people's problems—it is always the disability. Third, people assume that persons with disabilities are victims and that they see themselves as such. Persons with disabilities are not in control and can never have a viable, rich life; they are victims of a great and all-encompassing tragedy. Fourth, related to the preceding assumption, people assume that disability is the center of life for people with disabilities. It is central to their self-definition, to their patterns of friends, and to their comparisons of themselves to others. Persons with disabilities have no other basis on which to establish a social reference group than other people with disabilities. The fact that they may be male or female, a member of an ethnic minority group, or part of a professional interest community has little or no bearing on their associations. Only the disability is a factor. And fifth, people assume that terms such as *person with a disability* and *disabled person* are synonymous with the phrase "I need help." Disability means helplessness. A wheelchair user needs the door opened for her. A person who is blind needs to be helped across the street. It is the disabled equivalent of the "white man's burden." Help is always given with the expectation of the reward of feeling good and being thanked, much the same as the white colonialist missionaries' expectations in eighteenth- and nineteenth-century Africa toward native people.

Bogdan and Biklen (1977) discuss the concrete results of stereotypes and assumptions or prejudices about persons with disabilities. Persons with mobility disabilities are generally portrayed in a negative light by the media. Physical differences are associated with crime and horror. Humor is presented at the expense of persons with mobility disabilities. The lives of persons with mobility disabilities are depicted as tragic. Telethons present pathetic images of persons with disabilities in order to raise money. Persons with disabilities are portrayed as noble for choosing to live rather than commit suicide in the wake of such tragedy and pathos. Yet death is portrayed as a natural wish of persons with disabilities.

Another major result of stereotyping and prejudice is the discrimination in physical access for persons with mobility-related disabilities. Wheelchair users are denied access to public toilets, sidewalks, places of commerce, public telephones, housing, parking, parks and recreation, private and public transportation including buses and airplanes, and places of worship.

Persons with mobility disabilities are also denied access to education. School buildings and many classrooms are not designed to accommodate wheelchair users. Libraries are not designed to allow access to wheelchair users. Many college and university campuses remain inaccessible, with steps, steep inclines, no parking, broken sidewalks, and so on. In 2004, the Rehabilitation Research and Training Center on Disability Demographics and Statistics found that the percentage of persons with disabilities with bachelor's degrees had increased slightly between 2003 and 2004. But in 2004, 25.4 percent of persons with disabilities did not have a high school diploma, while 11.8 percent of the aggregate working age population did not possess a high school diploma or its equivalent, And 28.1 percent of persons with disabilities had some college education, while 30.3 percent of the aggregate working-age population had completed some college. And the percentage of persons with disabilities receiving a bachelor's degree (12.7 percent) remained well below the percentages within the aggregate working-age population (29.8 percent). The only positive comparison centered on those with high school diplomas: 33.7 percent of persons with disabilities had a high school diploma, while in the aggregate working-age population, 28.1 percent had a high school diploma (Rehabilitation Research and Training Center on Disability Demographics and Statistics, 2004).

Persons with physical disabilities that affect their mobility are denied access to service delivery in both the public and private sectors. An important aspect of the inaccessibility of service delivery is the segregation of persons with mobility disabilities. In public auditoriums and movie theaters, wheelchair accommodation is separate, usually in the back, and never equal. Wheelchair seating in restaurants is sometimes out of the way, near the kitchen. They are permitted to participate in "special education" programs and "special" sports events for persons with mobility disabilities, rather than being integrated into professional and amateur athletic events and games.

Casey Martin discovered the extent of this discrimination when he was denied the use of a golf cart in a Professional Golfers' Association tournament in the late 1990s. He sued. Martin has Klippel-Trenaunay-Weber syndrome, which limits his ability to walk. In commenting on the case, PGA commissioner Tim Finchem revealed the central stereotypes surrounding athletics and disability: "As we [the PGA] have said from the outset of this lawsuit, we believe firmly in the basic premise of any sport, that one set of rules must be applied equally to all competitors. Additionally, we believe strongly in the central role walking plays for all competitors in tournament championship golf at the PGA Tour and Nike Tour levels" (qtd. in Cullity, 1998a).

He failed to mention the sanctioned use of golf carts on the Senior PGA Tour, in the PGA Tour Qualifying Tournament, and at the NCAA level (Cullity, 1998b). U.S. magistrate Thomas M. Coffin, citing the Americans with Disabilities Act, dismissed the PGA's request to dismiss the lawsuit; he went on to find in Martin's favor.

In 2007, Oscar Pistorius, a South African world-class sprinter, sought to become the first amputee runner to compete in the Olympics. A bilateral below-the-knee amputee because of a congenital lack of fibula bones, he runs with prosthetics and posts world-class times. He is a champion Paralympian; however, the international track and field governing body successfully barred him from competition. The Court of Arbitration for Sport in May of 2008 ruled that there was insufficient evidence that his prosthesis gave him any advantage over athletes with typically formed legs and feet (Weihenmayer, 2008). We find it ironic that when a person who would be considered unable to work and eligible for disability benefits in many countries attempts to compete against nondisabled athletes, he is deemed by some to be advantaged by his disability. These attempts to exclude disabled persons smack of ableism.

One of the most significant areas in which persons with mobility-related disabilities remain discriminated against is employment. The National Organization on Disability (2006) reports that only 32 percent of all Americans with disabilities of working age are employed. Two-thirds of those who are unemployed would prefer to work. The rate of employment of persons with disabilities appears to be decreasing (Rehabilitation Research and Training Center on Disability Demographics and Statistics, 2004).

Discrimination in hiring has historically been and remains a significant factor in this low employment rate. Balcazar, Bradford, and Fawcett (1993) found that 70 percent of the disabled population they surveyed experienced major problems in employment. These included a lack of accommodation in the workplace, lack of training and professional development, and work disincentives in Social Security. Data indicate that 72 percent of those surveyed felt that persons with disabilities were discriminated against in the workplace and were not given the same employment opportunities as persons without disabilities. The Americans with Disabilities Act was created and passed to prevent discrimination against persons with disabilities. This remains an unachieved objective (Russell, 2001).

Aging

Most persons with physical disabilities that affect mobility share not only the experience of prejudice and discrimination; they also share the development of secondary physical complications that may be exacerbated in the aging process. Wilkins and Cott (1993) examine the issue of the aging of persons with physical disabilities in detail. Persons with physical disability are living longer and thus aging. A primary factor in this increased longevity is the efficacy of new health care technologies.

Kilian and Binder (1998) find that there are certain needs that must be addressed concerning aging and disability. The issue of aging and disability is critical and needs to be addressed by study and research. Like post-polio syndrome, conditions that affect mobility need to be studied in terms of the aging process's impact on the primary disability. It appears that depression is a significant factor among people with mobility-related disabilities. Particularly in cases where the disability onset was at a young age, persons with mobility disabilities find themselves fighting battles thought to be won years ago. This requires extensive study. There needs to be a conscious effort to record symptoms in the aging process and then to categorize them so that they can be used in research and in medical care and treatment. The roles of family members with persons with mobility-related disabilities need more research and exploration. Lastly, societal accessibility and acceptance are critical to the quality of life of people as they age.

UNIQUE CONCERNS

Although persons with disabilities face the common concerns of stereotyping, prejudice, discrimination, and aging, there are points of difference. Wright (1983) discounts the idea that drastic identity or personality changes occur as the result of disabilities acquired later in life. Wright also sees no distinct advantages and disadvantages to having been born with a disability or acquiring one later in life. But acquiring a disability several years after birth requires a person to adjust to changes and integrate these with old ideas of self. The success of this integration depends on a number of variables, including personality development prior to the disability and the degree to which self-concept is associated with societal constructs of health and beauty. If self-concept has had many years to develop around Hollywood's standards of beauty, the integration of a physical disability that affects mobility becomes more difficult.

Zink (1992) concludes from personal experience and observation that the age at which a person acquires a disability affects how he or she accepts it—how it is integrated into the person's self-concept. She describes the difference between her own acquisition of a disability in her teenage years and someone whom she had just met with a disability acquired in his forties. She viewed disability as the normal state of being, whereas her new acquaintance viewed himself in his present state as abnormal. She accepted the accommodations necessary for movement as integral to her success, whereas he held onto an inaccessible house, crawling up and down stairs and refusing to utilize a power chair. It was evident that he did not intend to become a person with a disability. Disability would never be a part of him.

Zink (1992) attributes the ability of those who acquire mobility disabilities early in life to successfully integrate disability into their self-concepts to the energy of youth. Mackelprang and Altshuler (2004) have found that disabled youths perceive their quality of life as similar to the quality of life of nondisabled youths of similar age. The aging process lessens the vast amount of energy required to integrate changes in self-perception and status. Also, when one has spent more years with a disability, one has had more opportunities to be exposed to role models, leaders, and cultural and political movements centered on the strength, power, and beauty of disability and difference.

SUMMARY

We believe that human service practitioners need to be aware of the different kinds of physical disabilities related to mobility. Each of these kinds of disability manifests in different ways and may require different approaches to life processes, including accommodation for mobility, activities of daily living, and certain basic biological functions.

Human service practitioners need to know that all persons with mobility disabilities have faced and experienced stereotyping, prejudice, and discrimination. While this needs to be acknowledged with the person being provided a service, the main intervention in eradicating this barrier centers on advocacy and political action. (This will be explored more later.)

Finally, the human service practitioner needs to be aware that a mobility disability acquired later in life may affect a person differently than one acquired before or at birth. "May" is the important word here. Practitioners cannot assume anything—they must seek knowledge from the individual. It is the responsibility of human service practitioners to be aware of possibilities but not to presuppose them.

PERSONAL NARRATIVE: KAREN PENDLETON

Karen Pendleton was a mainstay in the homes of millions of children during the 1960s as an original member of the Mickey Mouse Club. At age thirty-six, she acquired a spinal cord injury when she was in an automobile accident. Since then, she has become very involved in the disability movement. Currently, she is retired from the presidency of the board of directors of the Center for Independent Living in Fresno, California.

When I was eight, I was chosen to be one of the original Mouseketeers at the Walt Disney Fan Club. It was an absolutely fantastic experience. It was fun when I was doing it. I was so young, I didn't realize how important it was and how special it was going to be. I don't think anybody realized it was going to take off like it did.

It was a healthy show. They taught nice things and it was morally a good show. None of us were very professional, so kids watching could identify with us. I had never done anything professional in my life before that. I always capitalized on my mistakes on the show. I was the youngest; people thought I was cute because I was always screwing up.

The Mouseketeers ended when I was twelve. I had to go back to being a "regular person," and life got tough. I went right back into junior high school and other kids were really mean to me. For four years, I hadn't had a lot of contact with anybody but the Mouseketeers and had no idea that so many people knew who I was.

My first week in junior high was horrible. Kids would group around me every day at lunchtime and do things like ask me for my autograph and then tear it up. They would say, "Mickey Mouse, wiggle your ears and I'll give you some cheese." I was very shy and insecure. I thought nobody liked me. My self-esteem went down to the floor. From that time on, I really had a hard time thinking I had any value at all. I thought everybody hated me. I went through junior high and high school like that.

In my early adult years, I really wasn't into the Mouseketeers at all. The only contact I had with Disney until after I had my accident was in 1980, when we did a reunion, and that was really fun. But by that time I was married and had my daughter, Stacey. The Mouseketeers didn't have any contact with the public. We just went to the studio and did the reunion show, and then I headed back home.

When I was thirty-six, I became disabled in an automobile accident. I have T-2 paraplegia, which is pretty high up. I feel very lucky I've got my arms. Ha, God knew that if I didn't have my arms I couldn't put my makeup on and I would be miserable. He knows how much I can take.

When I got in the accident, I must have gone into shock because I didn't realize that there was anything wrong with me. As I think back now, when I first got out of the car I could sit up, which is something I can't do anymore. I should never have done that, but I didn't know what a spinal cord injury was then. It seems ridiculous now that, as a grown adult, I had no idea what a spinal cord injury was. My husband picked me up, put me in the car, and drove me to the hospital, which he should never have done. I even told him to take me home; I'd be fine in the morning. I was probably in shock. I think that if I hadn't done those two things, my injury wouldn't have been as severe as it is.

The doctor never told me I would never walk again. I remember that on about my fifth day in the hospital, I said, "So what's the deal here, doctor?" He said, "Let me put it this way, Karen: you and I will both be able to go to McDonald's someday, but it will take you a little bit longer than it will me because you'll either be in a wheelchair or on crutches." Still, I had this totally positive attitude at that time, thinking, "I'm going to walk again!" And each time I would come out with this positive attitude, my doctors or my therapist would say, "Well, that's a really nice attitude, *but. . . .*" Eventually I got it, like everybody else who's been through this.

Before my accident, my husband and I were having problems. He had an affair, so my self-esteem was really low, and I was trying to keep the marriage together. Sex was a very important part of our relationship; because it was important to my husband, I placed a lot of my self-esteem in my sexuality. After my accident, I felt like, "OK, that went right out the window." I basically said to my husband, "Well, I'm worthless to you, so whatever you want to do, you do it." Well, he took me up on my offer. He said, "There's no way I can take care of you." He dropped me right then and there. He was afraid to drop me publicly because he didn't want to look like the bad guy, so eventually I had to file for divorce.

The way I saw my life then was, "I've lost my marriage, my home, and my ability to walk. Everything has gone right out the window." It was really tough.

Since my marriage was ending, I went from the hospital right to my mom and dad's home. Oh boy, did things get interesting.

For my parents, I had been an independent married woman with a child. All of a sudden I was their baby again. I let them take care of me because it was much easier on me. I felt guilty about that.

If I had gone home with my husband, I would have become independent a lot faster. But everything happens for a reason. After a year with my parents, I moved out. I finally decided living with them was not good for me, and I started becoming independent. Finally, Stacey and I moved out by ourselves. That was the very first time in my life that I had ever been on my own.

.   Stacey was only nine when I became disabled. On the night of my accident, Stacey overheard my mother say, "They took Karen away," when they were taking me to the operating room. When Stacey overheard my mom say that, she interpreted it to mean that I had died. She was so relieved when she found I wasn't dead, I think she concluded that whatever was wrong with me was unimportant as long as I was still around.

Stacey was absolutely my rock. She was the only one who didn't treat me any differently. She would still get mad or frustrated with me when she didn't get her way. I was still her mommy. It didn't matter that Mommy had a disability. She didn't pamper me, and that was comforting.

Stacey would stand on the wheelchair and she would sit on my lap. The wheelchair didn't bother her like it did my mom and dad. She and I did just great together. One of the best things this disability has done for me is give me the opportunity to be with and watch my daughter grow up. I have been at home for her and can give her advice; we have an absolutely great relationship because of that. I could never have been there for her like that had I not been able to be home. Our closeness was a very positive outcome from all this.

Because I was already having problems with my husband, one of the first things I asked for when I was in the hospital was to see a psychologist. With therapy, I started to see my husband differently, and I started to change myself, but I wouldn't admit it to myself. After three years, I stopped therapy, believing I hadn't changed at all. Now I realize I had really gotten a lot out of it but didn't know it at the time.

Over time, I figured out that old Karen was no more. It's like I had to bury her and get to know the Karen that was left here. I found that I liked the new Karen a lot better than the old one! The old Karen had been a big phony. I tried to be everything I thought other people expected me to be. I was what my husband wanted me to be. I was what my parents wanted me to be. I was what my friends at the country club wanted me to be. It wasn't me.

Now all I have left is me. And I like me a whole lot better than I did that other me. That's where my self-confidence came from. It's not being conceited, because I believe conceited people have no self-esteem. This disability helped me become more assertive. I've had to take risks. I've had to ask for help, which I never would have done before. Like, when I'm at the grocery store, I will ask strangers, "Excuse me, could you reach that for me?" I would have never done that before and, believe me, at four feet ten, I needed help reaching things. I'm willing to take risks that I would never have taken before my disability. I like it, and I keep trying to teach the same thing to my clients.

I didn't even consider myself disabled for a long time. When I saw the shadow of my wheelchair, I would think it was creepy. I remember once going to a presentation on the electric stimulation of muscles. I was sitting in this roomful of people, and all of a sudden I realized these were all people with disabilities. And I thought to myself, "I do not belong here."

For the most part, I had never hung out with anybody with a disability, and I didn't even know anybody with a disability. I tried to gracefully embrace people with disabilities, but it was hard. I thought, "I don't know anything about you. I only know about my disability."

It seems weird now, but it took me awhile to become really accepting of others with disabilities. A really good eye-opener for me was a college course I took on the psychological aspects of disability. I took the class thinking I would know everything and get an easy A. But I really learned a lot in the class about other disabilities. Since then, I've learned a lot from other people with disabilities.

I'm much more accepting of people with disabilities and of myself with a disability. Some really neat things have happened to me only since I've been disabled. It wasn't until after I was disabled that I actually went out into the public as a Mouseketeer again. I was shocked when I saw how much people loved me after all those years. One time I did a Miss Wheelchair pageant. I'll never forget a young woman from Arizona. She said to me, "When I was growing up, you were the one thing that made me have some kind of happiness in my life. My parents abused me, and the only thing I ever had to look forward to was at five o'clock I could watch *The Mickey Mouse Club*." It profoundly affected me when she told me that story. All of a sudden I started to realize I had the ability to get some messages out, that people might be listening to me.

I am very grateful for some of my role models after I had my disability. One was Richard, who worked at the independent living center. He talked me into going back to school. I remember him telling me that I had three choices: I could get into commercials, I could start doing wheelchair pageants and make a job for myself doing that, or I could go back to college. I would never have gone back to college before that.

I remember doing a Barrier Awareness Day in Washington, D.C., which was a really neat event. The woman who put that together was phenomenal. She had severe muscular dystrophy. She was probably in her early twenties when she put this thing together. She got President Reagan to sign a National Barrier Awareness Day proclamation. She had half of Congress there. She had Jim Brady there and all the movie stars she could get. It was great. She was a really neat person, and that day was an eye-opening experience for a lot of people.

Disability is a subject that people don't want to talk or hear about. Some people have drawn an analogy between the disability movement and the civil rights movement. There were a lot of white people who went out and supported the civil rights movement, knowing that they would never be black. Still, they supported that movement. It's really hard, though, to get people involved in disabilities. Since anybody can become disabled, it's very scary for people to think about. I think disability is an unpleasant subject because people know it could possibly happen to them or to someone they care about. I think it makes some people hesitant to support disability rights.

I remember being extremely put off by people with disabilities as a child. I was never exposed to them. I didn't understand it. I was made to think disability was bad. I was taught, "Oh, don't look at that poor person" and "How sad that she has a disability." It was a totally negative thing. That's why I think mainstreaming is so great. One way to change attitudes is for nondisabled kids to grow up alongside people with disabilities. That way people won't be afraid of them or think of them as being different. I think we are becoming more mainstream, and that's good. Every time I go to the mall, I run into six or seven people in wheelchairs, whereas I never saw people in wheelchairs when I was young.

With exposure, children handle disabilities well. Kids at work love me. I'm down at their level in my wheelchair. Kids like that. They jump up on my lap and they ask me all kinds of questions. Sometimes I joke with them and I say I'm just really lazy so I don't want to stand up and walk. Sometimes it's hard for a four-year-old to understand that my legs don't work, but I explain it anyway. I find that if I treat kids well, they're not going to think twice when they talk to someone else with a disability. They're just going to be totally comfortable with that person. I try to be really good to kids. I love to teach them about disability.

When I was first in a wheelchair, I was terrified that people were going to stare at me. I found people reacted in a completely opposite manner. People turn their eyes away from me; they won't look at me. It sounds strange, but I've gotten to the point now where I'll stare someone down to make them look at me. It's like I'm saying, "I'm here, I'm a person, I'm alive!" People seem so afraid that they don't want to look.

I think familiarity is really important. My nondisabled friends include me in everything, and they sometimes forget that I'm disabled. However, they are also very sensitive to the fact that I am in a wheelchair and plan accordingly. I like to be able to open people's eyes about disabilities. Unfortunately, there are those who will never ever have their eyes opened, no matter what.

When I wake up in the morning, I have to roll around in bed for forty-five minutes just to get dressed. Because of my injury, I sometimes get all sweaty and I can't get cool. By the time I get to work in the morning, my hair is combed and my makeup is on and I'm dressed nicely, and people have no idea what it took to get ready. At my former job, some people complained, "Karen's been getting here five minutes late every day." I thought, "I'd like to strap your feet together, young lady, and have you get dressed. Then we'll see what time you get here." Ha, but I don't say those things because I'm too nice.

I'd like some people to sit in a wheelchair for a day and try to park the car in the driveway. I get really angry at that. For example, at my former job, I spoke to the entire staff at work about disability awareness. But I got really frustrated when people still parked in the driveway and I had to go on the grass. It's dangerous; I almost fell several times. I called and left notes for people, asking them, "Please do not park in the driveway," but sometimes people still parked there. I think that's extremely rude. They knew that was the only way I had to get into the building.

I've had other experiences too. Lots of people use disabled parking stalls. Sometimes people park so close to my car door that I can't get into the car because of my wheelchair. Sometimes people leave the parking space open but they park over the ramp. I've got a place to park, but I can't get into the building anyway because I don't do well hopping curbs. I'll never forget the time I got out of an upstairs class late and someone had turned the elevator off. I was almost stuck in the building all night. Fortunately, some other students carried me down the stairs. (I think I gave somebody serious back problems.) I hate to think what would have happened if I used an electric wheelchair.

Most people don't think about those things because they don't know any better. It's just a lack of awareness. When I'm with another person with a disability, there's an understanding that goes beyond what someone without a disability would ever know. There's a lot more to disability than what the general public sees. We just share that understanding.

I feel like I became disabled at a good time, because things are starting to change. We still have a long way to go, but things are a lot better than when I was a child. I believe things are different for people with disabilities now than they were back then. We have laws and are getting more opportunities.

If I were to offer advice to nondisabled people, I would say to treat a disabled person like a person, first. Second, try to learn as much about a person's disability as you can. For example, if the person is in a wheelchair, sit down in a wheelchair and see what it feels like. Experience the wheelchair to some extent. People without disabilities have no idea what it's like with a disability.

Truly, having a disability has not been the horrible experience that people might think. There's some negative stuff that goes along with it, like daily living skills, which are a pain. I also get nervous about getting older, because things are not going to get easier. But I would not be where I am right now, personally or professionally, had it not been for this disability. I've got to say a lot of positive things have come from it. Because I had no place else to go, I had to get to know the real me.

I would never have met so many important people in my life had I not been disabled. There are so many great people with disabilities, yet a lot of people without disabilities don't even give them the time of day. But it's changing, I think. We're coming out of our closet.

DISCUSSION QUESTIONS

1. What are some of the major issues in defining persons with mobility disabilities?
2. How does a medical model orientation influence the definition and discussion of disability?

3. What are some of the advantages of defining a mobility disability from a social model perspective?
4. Discuss in detail some of the primary issues facing all persons with mobility disabilities.
5. What are some of the primary differences between those who acquired disabilities early in life and those who acquire disabilities later in life?
6. Would knowledge of when a person with a mobility disability acquired that disability influence professional assessment and the plan of intervention?
7. How could you utilize the information provided in the above chapter in your future human services work?

SUGGESTED READINGS

Berger, L., Lithwick, D., & Campers, S. (1992). *I will sing life: Voices from the Hole in the Wall Gang Camp*. Boston: Little, Brown.

Crewe, N. M., & Zola, I. K. (1983). *Independent living for physically disabled people*. San Francisco: Jossey-Bass.

Noble, V. (1993). *Down is up for Aaron Eagle: A mother's spiritual journey with Down syndrome*. San Francisco: Harper.

Rehabilitation Research and Training Center on Disability Demographics and Statistics. (2004). *2004 disability status reports: United States*. Retrieved August 16, 2006, from http://www.ilr.cornell.edu/ped/disabilitystatistics/StatusReports/2004-html/US.html?CFID = 2550131&CFTOKEN = 33945622#top

Shapiro, J. P. (1993). *No pity: People with disabilities forging a new civil rights movement*. New York: Times Books.

Wright, B. (1983). *Physical disability—a psychological approach* (2nd ed.). New York: Harper & Row.

REFERENCES

Balcazar, Y., Bradford, B., & Fawcett, S. (1993). Common concerns of disabled Americans: Issues and options. In M. Nagler (Ed.), *Perspectives on disability: Text and readings on disability* (2nd ed., pp. 5–15). Palo Alto, CA: Health Markets Research.

Barker, E., Saulino, M., & Caristo, A. M. (2002). Spina bifida. *RN, 65*(12), 33–39. Retrieved August 15, 2006, from Expanded Academic ASAP via Thomson Gale.

Beers, M. H. (Ed.). (2003). *The Merck manual of medical information* (2nd ed.). New York: Simon & Schuster.

Black, G. S., Tyler, J. A., & Kabat, A. G. (2006). Arthritis as seen through the eyes: About one in four patients with rheumatoid arthritis reports ocular symptoms. *Review of Optometry, 143*(1), 39. Retrieved August 10, 2006, from Expanded Academic ASAP via Thomson Gale.

Blumenthal, S. (2006). Multiple sclerosis. *Radiologic Technology, 77*(4), 309–321. Retrieved August 10, 2006, from Expanded Academic ASAP via Thomson Gale.

Bogdan, R., & Biklen, D. (1977). Handicapism. *Social Policy, 7*(4), 14–19.

Centers for Disease Control and Prevention. (2007). Progress toward poliomyelitis eradication: Nigeria, 2005–2006. *Morbidity and Mortality Weekly, 56*(12), 278–281.

Chen, H. (2006, February 13). *Arthrogryposis.* Retrieved August 9, 2006, from http://www.emedicine.com/ped/topic142.htm

Cleveland Clinic Health Information Center. (2003, December 12). *The spinal cord and injury.* Retrieved August 10, 2006, from http://www.clevelandclinic.org/health/health-info/docs/2000/2036.asp?index=8720

Cullity, M. (1998a). Judge gives Martin his ticket to ride. *Golfweek, 24*(7), 31.

Cullity, M. (1998b). Ruling sets up additional drama: Impact to be felt on tour, on other sports and in legal circles. *Golfweek, 24*(7), 31–35.

Dillingham, T. R., Pezzin, L. E., & MacKenzie, E. J. (2002). Limb amputation and limb deficiency: Epidemiology and recent trends in the United States. *Southern Medical Journal, 95*(8), 875–883. Retrieved August 9, 2006, from Expanded Academic ASAP via Thomson Gale.

Emery, A. (2002). The muscular dystrophies. *The Lancet, 359*(9307), 687–695. Retrieved August 10, 2006, from Expanded Academic ASAP via Thomson Gale.

Fine, M., & Asch, A. (1993). Disability beyond stigma: Social interaction, discrimination, and activism. In M. Nagler (Ed.), *Perspectives on disability: Text and readings on disability* (2nd ed., pp. 61–74). Palo Alto, CA: Health Markets Research.

Fries, J. M. (2005). Critical rehabilitation of the patient with spinal cord injury. *Critical Care Nurses Quarterly, 28*(2), 179–187.

Genetics Home Reference. (2007). *Diastrophic dysplasia.* Retrieved September 7, 2007, from http://ghr.nlm.nih.gov/condition=diastrophicdysplasia

Grewal, R. P. (2004). A simple and rapid quantitative method of detection of the common achondroplasia mutation: Analysis in mismatch repair deficient cells. *Indian Journal of Human Genetics, 10*(1), 13–17. Retrieved August 15, 2006, from Expanded Academic ASAP via Thomson Gale.

Hahn, H. (1988). The politics of physical differences: Disability and discrimination. *Journal of Social Issues, 44*(1), 39–47.

Hekmatnia, A., McHugh, K., Basiratnia, R., & Offiah, A. (2007). *Juvenile rheumatoid arthritis.* Retrieved September 2, 2007, from http://www.emedicine.com/radio/topic836.htm

Henningsen, C. G., & Smith, S. L. (2005). Arthrogryposis multiplex congenital. *Journal of Diagnostic Medical Sonography, 21*(6), 497–501. Retrieved August 9, 2006, from Expanded Academic ASAP via Thomson Gale.

Kilian, J., & Binder, T. (1998, March). *Aging with a disability: Conclusions after a visit to the USA.* Retrieved August 18, 2006, from http://www.jik.com/awdnor.html

King, R. W. (2006, July 13). *Rheumatoid arthritis.* Retrieved August 10, 2006, from http://www.emedicine.com/EMERG/topic48.htm

Kramasz, V. C. (2005). Polio patients take a second hit. *RN, 68*(11), 33–37. Retrieved August 10, 2006, from Expanded Academic ASAP via Thomson Gale.

Krigger, K. W. (2006). Cerebral palsy: An overview. *American Family Physician,* 73(1), 91. Retrieved August 9, 2006, from Expanded Academic ASAP via Thomson Gale.

Lazoff, M. (2005, October 31). *Multiple sclerosis.* Retrieved August 10, 2006, from http://www.emedicine.com/emerg/topic321.htm

Little People of America. (2006a). *Frequently asked questions.* Retrieved August 15, 2006, from http://www.lpaonline.org/resources_faq.html

Little People of America. (2006b). *Welcome to LPA.* Retrieved August 16, 2006, from http://www.lpaonline.org/lpa_intro.html

Mackelprang, R. W., & Altshuler, S. (2004). A youth perspective on life with a disability. *Journal of Social Work in Disability and Rehabilitation, 3*(3), 39–52.

Macko, R. F., Ivey, F. M., & Forrester, L. W. (2005). Task-oriented aerobic exercise in chronic hemiparetic stroke: Training protocols and treatment effects. *Topics in Stroke Rehabilitation, 12*(1), 45–57.

Marlowe, A., Pepin, M. G., & Byers, P. H. (2002). Testing for osteogenesis imperfecta in cases of suspected non-accidental injury. *Journal of Medical Genetics, 39*(6), 382–386. Retrieved August 15, 2006, from Expanded Academic ASAP via Thomson Gale.

Mitchell, L. E., Adzick, N. S., Melchionne, J., Pasquariello, P. S., Sutton, L. N., & Whitehead, A. S. (2004). Spina bifida. *The Lancet, 364,* 1885–1895. Retrieved August 15, 2006, from Expanded Academic ASAP via Thomson Gale.

Myer, G. D., Brunner, H. I., Nelson, P. G., Paterno, M. V., Ford, K. R., & Hewett, T. E. (2005). Specialized neuromuscular training to improve neuromuscular function and biomechanics in a patient with quiescent juvenile rheumatoid arthritis. *Physical Therapy, 85*(1), 791–802.

National Organization on Disability. (2006). *Economic participation.* Retrieved August 18, 2006, from http://www.nod.org/index.cfm?fuseaction = Page.viewPage&pageId = 12

Parikh, S., Batra, P., & Do, T. (2007). *Diastrophic dysplasia.* Retrieved September 1, 2007, from http://www.emedicine.com/orthoped/topic632.htm

Parikh, S., & Crawford, A. H. (2003). *Spondyloepiphyseal dysplasia.* Retrieved August 9, 2006, from http://www.emedicine.com/orthoped/topic630.htm

Plotkin, H. B., & Pattekar, M. A. (2006). *Osteogenesis imperfecta.* Retrieved August 8, 2006, from http://www.emedicine.com/ped/topic1674.htm

Rauch, F., & Glorieux, F. H. (2004). Osteogenesis imperfecta. *The Lancet, 363*(9418), 1377–1385. Retrieved August 15, 2006, from Expanded Academic ASAP via Thomson Gale.

Rehabilitation Research and Training Center on Disability Demographics and Statistics. (2004). *2004 disability status reports: United States.* Retrieved August 16, 2006, from http://www.ilr.cornell.edu/ped/disabilitystatistics/StatusReports/2004-html/US.html?CFID = 2550131&CFTOKEN = 33945622#top

Rollins, J. A. (2003). Congress allocates $2 million for national spina bifida program. *Pediatric Nursing, 29,* 231. Retrieved August 15, 2006, from Expanded Academic ASAP via Thomson Gale.

Russell, M. (2001). Disablement, oppression, and the political economy. *Journal of Disability Policy Studies, 12*(2), 87–116.

Tierney, L. M., McPhee, S. J., & Papadakis, M. A. (Eds.). (2006). *Current medical diagnosis and treatment.* New York: Lang Medical Books/McGraw-Hill.

Trotter, T. L., & Hall, J. G. (2005). Health supervision for children with achondroplasia. *Pediatrics, 116,* 771–783. Retrieved August 9, 2006, from Expanded Academic ASAP via Thomson Gale.

Vincent, A., Palace, J., & Hilton-Jones, D. (2001). Myasthenia gravis. *The Lancet, 357*(9274), 2122–2128. Retrieved August 10, 2006, from Expanded Academic ASAP via Thomson Gale.

Weihenmayer, E. (2008). Heroes and pioneers: Oscar Pistorius. *Time.* Retrieved October 4, 2008, from http://www.time.com/time/specials/2007/article/0,28804, 1733748_1733756_1735285,00.html

Wilkins, S., & Cott, C. (1993). Aging, chronic illness and disability. In M. Nagler (Ed.), *Perspectives on disability: Text and readings on disability* (2nd ed., pp. 363–376). Palo Alto, CA: Health Markets Research.

Wright, B. (1983). *Physical disability—a psychological approach* (2nd ed.). New York: Harper & Row.

Wright, B. (1988). Attitudes and the fundamental negative bias: Conditions and corrections. In H. E. Yuker (Ed.), *Attitudes toward persons with disabilities* (pp. 3–21). New York: Springer.

Wyndaele, M., & Wyndaele, J.-J. (2006). Incidence, prevalence and epidemiology of spinal cord injury: What learns a worldwide literature survey? *Spinal Cord, 44*(9), 523–529.

Zink, J. (1992). Adjusting to early- and late-onset disability: A personal perspective. *Generations, 16*(1), 59–61.

7

Deafness and Hearing Impairments

When my parents and siblings saw what an important and positive transition I had made and how much signing had opened up for me, they all learned to sign, and communication in our family became much more effective and easier for all of us. I believe my parents were greatly relieved when they saw how much signing and my acculturation into the Deaf community had done for me.

—Martha Sheridan, Gallaudet University

STUDENT LEARNING OBJECTIVES

1. To understand and be able to contrast medical, social, and political definitions of being deaf and hard of hearing
2. To understand how using different definitions of hearing loss leads people to reach different conclusions about the meaning of hearing loss in people's lives
3. To identify elements of Deaf culture and how Deaf culture contrasts with mainstream American culture
4. To identify the implications of being Deaf, deaf, and hard of hearing
5. To understand the implications of prelingual and late-onset hearing loss

The frequency of deaf and hard-of-hearing people in the population is difficult to ascertain, due to the multiple definitions of deafness and hearing impairments as well as the lack of population data collection. Thus, figures are based on estimates rather than actual counts. According to Gallaudet University, the worldwide population of deaf persons is approximately .1 percent of the total population (Harrington, 2004). The World Federation of the Deaf (2005) estimates that there are 70 million deaf people worldwide, approximately 80 percent of whom live in developing countries. According to the National Institute of Deafness and Communication Disorders (2007), there are 28 million deaf and hard-of-hearing people in the United States (about 8.5 percent of the population). The prevalence of hearing loss increases steadily with age. About 2 to 3 per 1,000 children are born deaf or hard of hearing, and nearly one-third of the population age sixty-five years and older have hearing loss. Of the approximately one to one-and-a-half million deaf persons in the United States, about 15 percent have prelingual deafness, about 9–10 percent became postlingually deaf as children, and about 75 percent became deaf as adults (Harrington, 2004; Mitchell, 2006; Reis, 1994; Schein, 1996). Mitchell (2005) estimates that between 2 and 4 in 1,000 people are "functionally deaf," and about four to ten times that number have severe hearing impairment. Up to 14 percent of the total population has some kind of hearing loss, and a large share of them are at least sixty-five years of age.

Hearing loss can be categorized into three types: conductive, sensorineural, and central. Mixed hearing loss involves a combination of sensorineural and conductive components. Each of these can result in hearing disabilities ranging from mild hearing loss to profound deafness. Most deaf people have some residual hearing.

Conductive deafness occurs as a result of changes in the middle ear mechanisms that conduct sound. Middle ear infections and injury to the small bones of the middle ear are common causes. Hearing aids are used by people with conductive hearing loss and deafness who desire to enhance their ability to hear sounds and discriminate speech (Friedlander, 1996; Guyton, 1971; Jackler & Kaplan, 1990). *Sensorineural* deafness results from damage to the inner ear, specifically the cochlea or auditory nerve. Many adults have sensorineural deafness as a result of congenital rubella. Infections and exposure to loud noises are other common causes. In addition, several genetic conditions lead to sensorineural hearing loss; these account for deafness in most of the 10 percent of deaf children born to deaf parents. Hearing aids are generally ineffective in enhancing intelligible hearing for people with sensorineural deafness since they enhance sound, but generally not speech discrimination. In recent years, cochlear implants have been used to enhance hearing for people with bilateral total loss of hearing, severe deafness, and sentence recognition hearing loss (Zeng, 2004). Cochlear implants require surgery and are extremely controversial in the deaf community because of surgical risks, disputed effectiveness, and concerns of people who are part of Deaf culture that cochlear implants fit the clinical corrective view of deafness (Bendict & Sass-Lehrer, 2007; Friedlander, 1996; Guyton, 1971; Jackler & Kaplan, 1990). *Central* deafness is relatively rare and occurs as a result of conditions involving the brain, such as multiple sclerosis, cerebrovascular disease, and tumors.

The age of onset of hearing disability is important. Prelingual and postlingual hearing loss are age-based terms that have to do with the acquisition of spoken language and that were coined before the acceptance of signed languages such as American Sign Language (ASL) as true languages. *Prelingual* deafness is deafness that occurs prior to three years of age, the usual age of language acquisition. Prelingually deafened individuals do not become fluent in auditory language prior to the onset of their deafness. *Postlingually* deafened individuals experience hearing loss after acquiring spoken language, usually at three years of age or later. Spoken language is the first language for most persons with postlingual deafness. The later the onset of deafness, the greater the person's integration of spoken language is. Visual/manual language that may be learned after the onset of deafness becomes a second language. Prelingually deafened individuals, especially those who are profoundly deaf, are likely to experience language visually and manually. The native languages of many deaf individuals are signed/visual languages such as ASL, Russian Sign Language, and British Sign Language, which are unique and different from verbal languages. Even typically verbal languages such as English, Spanish, and Japanese are learned visually and manually by people who are deaf.

Zak (2008) suggests using two other terms in discussing language and deafness. *Nonlingual* deafness occurs when a deaf child does not acquire language (manual or spoken) at a typical developmental age. *Lingual* deafness occurs when a person, whether prelingually or postlingually deafened, develops language at a typical age. The important distinction is the time of the development of language, whether spoken or manual. *Presbycusis*, or deafness that occurs in adulthood, produces communication problems that impair deafened individuals' abilities to communicate in their native oral language; thus they have communication abilities that are different from those of the hearing population, not language differences.

The criteria used to define deafness and hearing disabilities are guided by the assumptions and beliefs of those doing the defining. Though deaf and hard-of-hearing people have traditionally been defined from an individual deficiency perspective, more recent models have focused on cultural and political realities. Foster (1996) describes three models of understanding deafness. The *medical model* assumes deafness is caused by the failure of a critical sensory system, which results in personal deficiencies. According to the medical model, people who are deaf need professionals to help them cope with their problems. According to the *social cultural model* of deafness, the experiences of deaf people "can be best understood as a function of interaction between the individual and society" (Foster, 1996, p. 5). Barriers experienced by deaf persons result from social, language, and cultural differences between majority and minority groups. The *political model* of deafness focuses on the power differences between hearing and deaf persons. Sociopolitical institutions are controlled by hearing persons, who impose their definitions of the meaning of deafness on deaf persons. As a result, deaf people must fight for their civil rights to overcome devaluation and oppression by the dominant society.

In keeping with the emphasis of the book, this chapter focuses on the social and political conceptualizations of hearing loss and deafness.

Certainly, hearing loss affects the roles of sound, hearing, and speech in people's lives; however, the sociocultural and political contexts in which people with hearing disabilities live greatly influence their life courses and quality of life. For example, deaf and hard-of-hearing people are more likely than hearing people to experience problems in transitions from school to work, social integration, self-concept, and overall life satisfaction (Israelite, Ower, & Goldstein, 2002; Kent, 2003; Moore, 2001; Punch, Creed, & Hyde, 2006). These difficulties are present in multiple countries and cultures. Historically, difficulties associated with hearing disabilities have been assumed to result from individual deficits; however, this flawed notion has been challenged in recent years. No challenge is more significant than the 1988 Deaf President Now movement at Gallaudet University, in Washington, D.C. For more than one hundred years, Gallaudet, a university established by the U.S. Congress for the education of the deaf, was run by a succession of hearing presidents. When yet another hearing president was hired by the board of trustees, alumni, students, and faculty refused to accept the appointment. The protestors asserted that ableism, not lack of qualification, was the primary reason that a deaf person had not been hired as president. I. King Jordan, a deaf professor, was finally hired for the position The refusal of a deaf university to hire a deaf president was analogous to hiring only white presidents to lead traditionally black universities, or male presidents to administer traditionally female universities.

Deafness is unique among disabilities because deaf people have their own languages unique from those of their hearing families and the communities in which they reside. These unique languages have led to the development of unique identities and cultures. Deaf identity and the Deaf civil rights movement have been revolutionary, and we believe understanding the development of Deaf culture provides a lens through which to understand the identity and civil rights movement for all people with disabilities.

TERMINOLOGY

As we discussed in chapter 1, terminology is an important element of discussions on disabilities. Whereas many persons with disabilities have traditionally embraced person-first language, deaf people have been more likely to embrace deaf-first language. Martha Sheridan (personal communication, 1997), a deaf social worker, explains this preference: "Using [person-first] language puts deafness and deaf people in a disability framework. Deaf people do not see themselves in that context and do not advocate that language for themselves. 'People with deafness' is not an acceptable phrase. 'Deaf people,' 'deaf,' and 'hard of hearing' are all acceptable. Deaf people view phrases such as 'people with deafness' and people-first language as a reflection of society's lack of acceptance of deafness. I'm deaf, say it, there's nothing wrong with being deaf, I'm not some hot potato you have to be careful with."

Sheridan clearly rejects the conceptualization of disability as individual pathology. Janet Pray (personal communication, 1997), former director of the social work program at Gallaudet University, echoes Sheridan's uneasiness with terms such as *hearing disabilities*. She also prefers the term *hearing loss* rather than *hearing impairment*, though she acknowledges the controversy over its use. Language relative to deaf and hard-of-hearing people (as well as other devalued groups) is constantly evolving and potentially controversial. In fact, as we discussed in chapter 1, the deaf community's emphasis on deaf-first rather than person-first language is being adopted by some other disability groups. The language we use in this chapter is an attempt to reflect terminology that is acceptable within the deaf and hard-of-hearing communities.

Hard-of-hearing individuals are people who have reduced hearing ability but who are not deaf. People with mild to moderate hearing loss have some difficulty hearing the full range of sounds, often in conversation. More severe hearing loss results in significant difficulty hearing and understanding oral communication. Schein (1996) defines deafness as "the common outcome of diverse causes resulting in an inability to hear and understand speech through the ear alone" (p. 22). Some people who are deaf can hear, but they do not understand speech through the ear alone. Some people with hearing loss choose to identify as deaf, whereas others with more hearing loss identify themselves as hard of hearing. Thus, the terms *deaf* and *hard of hearing* are defined as much by how individuals define themselves as by the amount of their hearing loss.

DEAF CULTURE

In 1965, Stokoe, Croneberg, and Casterline offered a unique view of deafness by emphasizing social and cultural characteristics of deaf people, particularly those who use sign language as their first language. In the generation since, Deaf people have redefined deafness in a number of ways. As we have noted, the traditional definition of deafness relates to audiological impairment. Since 1965, *deaf* and *Deaf* have taken on different meanings. In an anthology edited by Wilcox (1989), contributing authors differentiate between deaf and Deaf. The uppercased Deaf is used to describe Deaf people as a cultural group. The lowercased deaf refers to noncultural elements of deafness, such as medical conditions or proximity of residence. For example, Padden (1989) defines the "deaf community" as consisting of hearing and deaf people as well as culturally Deaf people. Deaf communities, like other communities, experience frequent interactions and have common concerns. In contrast to the deaf community, members of the Deaf culture "behave as Deaf people do, use the language of Deaf people, and share the beliefs of Deaf people toward themselves and other people who are not deaf" (Padden, 1989, p. 5). People who may be part of a deaf community are hearing family and acquaintances of Deaf people and people who become deaf later in life who do not participate in Deaf culture.

The definitions of who is a part of Deaf culture vary. According to the broadest definition, Deaf culture includes "all those who embrace ASL and other characteristics of Deaf culture, including hearing children of Deaf parents for whom ASL is the first language and others who use ASL as their primary language" (Pray, personal communication, 1997). Pray states that the most narrow view of Deaf culture is that taken by "those who say the only 'true' members of Deaf culture are the 10 percent of Deaf who are from Deaf families." We use a broad view of Deaf culture in this book. This definition includes people who have become acculturated into Deaf culture.

Stokoe (1989) uses a hundred-cell "map of culture" to present elements of culture and contrast mainstream American culture (MAC) with Deaf American culture (DAC). He states that "the use of vision instead of hearing for getting vital and incidental information is the fundamental difference between MAC and DAC, and it shows up in every cell" of the cultural map (Stokoe, 1989, p. 55). Stokoe discusses how MAC has attempted to force Deaf people to act as if they hear. He discusses how deaf people who try to pass as hearing in an attempt to gain full membership in MAC often fail to achieve full membership in either MAC or DAC. He cites the fact that more than 90 percent of deaf people marry other deaf people. He acknowledges the sociopolitical discrepancies between Deaf and hearing cultures, noting, "Deaf Americans who marry one another, who form their own clubs and associations, and who interact largely with their own kind, are seen erroneously by some sociologists as Americans with a physical impairment, a disability, a handicap, who have not been able to achieve the full status accorded to hearing persons" (Stokoe, 1989, p. 56).

Stokoe describes ways that Deaf Americans cope with life using strategies common to all cultures. He asserts that the culture and lives of Deaf Americans are different from but not inferior to those of mainstream Americans. Deaf persons may be affected by societal actions and policies that define them as disabled (e.g., the 1990 ADA, the 2007 UN Disability Convention and Protocol); however, they reject the disability label. This view is different from that of other disability advocates who embrace disability language and identity. We believe that Deaf culture may serve as a model for the development of general disability culture. Deaf culture advocates do not consider deafness a deficiency-based disability. We suggest that disability culture advocates make a similar differentiation, in which little-*d* disability is used to connote characteristics, whereas big-*D* Disability is used when one is referring to the cultural aspects of disability.

Deaf culture is not unique to the United States. The Canadian Cultural Society for the Deaf (2005) was created in 1973 to help preserve and promote Canadian Deaf culture. It supports a Deaf heritage museum and an art center that celebrates Deaf life as a form of diversity. British Sign Language is used by British Deaf. Australia's sign language, Ausian, and New Zealand's sign language are considered dialects of British Sign Language. Each has grammar, syntax, and other language characteristics that differ from those of oral language and contribute to the cultures of Deaf populations. Russia's Deaf developed strong cultural ties during the Tsarist era that continued through the Soviet era and still exist today. As in other countries, much of the impetus for Russian Deaf cultural development occurred in schools for the Deaf that used Russian Sign Language (Burch, 2000). Norwegian sign language and Deaf culture have been nurtured for nearly two hundred years, transmitted primarily through schools for the Deaf. Interestingly, Norway has two signed dialects. One, developed in Trondheim, is based on the French technique that makes it possible to communicate with French, Danish, Swedish, and American signers. The other, developed in Oslo, is similar to British Sign Language (Greftegreff, 1992). Internationally, Deaf unity is manifested in events such as the Deaflympics, which originated in 1924 and has been staged every four years since. The World Federation of the Deaf (2005), a United Nations–affiliated organization, is devoted to ensuring "that Deaf people in every country have the right to preserve their own sign languages, organizations, and cultural and other activities." Similar to the cultures of hearing people, different countries and regions throughout the world have unique Deaf cultures. Concomitantly, Deaf people share commonalties based on similar life experiences, societal reactions, and treatment by mainstream societies and cultures.

LANGUAGE

Language development is a critical task for young children that, in turn, leads to increasingly sophisticated cognitive skills. The use of language produces significant controversy for deaf people. A primary conflict has been the use of oral versus manual language. One school of language acquisition for deaf people is the "oral" school. Oralists believe that the primary language learned by deaf people should be lip reading (speech reading) and speech. Much emphasis is placed on learning oral language and pronouncing words verbally. Signed language is discouraged (or forbidden), while mastery of spoken language is strongly emphasized. Proponents of oral language as a first language argue that deaf people need to function in a hearing world and, therefore, need to learn the language of the hearing population. One problem with deaf people relying on oral communication is that even the best speech readers understand only about 40–60 percent of what is spoken. Therefore, people who rely on oral language can have significant difficulty becoming fluent in their primary language. This is especially critical in the first three to four years of life, when people are most capable of learning language. Ironically, an increasing number of hearing parents of hearing children teach their infants and toddlers rudimentary sign language, which they are able to master faster than oral language. With infants as young as four to six months of age developing signed language skills, we suggest that the cognitive development of all children would be enhanced if sign language were adopted as a primary language from birth. Further, we wonder if rather than being at a disadvantage, deaf children of Deaf parents may have the greatest advantage of all children in terms of early language and cognitive development.

Some language methods use a combination of English-based oral language and facilitative signing. One such method, cued speech, relies primarily on oral language but uses hand shapes around the face to represent sounds not easily distinguished visually (e.g., *t* and *d*). People using cued speech rely on lip shapes and hand cues to send and receive oral messages.

Other language methods are based on oral language but use manual rather than verbal methods. In the United States, these are signed English, Pidgin Signed English, Signed Essential English, and Signed Exact English. In Denmark, the Danish hand-mouth system, signed Danish, and Scandinavian pidgin sign language are used; in Estonia, signed exact Estonian; in Finland, signed Finnish and signed Swedish; in Iran, cued Persian; in Israel, manually coded Hebrew; in Luxembourg, signed-supported Luxembourgish and German; in Pakistan, signed Urdu; and in South Africa, signed Afrikaans (Harrington, 2007). These methods rely on oral language; however, they primarily use manual rather than verbal communication. Signing oral language in its various forms is time consuming and can take about twice the time to communicate as oral communication. These forms are not discrete languages but modifications of the respective oral languages; thus, people who learn these methods gain familiarity with their oral language in modified form. For example, they may use components of their respective sign language and grammatical shortcuts of the oral language. Since these communication methods are not languages, some claim they do not provide complete linguistic access (Zak, 1996). Some critics advocate that children learn their respective Deaf signed languages as a first language and variations of signed oral languages as a second language.

Within American Deaf culture, American Sign Language is the language of choice. Similarly, other countries use their own respective signed languages: Greek Sign Language; Guatemalan Sign Language; Guinean Sign Language and Ghanian Sign Language; Zimbabwe Sign Language, or Zimsign; and so on (Harrington, 2007). Unlike other English signing systems, which are based on English, ASL is a discrete language relying exclusively on visual and manual expression. ASL has unique syntax and structures separate from English. As a unique language, ASL is not understood by the vast majority of mainstream American culture; therefore, people who use ASL exclusively are limited in their ability to communicate with those who speak English or other verbal languages. Oftentimes, those whose native language is ASL become competent in written and/or oral languages such as English as a second language. Within Deaf culture, however, ASL is *the* language of choice.

It is important to note that signed languages are more than a way to communicate words. As languages, they are an influential component of Deaf culture and play an important role in shaping a Deaf worldview. Humor expressed using Deaf language such as ASL can be incomprehensible to English speakers (Rutherford, 1989). The ways in which Deaf people greet each other, engage in conversations, and depart are different from those in MAC. For example, Hall (1989) states that in Deaf American culture, people are often very direct in "getting to the point" when talking with others, which can be interpreted by people from MAC as rude and abrupt. On the other hand, in MAC, saying good-bye is often done quickly, whereas in DAC, lingering good-byes are common. In MAC, when large groups of people are in a room, private conversations are common, with people speaking softly to one another. In DAC, private conversations are difficult to have because signed language is visual; thus, cloistered discussions can be considered rude.

Language development is extremely crucial for deaf and hard-of-hearing people, just as it is for hearing people. Language is essential as children develop cognitively and as they interact with the world. Many language acquisition methods have been developed for people with severe hearing loss. It is critical that people develop fluency in at least one language. Therefore, if the hearing loss is severe enough that fluency in oral language is not viable, it is prudent to provide children with a manual/visual language such as ASL of which they can develop mastery. Then, as a second or supplemental language, verbally based languages can be learned to allow people to function well within the dominant hearing culture.

FAMILY RELATIONSHIPS

Deaf and hard-of-hearing children experience the world differently than hearing children. For example, deaf infants do not rely on environmental sounds that signify the presence of another. They do not hear sounds of comfort from parents. Deaf infants respond to nonvocal parental behaviors rather than their verbalizations. They do not recognize or learn to listen to parents' voices. Hard-of-hearing children may respond inconsistently to parental and other environmental auditory stimuli, depending on the nature and extent of the hearing loss. The lack of auditory responsiveness characteristic of hearing infants and toddlers alerts many hearing parents of deaf and hard-of-hearing children that something is atypical (Marschark, 1993). Unsuspecting parents can experience distress and feelings of rejection due to the child's lack of reciprocity (Harris, 1978), prompting them to seek help that can then lead to the discovery of their child's hearing loss.

Families into which deaf children are born have much bearing on their early life experiences. For deaf children born to Deaf parents, deafness is the norm. The birth of a deaf or hard-of-hearing child is not a shock, as it is when deaf children are born to hearing parents, who are usually ignorant of the needs of their child. Deaf parents are likely to communicate easily using visual language. They socialize their children based on their knowledge and personal experiences as Deaf people. They are aware of opportunities and obstacles their children face. Deaf parents are likely to have circles of friends who are deaf and may participate in communities comprised largely of other deaf people (Meadow-Orlans, 1996). Access to Deaf culture is common, and deafness is the norm. Similarly, hard-of-hearing parents may be attuned to the hearing loss, model multiple communication styles, and utilize optimal socialization strategies for their hard-of-hearing children.

For some deaf parents, the birth of a deaf child is a cause for celebration. Some have even sought genetic counseling to ascertain their "risk" of having a hearing child. Other deaf parents, concerned with the societal barriers that severely limit opportunities for deaf children, prefer to have hearing children. This issue is complex; people's views are influenced by pride in Deaf culture and by the devaluation of deaf and hard-of-hearing people in society (Pray, personal communication, 1997).

Only about 10 percent of deaf children are born to deaf parents. Most deaf and hard-of-hearing children are born into families in which their hearing loss is a shock. On average, children are about fifteen to sixteen months of age when diagnosed (Mace, Wallace, Whan, & Stelmachowicz, 1991; Meadow-Orlans, 1996). In reviewing research on deaf children, Lederberg (1993) found decreased social knowledge, decreased parent-child interactions, increased family stress, and parental grieving among hearing parents of deaf and hard-of-hearing children, and delayed language acquisition among the children themselves. Family grief over a deaf child results from the perception that deafness is a tragedy. Thus, chronic parental sorrow can result. Hearing parents most often have little or no experience with deafness or deaf people and can feel inadequate. Meadow-Orlans (1996) suggests that two problems arise for hearing parents when a child's deafness is diagnosed: "First, they must cope with the shock of the presence of an unexpected handicap. Second, they must face the difficulties of socializing their child in the absence of a common—that is, a spoken—linguistic system. This is the central feature of the socialization of deaf children by hearing parents: the easy, effortless, communication of skills, values, rules, and games, taken for granted by other parents, is not available to these families" (p. 72).

At least three factors can improve the quality of life for children born deaf or hard of hearing. First, early screening for hearing loss is critical to maximizing the language and social development of infants and young children. Along with screening, there must be effective early language and intervention programs for children with hearing loss. Third, hearing parents and families of children with hearing impairments need role models and supports to help them raise their children. Focusing on the social elements of deafness rather than on personal deficiencies is critical to the development of deaf infants and children. Parents who learn to focus on the social elements of deafness are equipped to raise their deaf children. Rather than focusing exclusively on developing oral language so they can be more "normal," parents focusing on social elements find ways to communicate with their children. This may require them to learn a signed language. Hearing parents need to learn that their deaf children must see them to communicate. They can learn that nurturing and socialization for deaf and hard-of-hearing children are different, not inferior, to nurturing and socialization for hearing children. And while hard-of-hearing children may not be raised to use signed language as their primary means of communication, they also benefit from supplemented communication and socialization strategies (Canale, Favero, Lacilla, Recchia, Schindler, Roggero, & Albera, 2006; National Association of the Deaf, n.d.; Nelson, Nygren, Walker, & Panoscha, 2006; Thompson, McPhillips, Davis, Lieu, Homer, & Helfand, 2002).

There are many drawbacks to the deficiency-based view of deafness. Wood (1989) suggests that parents are more reluctant to give up control of deaf children than hearing children because they expect their children to be less capable of exercising independence and autonomy. This, in turn, leads to poor self-image. Lederberg (1993) emphasizes that because deaf children do not develop the ability to communicate and socialize, they do not develop a critical understanding of the social world. She also emphasizes that deaf children of hearing parents experience social and cultural deprivation when they are not exposed to Deaf role models and Deaf culture.

Whereas research has traditionally focused on the problems and deficits that arise from hearing loss in childhood, attention is increasingly being given to normal parenting of deaf and hard-of-hearing children. Research focusing on children's needs rather than on problems can help parents develop parenting skills. For example, studies of deaf parents of deaf children show that they use touch to reinforce interaction, they make sure their infants are looking at them before interacting, and they use simplified sign language and mold their infants' fingers to form signing shapes (Erting, Prezioso, & Hynes, 1990; Spencer, Bodner-Johnson, & Gutfreund, 1992). Parents who are aware of these strategies can help children develop communication skills very early in life. More strengths-based research is important to our understanding of the specific needs and skills involved in parenting children with hearing loss. Increasingly, sign language is being used to teach infants and toddlers to communicate, as evidenced by the creation of organizations such as Sign Babies (created by Nancy Cadjan), which teaches hearing infants sign language to jump-start language and social development.

Research that attends to social issues rather than focusing on individual deficits can teach parents and others how to remove social barriers that impede deaf and hard-of-hearing children. Full development of young children can be enhanced in several ways. All children need parents and others who can communicate with them. This often requires parents of deaf and hard-of-hearing children to learn signed language. In addition, parents can be aware of their children's rights and help remove obstacles that limit those rights.

Views of deaf and hard-of-hearing people as less competent than others are stereotypical and inaccurate. Deaf and hard-of-hearing children may develop competence in alternate ways that are isomorphic and not inferior to others. Infants and toddlers may not respond to auditory cues, but they do respond to visual and tactile stimulation. Social development of deaf and hard-of-hearing children and youths is enhanced by exposure to peers, role models, and, for some, Deaf culture. Parents can create environments that help their deaf and hard-of-hearing children fully develop socially, emotionally, and intellectually.

EDUCATION

The first recorded school for the deaf was established in the mid-1500s in Spain by Pedro Ponce de León, a Catholic monk. Deaf schools were established in England in 1760 and in France in 1771 (Savitt, 2007). Schools for the deaf have been a primary means to educate deaf children in developed countries for decades. In the United States, there are more than one hundred schools for the deaf. A generation ago, large numbers of children with hearing disabilities were educated in residential schools for the deaf, sometimes far from home. A 1976 U.S. national study by Karchmer and Trybus (1977) of nearly 50,000 school-aged deaf children revealed that 38 percent were in residential schools, 11 percent were in day schools for the deaf, 22 percent used full-time special education classrooms, 19 percent used resource rooms, and 10 percent were in other programs. The study's authors found that people with more severe hearing loss tended to reside in residential schools, with 59 percent of "profoundly deaf" subjects and 41 percent of "severely deaf" subjects attending these schools.

In recent decades, public attitudes, laws, and policies relative to deaf and other disabled persons have led to decreases in self-contained deaf education. For example, Karchmer and Trybus (1977) noted that the proportion of deaf students who used U.S. residential schools had decreased in the years prior to their study. The 1976 passage of Pub. L. No. 94–142, the Equal Education for All Handicapped Children Act, and the 1986 passage of Pub. L. No. 99–457, now known as IDEA (the Individuals with Disabilities Education Improvement Act), have forced public schools to take responsibility for educating children with disabilities. Other countries' disability rights emphases have had similar effects. Subsequently, the proportion of deaf and hard-of-hearing children living at home and being educated in neighborhood schools has increased, and enrollment at residential schools has decreased dramatically (Calderon & Greenberg, 1993; Meadow-Orlans, 1996; Moores, 1987). Another significant factor in decreased deaf school enrollments is the decreasing number of deaf children as a result of medical advances. For example, immunizations today prevent maternal rubella, which was much more common during the 1960s.

For generations of deaf people, residential schools became "home and family" from early childhood. Children in residential schools had two families—their biological families and their school families. Many others were educated in day schools devoted exclusively to deaf people. These special programs had many effects. Although fewer in number today, residential programs segregate deaf people from hearing people. Some believe that academic standards are lower in deaf-exclusive programs. Separation from hearing people can hamper speech reading and speech skills. Social isolation from the mainstream also occurs. In addition, residential schools produce long-term separation from biological families (Calderon & Greenberg, 1993; Meadow-Orlans, 1996; Moores, 1987), who have less influence, and less ability to nurture and teach the children from whom they are separated. Some advocate mixed educational settings in which deaf students attend both self-contained and mainstreamed schools (Eriks-Brophy, Durieux-Smith, Olds, & Fitzpatrick, 2006; Wilson, 1997).

On the other hand, residential schools have created many opportunities within the deaf community. Students are raised in school communities of people like themselves, rather than as different and isolated individuals in hearing communities. Deafness is the norm rather than an aberration. Younger deaf children have role models in deaf adults and older deaf children. They have not had to face the language and communication barriers students face in schools made up of primarily oral English users. Learning environments using ASL can also help students achieve at levels beyond what they do in mainstream inclusion programs (Pray, personal communication, 1997).

Within programs devoted exclusively to deaf people, a culture of deafness has developed over the years. This culture has been built upon language, shared experiences, and a sense of identity. As deaf children grow up, they establish lifelong friendships and a world of Deaf culture. Deaf clubs provide opportunities to further Deaf culture, and national associations for Deaf people have given them political voice. Relationships that preserve and enhance Deaf people as a group flourish.

Ironically, deaf schools have had the exact effect of what was most feared by people such as Alexander Graham Bell, who a century ago was touted in hearing society as a champion of deaf people. Bell and other deaf "experts" of the day believed in eugenics. Though we know today that only 10 percent of deafness is hereditary (Pray, personal communication, 1997), Bell and his contemporaries sought to forbid marriage between deaf persons in order to prevent the perpetuation of a defective race of people. He had a profound influence on the denigration of signing, which has had lasting effects. As Shapiro (1993) states, "For ninety years after . . . 1880 . . . the use of sign language was banned from American schools. Students who disobeyed got their hands slapped or tied down. Deaf teachers—who by 1869 totaled 41 percent of instructors of the deaf—were driven from the classroom. By the turn of the century, that percentage had dropped to 25 percent and to only 12 percent by 1960" (p. 95).

Though deaf students who learned ASL were as literate as hearing people in the 1850s, Bell's contemporaries insisted on teaching oralism exclusively and eradicating deaf culture and ASL. However, despite the efforts of the "experts," most of whom were hearing persons, ASL was not eradicated in favor of oralism. Deaf people preserved their language, and in recent years Deaf culture has flourished. In part, this is attributable to residential schools and other programs that have brought Deaf people into intimate contact with each other.

Today, one of the largest social and political controversies in the deaf community and about deaf people is the proper forum for the education of deaf people. Cohen (1994) outlines the influences of public policies and summarizes some of the concerns relative to the diminishing numbers of students attending specialized schools:

> Confusing equality with sameness, they believe in doing away with special schools and educating all children together. How, then, to explain that their interpretation of the law may sever deaf children from a culture that offers them strength? Deaf people, unlike members of other disabled groups, have their own language. They have their own social clubs, their own theater companies and television programs, their own university, their own periodicals, and their own international Olympics. Unlike members of ethnic minority groups, they do not receive their culture through their parents. Cultural transmission, formally and informally, has been carried out by schools for the deaf. (p. 55)

Ironically, traditions that can be most oppressive to many groups—segregation, removing people from families, and institutionalization—have been essential components of the development and fostering of a rich Deaf culture and heritage. Conversely, civil rights laws for persons with disabilities, while providing increased opportunities for people with disabilities, are also affecting deaf and hard-of-hearing people in ways that many consider destructive to Deaf culture (e.g., fewer students are being educated in deaf schools).

HEARING FAMILIES OF DEAF CHILDREN

Many factors converge to influence the relationships of deaf children with their families. More and more, deaf children are raised with their hearing families. Increased familial stress, altered parent-child relationships, and other difficulties that occur when deaf children are born to hearing parents have been documented (Calderon & Greenberg, 1993). However, changing attitudes about deafness can mitigate negative consequences. If deafness is not perceived as a tragedy, having a deaf child is not perceived as devastating. Recent research demonstrates that language, cognitive, and educational deficits in deaf children "can most likely be attributed to limitations in the availability for deaf children of learning opportunities that allow fully for their hearing loss" (Nelson, Loncke, & Camarata, 1993, p. 124). Fortunately, past attitudes are being replaced by enlightened knowledge that deaf children are not multiply deficient. Access to manual language such as ASL allows parents to learn a second language and to communicate effectively with their young children. Social and learning strategies are available to meet the needs of deaf children so that children do not have to be forced into hearing modalities that can be extremely limiting.

Though lack of knowledge of children's hearing disabilities for the first months of their lives can negatively affect early development and attachments, research with deaf children of deaf parents indicates that hearing loss itself is not the source of decreased interactions and lack of bonding, language acquisition, and cognitive development. When parents of deaf and hard-of-hearing children are sensitive to their children's needs, attachments and relationships are of high quality. Early intervention programs for parents that include language training, counseling, and contact with other deaf and hard-of-hearing people can be critical to providing parents with the knowledge and skills to communicate with, bond with, and nurture their children (Bonvillian & Folven, 1993; Gilman, Easterbrooks, & Frey, 2004; Lederberg, 1993; Siegel, 2006).

With increased numbers of deaf children being raised in family homes rather than residential schools, parents and families are exerting an influence greater than ever on a new generation of deaf children. Parents who become bilingual in signed and spoken language create nurturing atmospheres for their children. Parental involvement in children's schools and community environments can positively influence children's education and socialization (Sheridan, personal communication, 1997). Parents may need support and education from deaf people, professionals, and others. This support can help them navigate bureaucracies and systems to ensure access to opportunities for their children.

Parents and students may become advocates with teachers and school administrators in integrated schools. The responsibility to dispel the myths that deaf people are academically and socially inferior often falls to parents. Parents must also take on the role of advocates for accessible learning environments. Ongoing parental involvement may be critical to ensure a goodness of fit between learning needs and the resources allocated to meet those needs.

Parents have become more involved in the lives of their deaf and hard-of-hearing children than in the past. They have more opportunities to transmit their values and culture to their children. Involvement of the larger deaf community varies among families based on various factors, including proximity and access to other deaf people and family attitudes. Parents must balance the various influences in rearing children and youths. However, parents have better access to positive images of deaf people and deaf role models. Greater opportunities also present the necessity of balancing various family, community, and cultural involvement and identities for their children.

MULTICULTURALISM

In recent years, signed languages have gained acceptance as distinct languages, and Deaf culture in multiple countries is thriving. Within the deaf community, there are widely differing beliefs about relationships with the hearing world. Some call for Deaf separatism, essentially disengagement from hearing culture. Others advocate assimilation into the hearing world. A multicultural view seems the most rational approach for Deaf people in society. In the United States, Humphries, Martin, and Coye (1989) argue for a bilingual, bicultural approach to teaching English to Deaf people: "We believe that ASL can and does have for many deaf people, the same function English has for English speakers—the capacity to transmit a culture, a way of life and happiness. We know that English can add to this happiness" (p. 123).

A bicultural approach acknowledges the importance of Deaf culture and sign languages such as ASL in the United States. This approach may be especially important as deaf people become increasingly involved in MAC. For example, the widespread placement of deaf and hard-of-hearing students in public schools can cause these deaf students to experience isolation, especially when there are communication problems (Stinson & Kluwin, 1993). Discrepancies between hearing and deaf people in education, occupational attainment, and income (Barnartt & Christiansen, 1996) may also be reduced with increased biculturalism and bilingualism (Eriks-Brophy et al., 2006; Siegel, 2006).

It is a reality that deaf people are a small minority and that societal structures and institutions are controlled by the hearing majority. In order for most Deaf people to gain full access to MAC, knowledge of both oral and signed language is critical. Conversely, increased access to telecommunications such as TTYs, e-mail, instant messaging, phone text messages, the Internet, and captioned television programming is providing new opportunities. Passage of civil rights laws in recent decades has opened up opportunities in education and employment. Opportunities for integrating deaf and hearing worlds are great.

Multiculturalism honors the roots of an individual's culture while acknowledging the intersections with the larger society. This is true for Deaf people as well as other cultural groups. Being from a cultural background different from the majority *and* being deaf can complicate matters. In a work edited by Christensen and Delgado (1993), the complications for people who are deaf and from different countries and ethnic backgrounds are discussed. For example, Latino deaf people in the United States may be forced to deal with two oral languages, English and Spanish, as well as ASL. Deaf people emigrating from the United States to England may need to learn British Sign Language in addition to ASL. As the amount of diversity increases, so do the intricacies of promoting multiculturalism.

HARD-OF-HEARING PERSONS

Much of this chapter has focused on Deaf culture and identity. However, Deaf people are the minority in the total population of deaf and hard-of-hearing people. The majority of people with hearing loss self-identify as hard of hearing rather than deaf. We believe it is important that deaf and hard-of-hearing people be identified based on social rather than audiological definitions. In general, Deaf people identify themselves as deaf; conversely, deaf and hard-of-hearing people who use spoken language or use their hearing in everyday life have a stronger identity with the hearing community. In reality, some people who identify as Deaf have greater hearing capacities than people who identify as hard of hearing.

Hard-of-hearing people function with the hearing world as their primary identity group. They often use hearing aids to facilitate improved hearing. They use telephones, often with enhanced amplification. Spoken language is the first language for hard-of-hearing people. To communicate, they may rely on a combination of hearing, speech reading, and other visual cues. Their expressed language is also generally spoken. Visual and manual language may be learned to supplement communication, but not as a primary language.

Early developmental issues for hard-of-hearing children are similar to those for deaf infants and children. They are less stimulated by auditory stimuli than hearing children. Parents may need to place an emphasis on visual and tactile more than auditory stimulation. Mechanical devices such as hearing aids are important for helping hard-of-hearing children develop language and interact with hearing parents, peers, and others.

Hard-of-hearing children can find themselves in an "in-between" world, since they do not fit into Deaf culture, yet much of the hearing world is not accessible to them. People who are hard of hearing are more likely to feel socially, educationally, and occupationally isolated than hearing peers (Eriks-Brophy et al., 2006; Gilman et al., 2004; Israelite et al., 2002; Jones, 2004; Punch et al., 2006). They may also find only partial acceptance in the Deaf world. Interestingly, social opportunities and the richness of Deaf identity motivate some hard-of-hearing people to immerse themselves in Deaf culture even though they have the physical hearing capabilities necessary for the hearing world. Achieving fluency in sign language helps them achieve membership. Others, even some with severe hearing loss, prefer to identify primarily with the hearing community.

Hard-of-hearing people are more likely than Deaf people to view deafness as a loss. People immersed in Deaf culture are on par with others in their culture, whereas hard-of-hearing people who live in and identify with the hearing community are different and disadvantaged in their community of choice. Technology can be extremely important in providing them with access to education, socialization, and work. For example, hearing aids have been miniaturized, and their quality has greatly increased. The Internet and other electronic "curb cuts" allow people to communicate without difficulty.

With expanded mainstreaming, more deaf and hard-of-hearing people are being educated in mainstream public schools than ever before. Residential placement has decreased markedly, and everyday involvement in the hearing community has increased. This may add to the numbers of people who identify as hard of hearing rather than Deaf. Technological advances, greater civil rights, and positive attitudes about disabled people are leading to increased opportunities for hard-of-hearing people. Heightened attention to the needs of hard-of-hearing people is critical to understanding them as a distinct group in a pluralistic society.

LATE-ONSET DEAFNESS

Late-onset or postlingual deafness refers to the occurrence of deafness after a person has developed spoken language. For this population, early language and cognitive orientation are based on spoken language. The earlier the onset of deafness, the more likely people are to assume a deaf identity. Young children with acquired deafness become involved in language training at an early age. Their exposure to other deaf children is increased. Given the chance to learn ASL, they have greater opportunities to become bilingual and bicultural. The greater their exposure to deaf people and culture, the more likely they are to identify strongly with the deaf community.

People who become deaf in adolescence and adulthood are more likely to retain their identity with the hearing community. Spoken language is deeply ingrained in their identities. Their language and cognitive development occurred in a hearing context. Oral language continues to be the primary language for these people. Signed language based on the oral language they learned as toddlers may be easier to learn and may be preferable to signed language such as ASL, British Sign Language, and Ausian.

Postlingually deafened individuals experience loss and grieving that people with prelingual deafness who identify with Deaf culture may not experience. They feel a sense of loss of something they once had that now is gone. Though most continue to communicate orally, comprehension is diminished. Although they can no longer hear conversations, hearing people may assume they hear because they can speak. Environmental sounds such as music, doorbells, and telephone conversations are diminished or lost. The way they organize their world changes significantly. Oral conversations are more deliberate and may require written messages. Captioned televisions, telephone amplifiers, and hearing aids may be needed.

People who experience hearing loss later in life may need time and resources to adjust to their loss. Their emphasis in coping may be geared primarily toward coping in a hearing world in spite of hearing loss rather than immersing themselves in the deaf community and Deaf culture. They need to learn to compensate and adjust to the change in their lives. They also need to understand that they may be susceptible to discrimination and marginalization because of their hearing loss and develop self-advocacy skills to combat prejudice and inequities. Technology and legal protections to promote quality of life are more available than ever before. Over time, changing societal attitudes will also increase access.

SUMMARY

Though a small number of people in the United States are deaf, Deaf people have been a major influence in the civil rights movement for people with disabilities. The development of Deaf culture and Deaf pride have redefined deafness—what was once viewed as cause for the practice of eugenics is now seen as a distinct life condition. Increasingly, deafness is defined according to social and political definitions.

There is great diversity among deaf and hard-of-hearing people. Deaf activists have contributed greatly to a strong Deaf culture; however, large numbers of deaf and hard-of-hearing people do not identify themselves as members of Deaf culture. There are opportunities to participate in society, whether one is Deaf, hard of hearing, or bicultural. For some, deafness is a great source of pride and identity. For others, it means that they must make adaptations as hearing-disabled persons in a hearing world. In understanding people who are deaf and hard of hearing, it is critical to understand what hearing loss means to the individual, and the place of hearing loss in the individual's society. In the hearing community, it is important that the meaning of deafness change from a condition of deficiency to an attribute of diversity.

PERSONAL NARRATIVE: MARTHA SHERIDAN

Martha Sheridan, who became deaf as a child, is a social work professor at Gallaudet University. She is an active member of the Deaf community, and a mentor to deaf and hard-of-hearing students.

Writing about my childhood experiences as a deaf child in a hearing world is difficult for me to do. This is because it presents certain educational and social truths about my early life that were painful at the time and represented the "clinical" perspective on deafness. As I grew and learned more about myself as a d/Deaf person and about my options, I chose a new path, became acculturated within the Deaf community, and adopted a cultural perspective for myself (progressing from being deaf to Deaf). That journey has been quite transcending and empowering for me. Writing this is also difficult because I tend to want to protect my parents, whom I love, from those earlier truths.

In addition, I don't want to imply that my story is representative of every other d/Deaf or hard-of-hearing person. Each person's story should be viewed in the context of the individual variables that exist in his or her life. There is much diversity among people who are d/Deaf and hard of hearing, and much to be learned from the variety of life experiences that d/Deaf and hard-of-hearing people have. For example, my life experiences would have been altered greatly had I been profoundly deaf from birth, had a non-deteriorating hearing loss, attended a deaf education program from early childhood on, if ASL had been my first language, or if I had Deaf parents. Not all d/Deaf or hard-of-hearing adults would say their early educational and social experiences were painful. Some may have had the goodness of fit early in their educational experiences that I did not have.

Being the first in my family to be deaf, I began, with my parents, a slow and long winding search that would last from early childhood through adolescence before we found the answers we needed. I grew up in the 1950s through the early 1970s, when technology such as closed captioned television and e-mail, as well as professional and legislative advancements such as the interpreting profession, IDEA, 504, and ADA, did not exist. Hearing aids were bulky, awkward, and very visible devices, and TTYs were just being developed and were not commonly known. Historically speaking, the state of education for deaf children was undergoing a heated debate, and all the professionals my parents met advised against my learning to sign or transferring to a deaf education program. It was not until I was a sophomore in high school that they were advised to consider a deaf education program for the social benefits.

Another important variable in my story is that while I became deaf in early childhood, the severity of my deafness increased throughout those years from onset at age three to profound at age thirteen (approximately an 85 decibel loss) to what is now a 120+ decibel hearing loss, and I no longer use or benefit from hearing aids as I did in childhood and young adulthood.

Having a deteriorating hearing loss meant that my communication, social, and educational needs were constantly changing throughout my life. This variable and others (the hearing status of my family members and my upbringing in hearing schools) influenced my constantly changing self-image.

Looking back, I remember the struggles and challenges to achieve academically when I was the only deaf child in a hearing elementary school and had no communication supports (no interpreters, no closed captioning for films, no signing teachers, no special education resource personnel, no note takers). I saw myself fail test after test and did not understand why, no matter how hard I tried, I couldn't seem to get good grades like my classmates.

I remember being in a class of sixty students in the first grade before my hearing loss was officially diagnosed, and being punished for not following the instructions I did not hear. I remember being humiliated in front of my peers when a teacher forced me to stand up in front of class until I could understand (through lipreading) what a classmate was saying. I remember not fitting in and not understanding why. I remember a feeling of failure.

Things changed a bit when I finally repeated the fifth grade. With this, I began to achieve a much higher GPA. It was then that I discovered that I was actually an intelligent person who could enjoy school and high academic achievements. I had known that I was different from my classmates but wrongly attributed this difference to intellectual inability. The lack of educational supports available to me had not only given me a dangerously false perception of myself; it also contributed to an extended period of educational underachievement.

Yes, I considered myself different from the other children. In truth, we were different, but the unfortunate thing was that I misunderstood that difference, as did my peers and many of my teachers. Having d/Deaf peers and d/Deaf adult role models and communication supports could have prevented that.

Many things changed when I attended Gallaudet University in Washington, D.C. At Gallaudet, I finally learned American Sign Language, which I had wanted to learn since age eleven, when I began to wonder if perhaps my "fit" was with other d/Deaf children. At Gallaudet, I met my peers and learned what it means to be deaf in the context of both Deaf and hearing communities. There, I also learned about, and had the opportunity to begin using, the various technologies available (TTYs, flashing alarm clocks, door and phone lights) and experienced all the joys of an accessible environment. At last, I could understand my teachers and peers in a signing environment. Gallaudet and the Deaf community helped me to discover the person I really was and to discard that old image of myself as a failure. At Gallaudet, I discovered the tools I needed to continue to achieve.

When my parents and siblings saw what an important and positive transition I had made and how much signing had opened up for me, they all learned to sign, and communication in our family became much more effective and easier for all of us. I believe my parents were greatly relieved when they saw how much signing and my acculturation into the Deaf community had done for me.

At Gallaudet, I majored in social work and went on to acquire an MSW at the University of Maryland and a PhD in social work from Ohio State University in 1996. My career focus has been generalist social work practice with people who are Deaf, deaf, and hard of hearing and people with disabilities. I believe my career also represents a goodness of fit in that I have never had a problem getting a job.

As a child and now as a mother, my role model was my own mother. In high school that expanded to include hearing friends of mine who were highly accomplished. Since that time, my role models have included my peers, particularly women, who are also d/Deaf, who are successful in their careers and as mothers. As a child or adolescent, I had no visible role models in women who were d/Deaf.

Yes, I have developed an identity as a Deaf person. I went from being a child in a hearing school who had "trouble hearing," felt I was different, and just couldn't seem to succeed in school, and not understanding what being deaf meant or even that I was in fact deaf, to readily identifying myself as Deaf, understanding what that means to me and others, and I embrace it comfortably.

As an adult, being Deaf has become a central and very positive aspect of my life. Although I still run into barriers, I now know what my rights and responsibilities are and how to use them effectively. I still have to struggle to get hospitals, doctors, and public accommodations to provide interpreters but usually succeed in those efforts. On the spiritual side, I grew up Catholic and have faced many barriers to participation in the church, as I know other people with disabilities have. I would like to see that change. Even though laws against discrimination do not apply to religious organizations, it is a moral and ethical responsibility that the church has to its members.

The things in life that contributed to my success include having a loving family that encouraged my postsecondary educational endeavors: attending Gallaudet University, learning to sign, and adopting a Deaf identity. Perhaps the most basic psychological aspect of this was those moments of epiphany and initial academic successes from the fifth grade on, when I realized that I was an intelligent person and I discovered I thoroughly enjoyed this newfound academic mastery. I also had successes in non-academic areas such as dance and athletics, which helped me develop a sense of achievement. My early educational experiences were my biggest obstacle—a huge struggle, and painful to recall. I was fortunate to have found my way through that to Gallaudet and beyond. I would not advocate those early experiences in a hearing school without proper communication and education supports for any other deaf child. Once I found my way through that early childhood maze, my later educational achievements became an empowering tool.

Professionally, I have worked as a direct service provider, macro-level change agent, and administrator in a variety of settings, including schools, community mental health agencies, and social service agencies. I've been fortunate to be in positions where I have been able to influence change in service systems and in social work education programs. The current joys in my life are my husband and son and my position on the faculty in the Department of Social Work at Gallaudet University.

On the macro level, I believe that laws such as the Rehabilitation Act of 1973 and the Americans with Disabilities Act have been a tool that people with disabilities have been able to use successfully. However, I think we are only beginning to see the positive results of these laws. There is much more to come. As awareness and access increase, people with disabilities will become increasingly visible. These laws would not have come about without the successful self-advocacy efforts of people with disabilities, and they will only continue to effect change in the same manner. Although it is important to know and understand your own disability and rights as a person with a disability, it is also important to know and understand how to effect change on the macro level. Skills in community organizing, grant writing, and research are important for social workers with disabilities and for those who work with people with disabilities to have.

DISCUSSION QUESTIONS

1. What are prelingual, postlingual, lingual, and nonlingual deafness?
2. Compare and contrast the medical definition of deafness with social and political definitions of deafness.
3. What are the elements of Deaf culture? How does Deaf culture compare to ethnic culture?
4. What are the social, cognitive, and emotional differences between being born deaf and becoming deaf as an adult?
5. What are the positive and negative consequences of disability civil rights legislation of recent years for deaf and hard-of-hearing people?
6. What are the social implications of being hard of hearing or deaf? Of being Deaf?
7. What are the commonalties of Deafness that transcend countries and cultures?

SUGGESTED READINGS

Christensen, K. M., & Delgado, G. L. (1993). *Multicultural issues in deafness.* White Plains, NY: Longman.

Cohen, L. H. (1994). *Train go sorry: Inside a deaf world.* New York: Houghton Mifflin.

Higgins, P. C., & Nash, J. E. (1996). *Understanding deafness socially: Continuities in research and theory* (2nd ed.). Springfield, IL. Charles C. Thomas.

Marschark, M., & Clark, M. D. (1993). *Psychological perspectives on deafness.* Hillsdale, NJ: Lawrence Erlbaum.

REFERENCES

Barnartt, S. N., & Christiansen, J. B. (1996). The educational and occupational attainment of prevocationally deaf adults: 1972–1991. In P. C. Higgins & J. E. Nash (Eds.), *Understanding deafness socially: Continuities in research and theory* (2nd ed., pp. 60–70). Springfield, IL: Charles C. Thomas.

Benedict, B. S., & Sass-Lehrer, M. (2007). Deaf and hearing the partnerships: Ethical and communication considerations. *American Annuals of the Deaf, 152*(3), 275–282.

Bonvillian, J. D., & Folven, R. J. (1993). Sign language acquisition: Developmental aspects. In M. Marschark & M. D. Clark (Eds.), *Psychological perspectives on deafness* (pp. 229–265). Hillsdale, NJ: Lawrence Erlbaum.

Burch, S. (2000). Transcending revolutions: The tsars, the Soviets, and Deaf culture. *Journal of Social History, 34* (2), 393–421.

Calderon, R., & Greenberg, M. T. (1993). Considerations in the adaptation of families with school-aged children. In M. Marschark & M. D. Clark (Eds.), *Psychological perspectives on deafness* (pp. 27–48). Hillsdale, NJ: Lawrence Erlbaum.

Canadian Cultural Society for the Deaf. (2005). *Profile*. Retrieved August 29, 2007, from http://www.ccsdeaf.com/indexe.html

Canale, A., Favero, E., Lacilla, M., Recchia, E., Schindler, A., Roggero, N., & Albera, R. (2006). Age at diagnosis of deaf babies: A retrospective analysis highlighting the advantage of newborn hearing screening. *International Journal of Pediatric Otorhinolaryngology, 70* (7), 1283–1289.

Christensen, K. M., & Delgado, G. L (1993). *Multicultural issues in deafness*. White Plains, NY: Longman.

Cohen, L. H. (1994). *Train go sorry: Inside a deaf world*. New York: Houghton Mifflin.

Eriks-Brophy, A., Durieux-Smith, A., Olds, J., & Fitzpatrick, E. (2006). Facilitators and barriers to the inclusion of orally educated children and youth with hearing loss in schools: Promoting partnerships to support inclusion. *Volta Review, 106* (1), 53–88. Retrieved August 20, 2007, from Research Library database.

Erting, C. J., Prezioso, C., & Hynes, M. O. (1990). The interactional context of deaf mother-infant communication. In V. Volterra & C. J. Erring (Eds.), *From gesture to language in hearing and deaf children* (pp. 97–106). Berlin: Springer-Verlag.

Foster, S. (1996). Doing research in deafness: Some considerations and strategies. In P. C. Higgins & J. E. Nash (Eds.), *Understanding deafness socially: Continuities in research and theory* (2nd ed., pp. 3–20). Springfield, IL: Charles C. Thomas.

Friedlander, E. (1996). *Diseases of the ear*. Retrieved February 28, 1998, from http://worldmall.com/erf/lectures/earpath.html

Gilman, R., Easterbrooks, S. R., & Frey, M. (2004). A preliminary study of multidimensional life satisfaction among deaf/hard of hearing youth across environmental settings. *Social Indicators Research, 66* (1–2), 143. Retrieved August 20, 2007, from ABI/INFORM Global database. (Document ID: 718437941).

Greftegrefe, I. (1992). Orientation in indexial signs in Norwegian sign language. *Nordic Journal of Linguistics, 15* (2), 159–182.

Guyton, A. C. (1971). *Textbook of medical physiology* (4th ed.). Philadelphia: W. B. Saunders.

Hall, S. (1989). Train-gone-sorry: The etiquette of social conversations in American Sign Language. In S. Wilcox (Ed.), *American Deaf culture: An anthology* (pp. 89–102). Burtonsville, MD: Linstock.

Harrington, T. (2004). *Deaf statistics: Other countries*. Retrieved August 27, 2007, from http://library.gallaudet.edu/dr/faq-statistics-deaf-other.html

Harrington, T. (2007). *Sign languages of the world, by country.* Retrieved September 3, 2007, from http://library.gallaudet.edu/deaf-faq-world-sl-country.shtml

Harris, R. Y. (1978). Impulse control in deaf children: Research and clinical issues. In L. S. Liben (Ed.), *Deaf children: Developmental perspectives* (pp. 137–156). New York: Columbia University Press.

Humphries, T., Martin, B., & Coye, T. (1989). A bilingual, bicultural approach to teaching English (how two hearies and a deafie got together to teach English). In S. Wilcox (Ed.), *American Deaf culture: An anthology* (pp. 121–143). Burtonsville, MD: Linstock.

Israelite, N., Ower, J., & Goldstein, G. (2002). Hard-of-hearing adolescents and identity construction: Influences of school experiences, peers, and teachers. *Journal of Deaf Studies and Deaf Education, 7*(2), 134–148. Retrieved August 20, 2007, from Health & Medical Complete database.

Jackler, R. K., & Kaplan, M. J. (1990). Ear, nose and throat. In S. A. Schroeder, M. A. Krupp, L. M., Tierney, & S. J. McPhee (Eds.), *Current medical diagnosis and treatment* (pp. 124–150). Englewood Cliffs, NJ: Prentice Hall.

Jones, D. D. (2004). Relative earnings of deaf and hard-of-hearing individuals. *Journal of Deaf Studies and Deaf Education, 9*(4), 459–461. Retrieved August 20, 2007, from Health & Medical Complete database.

Karchmer, M. A., & Trybus, R. J. (1977). *Who are the deaf children in "mainstream" programs?* Washington, DC: Office of Demographic Studies, Gallaudet College.

Kent, B. A. (2003). Identity issues for hard-of-hearing adolescents aged 11, 13, and 15 in mainstream setting. *Journal of Deaf Studies and Deaf Education, 8*(3), 315–324. Retrieved August 20, 2007, from Health & Medical Complete database.

Lederberg, A. R. (1993). The impact of deafness on mother-child and peer relationships. In M. Marschark & M. D. Clark (Eds.), *Psychological perspectives on deafness* (pp. 60–70). Hillsdale, NJ: Lawrence Erlbaum.

Mace, A. L., Wallace, K. L., Whan, M. Q., & Stelmachowicz, P. G. (1991). Relevant factors in the identification of hearing loss. *Ear and Hearing, 12,* 287–293.

Marschark, M. (1993). Origins and interactions in social, cognitive, and language development of deaf children. In M. Marschark & M. D. Clark (Eds.), *Psychological perspectives on deafness* (pp. 7–26). Hillsdale, NJ: Lawrence Erlbaum.

Meadow-Orlans, K. P. (1996). Socialization of deaf children and youth. In P. C. Higgins & J. E. Nash (Eds.), *Understanding deafness socially: Continuities in research and theory* (2nd ed., pp. 60–70). Springfield, IL: Charles C. Thomas.

Mitchell, R. E. (2005). *Can you tell me how many deaf people there are in the United States?* Retrieved August 27, 2007, from http://gri.gallaudet.edu/Demographics/deaf-US.php

Mitchell, R. E. (2006). How many deaf people are there in the United States? Estimates from the survey of income and program participation. *Journal of Deaf Studies and Deaf Education, 11*(1), 112–119.

Moore, C. L. (2001). Disparities in job placement outcomes among deaf, late-deafened, and hard-of-hearing consumers. *Rehabilitation Counseling Bulletin, 44*(3), 144–150. Retrieved August 20, 2007, from Research Library database.

Moores, D. F. (1987). *Educating the deaf: Psychology, principles and practices*. Boston: Houghton Mifflin.

National Association of the Deaf. (n.d.). *Nationwide hearing screening for infants: Early hearing detection and intervention*. Retrieved September 2, 2007, from http://www.nad.org/infant

National Institute of Deafness and Communication Disorders. (2007). *Statistics about hearing disorders, ear infections, and deafness*. Retrieved August 27, 2007, from http://www.nidcd.nih.gov/health/statistics/hearing.asp

Nelson, H. D., Nygren, P., Walker, M., & Panoscha, R. (2006). Screening for speech and language delay in preschool children: Systematic evidence review for the US Preventive Services Task Force. *Pediatrics, 117*(2), 298–319.

Nelson, K. E., Loncke, F., & Camarata, S. (1993). Implications of research on deaf and hearing children's language learning. In M. Marschark & M. D. Clark (Eds.), *Psychological perspectives on deafness* (pp. 123–151). Hillsdale, NJ: Lawrence Erlbaum.

Padden, C. (1989). The Deaf community and the culture of Deaf people. In S. Wilcox (Ed.), *American Deaf culture: An anthology* (pp. 1–16). Burtonsville, MD: Linstock.

Punch, R., Creed, P. A., & Hyde, M. B. (2006). Career barriers perceived by hard-of-hearing adolescents: Implications for practice from a mixed-methods study. *Journal of Deaf Studies and Deaf Education, 11*(2), 224–237. Retrieved August 20, 2007, from Health & Medical Complete database.

Reis, P. W. (1994). Prevalence and characteristics of persons with hearing trouble: United States, 1990–91. *Vital and Health Statistics,* Series 10, No 188.

Rutherford, S. D. (1989). Funny in deaf—not in hearing. In S. Wilcox (Ed.), *American Deaf culture: An anthology* (pp. 65–81). Burtonsville, MD: Linstock.

Savitt, A. (2007). *Evolution of a language: American Sign Language*. Retrieved September 4, 2007, from http://www.lifeprint.com/asl101/pages-layout/evolutionof signlanguage.htm

Schein, J. D. (1996). The demography of deafness. In P. C. Higgins & J. E. Nash (Eds.), *Understanding deafness socially: Continuities in research and theory* (2nd ed., pp. 21–43). Springfield, IL: Charles C. Thomas.

Shapiro, J. P. (1993). *No pity: People with disabilities forging a new civil rights movement*. New York: Times Books.

Siegel, L. (2006). The argument for a constitutional right to communication and language. *Sign Language Studies, 6*(3), 255–272. Retrieved August 20, 2007, from Research Library database.

Spencer, P. E., Bodner-Johnson, B. A., & Gutfreund, M. K. (1992). Interacting with infants with a hearing loss: What can we learn from mothers who are deaf? *Journal of Early Intervention, 16,* 64–78.

Stinson, M. S., & Kluwin, T. N. (1993). Social orientations toward deaf and hearing peers among deaf adolescents in local public high schools. In M. Marschark & M. D. Clark (Eds.), *Psychological perspectives on deafness* (pp. 113–134). Hillsdale, NJ: Lawrence Erlbaum.

Stokoe, W. C. (1989). Dimensions of difference: ASL and English based cultures. In
S. Wilcox (Ed.), *American Deaf culture: An anthology* (pp. 49–59). Burtonsville,
MD: Linstock.

Stokoe, W. C., Jr., Croneberg, C., & Casterline, D. (1965). *A dictionary of American
Sign Language on linguistic principles.* Washington, DC: Gallaudet Press.

Thompson, D. C., McPhillips, H., Davis, R. L., Lieu, T. L., Homer, C. J., & Helfand, M.
(2002). Universal newborn hearing screening: Summary of evidence. *Journal of
the American Medical Association, 287*(5), 286–201.

Wilcox, S. (1989). *American Deaf culture: An anthology.* Burtonsville, MD: Linstock.

Wilson, C. (1997). Mainstream or "deaf school?" Both! deaf students say. *Perspectives
in Education and Deafness, 16*(2). Retrieved September 4, 2007, from http://clerc
center.gallaudet.edu/products/perspectives/nov-dec97/deafschool.html

Wood, D. (1989). Social interaction and tutoring. In M. H. Bornstein & J. S. Bruner
(Eds.), *Interaction in human development* (pp. 59–80). Hillsdale, NJ: Lawrence
Erlbaum.

World Federation of the Deaf. (2005). *Home.* Retrieved August 29, 2007, from http://
www.wfdeaf.org/

Zak, O. (1996). *Zak's politically incorrect glossary.* Retrieved October 10, 2008, from
http://www.zak.co.il/d/deaf-info/old/zpig.html

Zeng, F. (2004). Trends in cochear implants. *Trends in Amplification, 8*(1), 1–34.

8

Visual Disabilities

The first time I remember understanding that my vision was different from other people's was in the second or third grade, when I
realized other students could read the blackboard. Before then, I
couldn't understand why the teacher would bother to write on the
board. When it dawned on me that other kids could read the
board and I couldn't, it was one of those "aha" moments of life. It
was a new discovery. I knew I was different on some level
because I was in special education classes, but I hadn't known
that it was because I saw differently than others.

—Brenda Premo
Western University of Health Sciences

STUDENT LEARNING OBJECTIVES

1. To understand issues around defining blindness and visual impairment
2. To understand the many consequences of social stigma, stereotyping, and
   prejudice concerning persons who are blind and visually impaired
3. To understand that persons who are blind and visually impaired are limited by society's preconceptions of their abilities or lack of them
4. To understand the differences of opinion within the blind community
   regarding preferential treatment
5. To understand some of the unique problems of persons who are both
   deaf and blind

Stroman (1982) offers insight into the various nuances of the task of defining
blindness and visual impairment. Traditionally, the medical model has
served as the basis for defining blindness. The origins of the medical model
definition go back to at least 1868. Dr. Herman Snellen developed the eye-
test chart used today by most ophthalmologists and optometrists. Based on
nine lines of letters, visual acuity is determined as a fraction based on what
a "normal" eye can see at twenty feet. Thus 20/20 is considered normal.
Medically, an individual is considered visually impaired if vision in the eye
with the best sight is 20/80 or less when corrected. In the United States, the
medical profession defines a person who is legally blind as having visual

acuity for distant vision of 20/200 or less in the better eye with the best correction (Beers, 2003).

Based on the above definition, over one million Americans over age forty years are blind. In addition, 2.4 million have some form of visual impairment. It is expected that these rates will double in the next thirty years ("Number of Blind," 2004). Globally, the number of persons who are blind or visually impaired is not really known because of the inconsistencies in reporting, and, among other things, nonstandardized criteria for blindness. The estimate as of 1990 was around 38 million individuals (Thylefors, Negrel, Pararajasegaram, & Dadzie, 1995). As of 2002, the World Health Organization estimated that there were about 37 million blind in the world. Blindness from infection has decreased but blindness from conditions of aging has increased. These are conservative estimates at best, and their limitations point to the need for a current worldwide scientific survey of blindness and visual impairment based upon standardized definitions.

According to Stroman (1982), self-reporting and administrative determination are two other methods of defining visual disability. Self-reported definitions of visual disability classify visual acuity based upon visual levels established by medical authority or a federal agency. A visual problem would be defined, for example, according to a person's own report of whether he or she is able to read ordinary newspaper print with glasses. If not, the individual would be self-classified as severely visually impaired. Two problems are associated with this type of definition. First, because of the lack of objective criteria, a great deal of subjectivity in determining the degree of severity of blindness prevails. Second, because of the stigma associated with being blind, people are reluctant to self-disclose regarding the severity of their disability.

The administrative determination of visual impairment classifies visual loss based upon functional categories (Stroman, 1982). Many government agencies and service providers utilize this functional definition to determine eligibility for economic and educational benefits and services. Developed by the American Medical Association, this definition divides visual impairment into five categories. Category 1 encompasses total blindness, where the individual does not perceive any light at all. This is very rare. The second category centers on the ability to perceive whether or not light is present. Those in category 3, economic blindness, cannot do any kind of work for which sight is essential. This is the category usually thought of as legally blind. The fourth category, vocational blindness, includes individuals who are unable to do the work for which they have experience or training. The fifth category, educational blindness, is a level of impairment that would make it difficult, dangerous, or impossible to learn through usual and traditional methods of education.

Categories 3, 4, and 5 require a word of caution. The essentials of visual acuity required for work and education are relative. With reasonable accommodation, most vocational and educational activities can be mastered by a person with limited visual acuity. Those using the administrative definition of visual impairment should take into account that it is predominantly individuals who are sighted who establish descriptions of the various tasks involved in a position or job. Often they have difficulty differentiating the essential functions and tasks of a particular job from the nonessential functions. It can be easy to define nonessential functions as essential due to a lack of knowledge of the various types of accommodation available. An individual who is sighted may define reading a computer monitor as essential in computer programming. However, with the use of relatively inexpensive hardware and software, a person who has a visual disability can efficiently utilize a computer for all its input and output functions without being able to read the monitor. Often people who are sighted are unaware of simple techniques to accommodate complex tasks that seem to require sight.

CAUSES OF BLINDNESS AND VISUAL IMPAIRMENT

The National Federation of the Blind (n.d.) found that the most common causes of blindness today are glaucoma, cataracts, and diabetic retinopathy. Anything that inhibits the movement of light from the environment to the back of the eye or nerve impulses from the back of the eye to the brain will interfere with vision. Blindness is not an absolute condition. The variations are as numerous as the individuals who experience it. A person who is considered legally blind may be able to ascertain shapes and/or shadows (Beers, 2003).

The causes of blindness may be grouped into five categories. When light cannot reach the retina, infection, vitamin deficiency, or cataracts may be the cause. When light rays do not focus on the retina to allow detailed focusing, severe refraction changes may be the cause. When the retina senses light rays in an atypical manner, the cause could be a detached retina, diabetes, glaucoma, macular degeneration, or retinitis pigmentosa. When nerve pulses from the retina are transmitted to the brain in an atypical fashion, possible causes include brain tumors, primary disabilities such as multiple sclerosis, disrupted blood supply, or some kind of inflammation of the optic nerve. When the brain interprets information sent via impulses by the eye differently, the cause may be a stroke or brain tumor that affects the area of the brain that deals with visual messages (Beers, 2003).

SOCIAL STIGMA

Stroman (1982) and tenBroek (1993) discuss the specific elements of prejudice regarding persons who are blind and visually impaired. Many people perceive blindness and visual impairment as an impenetrable, terrible fate. This stereotype reinforces the notion that persons who are blind are miserable and innately depressed, that living "in the dark" is almost as bad as being condemned to hell. Because of its negative nature, many in society believe that persons who are blind should be pitied. This view reinforces the notion that persons who are blind are helpless and useless and therefore must be cared for. These views substantiate the misconception that persons who are blind are easily fooled and that, outside of established welfare, the only viable "occupation" for persons who are blind is begging.

TenBroek and Matson (1959) demonstrate that many people view being blind as the equivalent of being dead. Directly related to Judeo-Christian heritage, blindness is the symbol of death. In the historical and sacred writings of the Jews, there are many references to the blind man as one who is dead.

As discussed previously throughout this book, there is a societal sense that disability results from immorality and evil. This belief particularly plagues people who are blind or visually impaired. Again, this stereotype is directly related to the Judeo-Christian belief that evil and immorality result in disability and blindness: "The Lord shall smite thee with madness, and blindness, and astonishment of heart" (Deuteronomy 28:28). For persons who are blind or visually impaired, the ramifications of this belief are many. Persons who are blind are feared, at best avoided, and better yet rejected. If they or their families are sinful and immoral in some way, persons who are blind are to be ostracized.

Perhaps one of the more common stereotypes about persons who are blind or visually impaired centers on their maladjustment. Components of this stereotype include the belief that the lack of ability to see has led to poor psychosocial development, that persons who are blind are envious of sighted person and exist within the constant turmoil of wishing to be sighted, and that person who are blind live in constant depression concerning their loss. Many in our society believe that because of the nature of blindness, persons who are blind are "bored, idle, aloof, self-pitying, paranoid, prone to petty angers, unfriendly and hypersensitive" (Stroman, 1982, p. 95).

THE CONSEQUENCES OF STEREOTYPING

Newberry (1993) indicates that most persons who are blind or visually impaired view themselves as basically normal. To most, blindness or visual impairment is a physical nuisance at worst. Like the population in general, persons who are blind tend to be diverse. Some people who are blind have emotional difficulties such as overdependency, timidity, and depression. For those having emotional difficulties related to being blind, most of those difficulties result directly from the stereotyping and stigma in the socialization process: "The various attitudes and patterns of behavior that characterize people who are blind are not inherent in their condition but, rather, are acquired through ordinary processes of social learning. Thus, there is nothing inherent in the condition of blindness that requires a person to be docile, dependent, melancholy, or helpless; nor is there anything about it that should lead him to become independent or assertive. Blind men are made, and by the same processes of socialization that have made us all" (Scott, 1969, p. 14).

Large (1993) cites studies that indicate that some persons who are blind or visually impaired tend to comply with the social stereotypes imposed upon them. Thus, some persons who are blind take on some or all of the psychosocial characteristics of these stereotypes, much in the same way that some African Americans (Solomon, 1976), ethnic minorities, women, and gays and lesbians (Pharr, 1988) respond to their oppression.

Central to the process of inculcating stereotypes of persons who are blind are public and private agencies that "serve" persons who are blind. According to Scott (1969), with as low as 5 percent of normal vision, a person can function as a fully sighted person in most areas of life. Scott states that in spite of this fact, "one of the most important, but least recognized, functions performed by organizations of the blindness system is to teach people who have difficulty seeing how to behave like blind people" (p. 71). This happens at two levels. First, when an ophthalmologist diagnoses blindness, the social response is immediate. Prior to the diagnosis, the individual is treated like a person who can see and has difficulty with sight. After the diagnosis, the person is treated like a person who is blind but has some sight. Second, this redefinition of the person is maintained and reinforced once he or she becomes involved with an agency dealing with persons who are blind. The training techniques, the mobility strategies, the job training, and the counseling all attempt to socialize the person to conform to the stereotypes of persons who are blind. "The impaired person is thus under strong pressure to think of himself as blind and to redefine his visual impairment from a medical condition of attenuated vision to a kind of welfare problem requiring extensive social services. Accompanying this phenomenon is a strong emphasis on psychological adjustment to blindness and personal acceptance of this condition. The visually impaired person's readiness for the offered services is measured by his willingness to admit to himself the fact of his blindness and to show that he is resigned to the alleged permanence of his condition" (Scott, 1969, p. 74).

Thus, the very agencies designed to empower persons who are blind or visually impaired may in fact further their dependency and disenfranchisement by encouraging the inculcation of certain psychosocial characteristics. Albrecht (1992) states this paradox well: "Rehabilitation institutions and programs generally perpetuate dependency even though they purport to make people functionally independent" (p. 267).

Scott (1969) points out that human service professionals tend to use one of two approaches to "treat" blindness. The restorative approach seeks to restore persons who are blind to a level of performance that allows for their independence. The process usually involves a period of mourning and bereavement over the loss of sight. Many professionals consider the new blind state as similar to death, as the loss of the old sighted self must be mourned. Rehabilitation is a process of introspection around the loss, counseling, and skills training to establish a new kind of control of the environment as well as an understanding of self. Although much caution should be exercised concerning the equation of blindness to death (since this notion reinforces societal stereotypes), the end product of the restorative approach for the person who becomes blind or visually impaired is usually independent living and perhaps gainful employment.

The second approach, accommodation, also strives for the goal of independence but assumes that only a small percentage of persons who are blind have the capability of becoming truly independent. Professionals who use this approach create an environment free of physical, recreational, and educational barriers. Most job training and job acquisition are within the realm of sheltered workshop environments. Praise is used to reinforce dependency: "The general environment of such agencies is also accommodative in character. Clients are rewarded by trivial things and praised for performing tasks in a mediocre fashion. This superficial and over-generous reward system makes it impossible for most clients to assess their accomplishments accurately. Eventually, since anything they do is praised as outstanding, many of them come to believe that the underlying assumption must be that blindness makes them incompetent" (Scott, 1969, p. 85).

The end result of this approach is, of course, that persons who are blind organize their lives around the safe milieu of the agency. They can function effectively only within that agency milieu, thus depending upon it for work, leisure, and education. The larger community and their own independence are lost to them.

The medical model perspective pervasive in traditional rehabilitation agencies has led to open conflict between the professional fields of social services and rehabilitation services and organizations such as the National Federation of the Blind, which have a definitive social model perspective in looking at blindness as a characteristic rather than a disability or handicap (Richert, 2002). The conflict is real. Grassroots organizations such as the National Federation of the Blind represent more than 50,000 voices. They extol the views shared by the philosophical underpinnings of this text that much of the dysfunctional nature of blindness and visual impairment has to do with the pejorative social construction of visual disability. On the other hand, many of the approaches of professional social service and rehabilitation services are strongly influenced by the core values of the medical model. The professional is the expert. Peer intervention threatens the professional standing and marketability of the professional social service and rehabilitation worker. Educators, social service workers, and rehabilitation workers have personal and professional interests to protect. Agencies must compete for dollars from federal and state government sources based upon the tenets of the medical model (Vaughan, 1993). Arguably, the medical model relies on the dependence of blind and other disabled people to justify their roles and viability.

The approach we recommend in working with people who are blind or visually impaired is one that lessens the possibility of stereotyping. We believe that the human service professional should see blindness as difference rather than dysfunction and should not assume the need for a grieving process. In fact,\human service professionals should assume nothing about blind people but should wait to be informed by blind persons themselves\ We believe that human service professionals should act merely as consultants to blind consumers, who are in total control of the path they wish to take and direction in which they want to go. Our job as human service professionals is to work with individuals to explore the many paths and alternatives that exist for reaching their goals and then to provide help, if requested.

WHAT CAN PERSONS WHO ARE BLIND REALLY DO?

Newberry (1993) points out that the stereotype that persons who are blind and visually impaired are inferior, helpless, and dependent and cannot do physical labor or function in a fast-paced world has its origins in the social construction of blindness created by the people who can see: "The real problem of blindness is not the loss of eyesight. The real problem is the misunderstanding the general public has about blind people's abilities. We often assume that people who are blind cannot get along without their sight merely because we, with our sight, cannot imagine ourselves doing so" (p. 11).

In an effort to change the pejorative social construction of blindness, the National Federation of the Blind (n.d.) has compiled a list of questions that have been addressed to them by individuals across the United States who are concerned about being blind and visually impaired, and the answers to their questions reveal the nature of the independence of persons with visual disabilities. It is important for human service practitioners to understand the methods of independence used by persons with visual disabilities. These answers go a long way in refuting the myths and stereotypes concerning blindness and visual impairment.

Mobility

How do persons who are blind and visually impaired get around? There are a variety of techniques for facilitating mobility used by persons who are blind. Many use a white cane. This device allows the person to locate steps, curbs, streets, driveways, and most other obstacles that may present themselves in everyday living. The cane is a length that allows people to discern potential obstacles about two feet ahead. The length of the cane varies, depending on the height of the user.

Some persons who are blind or visually impaired use guide dogs. These are dogs that are specially trained to move around obstacles, go through doorways, and stop at curbs and stairs. The person using the dog is always in control and must tell the dog what to do. When the dog stops at a curb, the person using the dog must listen and determine when it is safe to proceed. Persons who are blind are able to cross a street safely by listening to the sounds of traffic and, more recently, traffic signals. They listen to ascertain when cars start to slow down and stop at a traffic light or a stop sign. When one hears cars to the side start moving, it is time to cross the street. If there is no light, the person listens to hear if any cars are approaching and waits until there are no vehicles or until vehicles stop before crossing streets. In recent years, traffic intersections have been equipped with auditory cues such as beeps and chirps that blind people can use in crossing streets.

Persons who are blind or visually impaired use a variety of cues to help them locate specific places and addresses. They determine where they are by using landmarks and directions such as north, south, east, or west. They keep in mind cues, such as a busy street or a lot that has no house or building or a noisy school yard. The story of a friend of one of the authors illustrates the degree of mobility of most persons who are blind.

Rev. David Williams (pseudonym) served as the executive director of Presbyterian House, which served the campus of a small university in western Pennsylvania. David has been blind since birth and graduated with honors from Harvard. The students, the campus community, and the general community loved him. He had doubled the income of the center, and the place was packed with students every day of the week. There was nowhere in the small college town that David could not go. One could see him anywhere on campus, run into him downtown, or come across him at one of several restaurants in the community. David used neither a cane nor a dog. He had memorized the sounds of the entire town and could go anywhere on his own. For one reason or another, Susan, David's wife, became concerned for his safety in getting about and insisted that he get a guide dog. After much resistance, David gave in and began the process. He went through the training and one day appeared on campus with a guide dog. The question was, "Who was guiding whom?" David could frequently be seen pulling the dog across the street. Students observed him trying to stop the dog at a curb. On occasion, students would encounter David trying to get the dog to go up a set of stairs. David certainly was in control, but for what purpose? Lack of mobility was never an issue for Rev. Williams, with or without the guide dog.

Reading

How do persons who are blind read? Most people who are blind read either by using books on audiotape or CD or by using Braille. Originally developed

FIGURE 8.1   Braille Alphabet

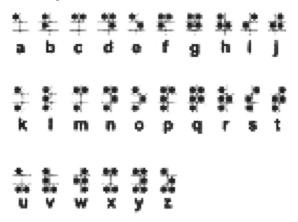

by Charles Barbier, an officer in Napoleon's army, as a military code that could be utilized in the dark, Braille was refined by its namesake, Lewis Braille, a student at the National Institute for the Blind in Paris in 1829 (Koestler, 1976). Braille simplified the complicated Barbier code into simple cells consisting of two parallel columns of raised dots of three dots apiece. The dots are numbered 1, 2, and 3 from top to bottom on the left side of the cell and 4, 5, and 6 from top to bottom on the right side of the cell. The code can be used for letters, numbers, or musical notes, depending on which dots are raised. For example, *a* is the first dot on the left column, *b* is the first and second dots on the left column, and so on (see figure 8.1).

Braille can be written with a Braille writing machine or with a pointed stylus and a Braille slate with rows of small cells, which are used to punch dots down through paper. There are also Braille computer monitors and printers. A person reads Braille by feeling the different dots in each cell and differentiating combinations of dots in relationship to the letter, number, or note that they stand for. There are libraries that provide Braille and recorded books and magazines for persons who are blind.

Technology is constantly improving access to written materials for blind and visually impaired persons. For example, voice recognition software such as Dragon Naturally Speaking, alt tagged Web sites, and screen readers provide access to written and visual information. Computers are also equipped with enlarged text programs, and programs such as Bobby Watchfire and Cynthia Says allow people to determine the accessibility of their Web sites.

Personal Grooming

How do persons who are blind maintain their personal appearance? How does a man who is blind shave or tie his necktie? Men who are blind or visually impaired shave and tie their neckties by feel. After doing these tasks over and over, they become routine and basically a habit. Many men who are blind prefer to shave in the shower. Generally, men can feel where there is a spot to be shaved and where there is not. Tying ties takes a bit of practice, but again by feel, the man who is blind can determine the length and the nature of the knot. Some men who are blind keep their ties tied when they take them off and hang them up already tied, ready for the next use.

How does a woman who is blind apply makeup and do her hair? The first step in this process is to work with someone who can demonstrate the various techniques of makeup artistry and hairstyling. A woman who is blind can feel the different ways of drying, curling, or styling her hair. Women learn to feel when their hair is right or when they have missed a spot. Women who are blind can apply makeup by touch, by feeling the different places where they want different kinds of makeup to be. A woman who is blind can learn which colors are best for her by asking friends or beauticians whom she trusts. As among sighted people, the decision to wear makeup is a personal choice.

How can persons who are blind know what clothes to wear? Most clothing has some unique characteristic that can be felt. Some shirts and jackets have different shapes of buttons or snaps. Fabric texture may also differ. Dresses or skirts have different kinds of belts or elastic at the waist. Jackets and shirts may have different sizes of pockets. By matching these different characteristics with colors, persons who are blind can coordinate design and color. For example, the person who is blind knows that the green shirt is the one with the unusually shaped buttons or the red pants are the ones with straight pockets. The blouse with the wide collar is yellow, which matches the green skirt with the elastic waistband.

If similar items feel the same, persons who are blind mark the clothes in order to tell them apart. Special tags are used to sew on Braille labels, and specially placed safety pins or buttons can be used to identify articles of a similar texture. Some persons who are blind create a list of their clothing articles that feel similar and match them with others, using Braille numbers and letters attached to the clothing. Whatever the material, persons with visual disabilities are able to dress with a few accommodations.

Preparing Food

How do persons who are blind shop for groceries? Many kinds of food can be recognized by feel and touch. Different kinds of fruits and vegetables have different shapes and textures. Certain meat items feel different. There is much difference between the feel of a hot dog and that of a chicken. But identifying wrapped meat items and items in cans or boxes by touch is difficult. Many persons who are blind go shopping with someone who can help them identify canned and boxed food items. Blind people often ask store employees to help them find groceries. Many blind people make two lists, one in Braille for themselves, and one printed for a friend, helper, or store employee.

How do persons who are blind cook? Persons who are blind can use all the fixtures found in the kitchen. Coded labels using Braille or other codes can be affixed to touch buttons and dials on microwaves, stoves, and ovens. Persons who are blind generally use measuring devices such as spoons or cups that stack so the relative size can quickly be determined. The smell, sound, temperature, time of cooking, texture, and consistency can help determine how the foods are cooking.

How do persons who are blind know which can or package to open in food preparation? Many different foods can be identified by the size and shape of the containers in which they come. Spaghetti boxes, ketchup bottles, tuna cans, bags of beans or rice, flour, sugar, coffee or tea, and butter are just some of the examples of the unique sizes and types of containers that can be used to identify the contents. Other items not so unique can be identified by Braille labels or other methods of coding. Some Braille labels are made in such a way that they can be used over and over again. Some persons who are blind or visually impaired label their foods right at the store. Some food can be readily identified by smell while still in containers.

School and Work

Where do children who are blind go to school? Although most states have "special" schools for children who are blind, the vast majority of children who are blind attend "regular" schools in their communities. Children who are blind or visually impaired participate in regular classrooms and move throughout school buildings using the techniques described previously. Most read and write Braille and use adaptive technology. Resource teachers facilitate the education of students who are blind, receiving textbooks and library books in Braille and on tape or CD. Most students type papers using computers. Students who are blind have the legal right to accommodation if needed, and technological advances have made access far easier than in the past.

Where do persons who are blind work? Persons who are blind work in a vast array of jobs. With necessary training and assistive equipment, people who are blind or visually impaired have the same range of abilities as people who are not. Persons who are blind or visually impaired work as artists, boat builders, politicians, computer programmers, lawyers, social workers, teachers, cosmetologists, auto mechanics, fashion models, accountants, and so on.

How do persons who are blind do their jobs? Access on the job for persons who are blind or visually impaired may be relatively simple and low tech or can involve the use of sophisticated computer hardware and software. Accommodation can take many forms. In human services, jobs can be restructured to accommodate transportation issues, particularly in rural settings. If people who are blind or visually impaired cannot make home visits because of lack of public transportation, they can be assigned specialized duties, such as doing new intakes, that involve remaining in the office. In urban areas where mass transit is more available, this particular accommodation would not be necessary. Additional examples of accommodation include using Velcro fasteners on protective clothing. A dot of silicon adhesive on switches or control knobs that need constant monitoring permits a person who is blind or visually impaired to use electronic machines with controls. Enlarged print or Braille labels make file folders readable, and soft drink selection on the soda machine possible. Striping codes using masking tape can be used to identify parts on shelves. High-tech accommodation usually involves computers. Hardware and software accommodations can include enlarged print on an enlarged screen, voice synthesizers, and Braille tactile boards. An optical scanner along with a voice synthesizer makes reading of regular print possible (Dickson, 1994).

Identifying Money

How do persons who are blind know what money to give when they are purchasing an item? Coins generally have textural difference to the degree that they can be easily differentiated by feel. They vary in size, and quarters and dimes have ridges around then, whereas pennies and nickels are smooth. To identify different denominations of paper money, some persons who are blind keep different bills in separate places in their wallets. Most persons who are blind develop a coding system based on folding. They fold different denominations in different ways. One method would be to fold a five-dollar bill in half the short way, and a ten-dollar bill in half the long way. A twenty could be folded twice, and a one not folded at all. When paper money is exchanged, persons who are blind ask which bill is which and fold them accordingly.

Telling Time

How do persons who are blind know what time it is? Generally, there are two ways persons who are blind tell time. Braille watches are open so a person who is blind can feel Braille dots at the different hour points. Other watches actually speak the time and have built-in alarms.

Games and Recreation

How do persons who are blind play cards and other games? Most games, including cards, can be easily modified. Braille can be put on decks of cards. Word games such as Scrabble can be played with Braille letters and a board with raised squares. Playing pieces can be made of different textures and shapes. Dice can be made to have dots that can be felt.

Team sports can be audibly modified so that persons who are blind or visually impaired can play. In baseball, a large ball or a ball with an audible buzzer inside can be used. The first-base coach can call to instruct the batter to the base. Playground balls can be cut open, and bells placed inside, and they can be resealed with bicycle tire patches. Making the playing area brighter through enhanced lighting makes playing easier for persons who are blind or visually impaired. In addition, the use of contrasting colored tape helps in play areas, particularly for gymnastics (Winnick, 2005).

THE ISSUE OF PREFERENTIAL TREATMENT

Berkowitz (1987) discusses the issue of persons who are blind historically receiving preferential treatment in relationship to other disability groups. Persons who are blind have historically held the position of the "worthy" poor in Western social welfare systems. The original U.S. Social Security Act held that only persons who were blind could qualify for welfare. The Randolph-Sheppard Act of 1936 allowed for the exclusive operation of snack bars and newsstands in federal buildings by blind persons. Many public transit systems have lowered rates for persons who are blind. More than thirty states have separate vocational rehabilitation programs for persons who are blind. No other disability group has these privileges to the extent the blind have.

There are several reasons why persons who are blind are recipients of this targeted treatment. People who are sighted fear blindness perhaps more than other disabling conditions and therefore respond to it with greater zeal. Persons who are blind have been a part of history and seem to have a greater impetus to involve themselves historically in the political process, resulting in legislation and policy favorable to persons who are blind. In Europe, blind people have held a special place due to the occurrence of blindness resulting from military service.

Within the blind community, a debate rages on the issue of whether or not persons who are blind should have preferential treatment. TenBroek (1993) argues that there are two kinds of preferential treatment. Preferential treatment based on irrational motivations, including prejudice or fancy, cannot be supported. There is no argument for giving to a blind-related charity out of pity. On the other hand, preferential treatment based upon the unique qualities or the particular needs of a group can be supported. The disabling component of blindness and visual impairment has mainly to do with the misconceptions of persons who are sighted. These misconceptions deny persons who are blind their full membership in society. Reaching full membership means removing the social, environmental, and economic barriers that prevent the full inclusion of persons who are blind. Programs that have these goals and involve preferential treatment certainly can be argued for and supported.

According to tenBroek (1993), programs that have preferential treatment components must have the following characteristics:

1. They must allow persons who are blind or visually impaired to have full autonomy in handling their own affairs.
2. The programs must encourage persons who are blind to develop to their full potential.
3. Programs must direct and encourage persons who are blind to seek opportunities, occupations, and professions.
4. Programs must use a wide range of incentives, including financial remuneration.
5. Programs must encourage the acquisition of private property, not just for consumption's sake but as a means of economic improvement.
6. Programs must reinforce the idea of the individual worth of persons who are blind rather than seeing them as a societal liability.

Other members of the blind community do not agree with tenBroek's position. Shore (1993) questions preferential treatment for persons who are blind or visually impaired. According to Shore, preferential treatment is, by its very nature, demeaning and unnecessary. Preferential treatment prevents persons who are blind from fulfilling the basic desire for financial independence. It reinforces the innate dependency built into the social welfare system and the stereotype that the blind must be cared for. Preferential treatment substantiates the myth that persons who are blind should be objects of pity and charity, that they are helpless, and that they can be little more than beggars. As long as preferential programs exist for persons who are blind, they will not have full equality with sighted persons. Persons who are blind must pay their way in full to be seen as equal and viable citizens.

The issues presented by these two perspectives sound very similar to the debate around affirmative action. Do programs that try to make up for historical inequities in the cases of gender, ethnicity, and disability have a positive or negative impact on how members of the general society view these groups? Do special programs reinforce negative stereotypes and invite backlash, or do they break down stereotypes by promoting increased interaction and economic parity? Do they compensate for racism, sexism, and ableism, or do they further discrimination? Or do they have little impact one way or the other?

People's answers to these questions depend on their ideological perspectives. Hopefully, continued empirical research and policy analysis will provide increased understanding. However, some cautions must be taken regarding this debate. First, opponents of preferential treatment assume that equal competition exists in both the labor and consumer markets. In our current economic system, preferential treatment for the wealthy in buying goods, acquiring an education, and competing for jobs is standard (Hogan, 2005). Stigma is not inherent in preferential treatment but, rather, in the negative stereotypes and low status of persons who are visually disabled. Second, the removal of preferential treatment would have little impact on the stereotypes, bias, and discrimination that are a part of the lives of persons with visual disabilities. Stereotypes around all disability exist for a variety of reasons. They run deep within American culture. The avoidance or refusal of preferential treatment by persons who are blind will not significantly affect these negative stereotypes. Third, many persons who are blind and who are in economic or political leadership positions attained their authority in part by using preferential treatment programs. Research that gives us a better understanding of which policies and what kinds of programs truly add to the economic and social independence of persons who are blind would greatly clarify the preceding issues.

PERSONS WHO ARE BLIND AND DEAF

Shapiro (1993) points out that medical professionals and teachers of persons who are both blind and deaf were the first to realize the importance of the integration of persons with disabilities into society and act upon this realization. Samuel Gridley Howe was an educator who opened the Massachusetts Asylum for the Blind·in 1832. His most noted success was Laura Bridgman, through whom he brought to the public the knowledge that persons who were blind and deaf could be educated. Laura had been blind and deaf from the age of two years as a result of scarlet fever. Howe's success with her brought notables such as Charles Dickens to his school to observe her progress. Perhaps the most famous person who was blind and deaf was Helen Keller. Growing up in the late 1800s, Helen Keller was taught by Anne Sullivan, a graduate of the Perkins School for the Blind. Helen Keller was the first person who was deaf and blind to receive a bachelor's degree, which she earned from Radcliffe College. She dedicated her life to advocacy for persons with disabilities across the world (Thompson & Freeman, 1995).

The causes of deaf-blindness in children can be grouped into four categories, although in many cases the cause is unknown. These four categories are genetic and chromosomal syndromes, congenital infections, environmental and fetal exposures, and postnatal etiologies (Holte, Prickett, Van Dyke, Olson, Lubrica, Knutson, et al., 2006). Many sources conclude that the primary causes of deaf-blindness are rubella and Usher syndrome (Sasse, 2006). Rubella is a systemic infection caused by a togavirus inhaled through infective droplets. It is generally only moderately communicable and has been virtually eliminated in the United States, with the exception of an outbreak in 1999 in Nebraska. Globally, more than 100,000 cases occur annually. Fetal rubella brings about changes that can result in both hearing and visual disabilities (Tierney, McPhee, & Papadakis, 2006). Usher syndrome refers to a group of conditions where hearing loss is combined with retinitis pigmentosa (Sasse, 2006). Retinitis pigmentosa is often an inherited condition that results in changes in the retina that eventually lead to blindness (Beers, 2003).

There are four basic categories of deaf-blindness. The first of these includes those who are deaf and blind at birth as well as those who lose both vision and hearing very early in life. Helen Keller represents this category. The second category includes those who either are born deaf or lose their hearing very early and later lose their vision; the third category includes people who are blind early in life and later lose a significant amount of their hearing; and the fourth category includes adults who, later in life, either through disease or accident, lose both their sight and hearing ("Meeting the Needs," 1994). Koestler (1976) presents a description of the fourth category given by an English businessman left blind and deaf after being involved in an automobile accident:

> What is it actually like to be deaf-blind? I can only tell you what it is like for me. What it's like for a person who has never seen or heard, I do not know. First, it is neither "dark" nor "silent." If you were to go out into a London fog—one of the thick yellow variety—and then close your eyes, you would see what I see. A dull, flesh colored opacity. So much for literal "darkness. . . ."
>
> Nor is my world "silent" (most of us wish it were so!). You have all put a shell to your ear as children and "listened to the waves." You may, at times— when dropping off to sleep perhaps—have "heard" the clang of a bell in your ear, or a sound like the shunting of railway wagons, or a shrill whistle, or the wind moaning round the eaves on Christmas Eve. All these have I perpetually. They have become part of the background. Cracklings, squeakings, rumblings—what I hear is the machinery of my being working. The blood rushing through my veins, and little cracklings of nerves and muscles as they expand and contract. In short, my hearing has "turned inwards." (p. 452)

Persons who are both deaf and blind experience a variety of unique problems. First, if the conditions develop sequentially, the initial diagnosis results in treatment for the earlier condition, generally leaving the later developing condition without consideration. The article "Meeting the Needs of the Deaf-Blind Child" (1994) discusses an example. Keri-Ann, attending sixth grade, had been deaf for several years before she began to lose her sight. Educational professionals planned her education based upon her hearing loss and did not take into consideration her visual limitations. As a result, Keri-Ann was doing poorly in school. The problem centered on the unknown fact that Keri-Ann was experiencing tunnel vision. When ASL interpreters signed to her, their signing was very broad, leaving many of the phrasings outside her field of vision. A second problem for those who are both deaf and blind is that services directed to the uniqueness of this condition are very limited. Most services, particularly educational services, are specialized either for persons who are deaf or for persons who are blind

("Meeting the Needs," 1994). And third, because society views blindness and deafness separately as being overwhelmingly devastating, when they are combined, persons who are both blind and deaf suffer the full force of prejudice and discrimination that are a part of ableism (Koestler, 1976).

The eradication of prejudice and discrimination, resulting in full and rich lives for persons who are both blind and deaf, starts with knowledge and then action. Prickett and Welch (1995) point out that total blindness and total deafness are very rare. So most people who are both blind and deaf have either some vision or some hearing, or both. The second piece of knowledge that is important is that language formulation exists for persons who are blind and deaf. And for those for whom language development is a difficult alternative, techniques of communication exist (Goode, 1994). Goode argues that the disability of deaf-blindness is, like all disabilities, a social construct. Therefore, with the removal of attitudinal barriers through education and association and of environmental barriers through techniques of accommodation, people who are deaf and blind can lead fulfilling, productive lives.

Prickett and Welch (1995) outline several significant educational modifications for inclusive classrooms, which are also applicable to home, community, and work. Lighting is crucial. Eliminating glare, particularly from the sun, is important. Seating in relation to the light and to the source of sound is also important so that persons who are deaf and blind can make use of any residual sight and hearing. In addition, proximity to fellow students or fellow workers is important so that touch can be used as a means of communication. Furthermore, an interpreter using tactile signing or hand signing may help facilitate communication. Originally used mostly in Canada, interveners, who help persons who are deaf and blind gather information for daily living, are becoming more common in other countries. Finally, various pieces of technology, including Braille computer equipment, can facilitate independence.

SUMMARY

As with most disabilities, the definition of blindness finds its roots in the medical model. Most ophthalmologists and optometrists use the eye-test chart to make the diagnosis of blindness. Self-reporting and administrative determination are two other methods of defining blindness. Self-reported definitions of blindness classify visual acuity based upon preestablished visual levels. The administrative definition of visual impairment classifies visual loss based upon functional categories.

Many people fear becoming blind. The idea of being blind depresses individuals, who then jump to the conclusion that people who are blind are miserable and are themselves depressed. These assumptions result in paternalism and pity toward individuals who are blind. On the contrary, most persons who are blind or visually impaired view themselves as basically normal. To most, blindness or visual impairment is a physical nuisance at worst.

Persons who are blind have historically held the position of the "worthy" poor in Western social welfare systems. Within the blind community, there is a debate over the issue of whether or not persons who are blind should have preferential treatment. Some say that preferential treatment based upon the unique qualities or particular needs of a group can be supported. Others say that preferential treatment is by its very nature demeaning and unnecessary. Empirical studies addressing the question of what kinds of programs truly add to the economic and social independence of persons who are blind would greatly clarify the issues.

Persons who are both deaf and blind experience a variety of unique problems. Blindness is feared by sighted individuals. Deafness is also misunderstood and feared. When blindness and deafness are combined in one individual, many people with typical sight and hearing reinforce the prejudice. They cannot comprehend how that individual can continue to live. The resulting discrimination can be tremendous. The eradication of prejudice and discrimination, along with techniques of accommodation, can result in full and rich lives for persons who are both blind and deaf.

PERSONAL NARRATIVE: BRENDA PREMO

Brenda Premo is legally blind and has albinism. She has been actively working for persons with disabilities throughout her adult life. Currently, she is associate professor at Western University of Health Sciences and director of Western University's Center for Disability Issues and the Health Professions. She formerly held the position of director of the California Department of Rehabilitation under Governor Pete Wilson.

I have about 10 percent of my vision, so I am legally blind because of a condition called albinism, which is genetic. I also have no melanin, a chemical that gives people pigmentation and allows them to tan. Thus, I am also very sensitive to the sun.

One early memory that sticks out for me is when I was about four years old. There were times I was supposed to be napping but wasn't. My mother would know that I wasn't napping, so I started thinking she had ESP. Finally, I asked, "Mom, how do you know that I'm not asleep?" She just said, "Mothers know these things." She didn't tell me, but I eventually figured out that she could see my eyes were open. I couldn't see whether her eyes were open or closed, so I couldn't understand that she would know whether or not my eyes were open. I thought that she had ESP, but the reality was that she could see my eyes.

When I was very young, my mother did not explain that I had a disability. There was no discussion of it. She was a single mother making $1.25 an hour as a waitress, so she couldn't work and keep me. She worked and had to give me up until she met my stepfather, to whom she was married for the rest of her life. So I had to live in foster homes from about age two until about age five. I did not realize my disability contributed to my having to live in foster homes. I knew that I was different, but I thought I was different then because I was living in homes where people were not my family. The foster families didn't treat me badly, but they didn't treat me like their children either.

As a child, I knew I couldn't go outside much. This was before they had sunblock, which is a very inexpensive way to keep from what I refer to as "having baked albino." I was severely burned on two occasions because of my sensitive skin. Once, I was put in the hospital for three days with third-degree burns because one of my foster parents put me on the beach for three hours.

I don't think I was aware that I was disabled until I was about five or six. Before then, I was conscious of some differences, but I wasn't aware that others saw me differently. My first vivid memory of my disability was when I was in second grade and children chased me and called me names. I had to dive under the playground merry-go-round to escape. I was in a multicultural school in the middle of L.A., and I was, because of the albinism, the only truly white person in the school. There were white, black, and Hispanic kids, and they all chased me. Being taunted by other kids is my first vivid memory of my disability or my difference. It wasn't my vision that caused them to taunt me; it was that I looked different.

The first time I remember understanding that my vision was different from other people's was in the second or third grade, when I realized other students could read the blackboard. Before then, I couldn't understand why the teacher would bother to write on the board. When it dawned on me that other kids could read the board and I couldn't, it was one of those "aha" moments of life. It was a new discovery. I knew I was different on some level because I was in special education classes, but I hadn't known that it was because I saw differently than others.

As a child, I knew I was different and that people treated me differently than other children. I knew I was perceived as "less than" other children. There were several elements involved in that.

At that time, I believe people treated me differently mostly because of my physical difference—the white eyebrows and the white hair, the pink skin, and the squinting. My physical appearance caused lots more reaction than my visual disability. In fact, many people did not even know of my visual difference unless they saw me read. I also felt different because I lived in foster homes.

The fact that I was born with my visual disability has had advantages. I have what my eye doctor calls "compensating skills." My brain has compensated and fills in the pictures of what I cannot see with my eyes. For example, I remember where steps are if I have been on them before. I see the steps because the brain is filling in what the eyes can't see. Sometimes I make mistakes, so I have to be careful, but my brain gives me the picture. It's easier for me than for someone who is blinded later in life.

Most people don't understand my compensating ability. When I was a child, the doctors told my mother and father, "You have a handicapped daughter who'll probably not be able to care for herself." They didn't understand. My mother was proud when we proved them wrong. When she was terminally ill, my dad cared for her physically, but I was responsible for facilitating her required treatments when she was in California. It was with pride that she announced to the family that I was taking care of her.

I began to understand that my difference from other kids was disability related in the fourth or fifth grade. This was before special education laws. I was in a special school, and the school district decided to experiment with letting us be in the regular schools. I was in a pilot project. It was frightening, and they didn't think things out too well. For example, they put me in a physical education class and had us playing softball out in the middle of the day in the sun. Softball is not something that a person with 10 percent vision does really well at. I noticed I was always picked last. It was obvious other people didn't really want me on the team. Early on, I figured out that I didn't really want to be rejected, so I got a teacher to agree to hit for me and then I began to get picked first.

I began to see two things as a result of this school experience. First, I saw that the classes the other kids were in were different from the classes I was in. I was in an integrated school but in separate classes and removed from other kids because they weren't sure if integration was going to work. Second, I noticed that less was expected of me than of other kids. I was expected to do less. I didn't understand it in words, but I knew that I was somehow expected to achieve less, to know less, and to be less than the other kids. It was a standard that people just accepted. I didn't like it. I knew it wasn't right. I don't know why, but I just didn't accept this. I understood I could do more, and I wanted to do more than they would let me.

Finally, in the sixth grade I told my mother that I wanted to go to a regular junior high school. I didn't want to go to special schools or be in special classes. We moved to Orange County, California, which, at that time in the sixties, had superb schools. By then, I had formulated in my mind that I was visually impaired. There were no special education laws at the time, and the school officials just about fainted dead away when I informed them I wanted to go to a regular school.

I remember this bullheaded psychologist who gave me a small-print IQ test and told my mother that I was retarded. What he had really tested was my ability to read small print. Even my mother knew that his diagnosis was not correct. After all, why would someone give me a small-print test when he knew I couldn't read small print very well? Because I was very determined to go to regular school, my mother told the resistant school officials, "You'll have to fight with her. She wants to go here." So this bullheaded psychologist then said to my mother, "Well, we'll let her go here so she can learn about failure." So my mother says, "Yeah, OK." She only had an eighth-grade education, but she understood intuitively that I was brighter than they gave me credit for.

In my first year in junior high, they didn't let me do anything extra. I had a counselor who believed I could actually communicate and reason, but others did not. My sewing teacher almost became a nervous wreck. I had to get so close to see what I was doing that she was afraid I would affix my nose to the fabric. One time my mother got called into the principal's office because I wouldn't use big-print books. Instead of just bringing me in and chatting with me, the principal brought my mother in. In the meeting, my mother turned to me and said, "Sweetheart, why don't you want to use big-print books?" I said, "Mom, it's like this. I've got four academic classes and all the teachers assign several chapters to read. In large-print books, chapters are in volumes. So if I have four academic classes and I have to have three volumes each, I need a wagon to take my books home." I told her I needed a magnifier, a $1.50 magnifier, but nobody had asked me. So my mother bought me a magnifier and the problem was solved. School helped my dad and me bond a lot because he helped me with lots of projects when I couldn't see well enough to do them alone. The school didn't like it, but my parents stuck up for me.

The second year they let me do everything. In PE, I did track. I didn't do volleyball because I kept getting hit in the face with the ball. We played volleyball outside, and when I saw the sun, I'd think the sun was the volleyball. I did basketball and I did a lot of after-school sports and volunteering because my way to achieve recognition was to do volunteer work.

I became a competitive speaker in the seventh and eighth grades. I was on varsity by the end of seventh grade, and I was one of the leading students on the debate team in spontaneous speaking. I went to the state contest and did very well. I got a lot second- and third-place awards. I think the reason I didn't get first place a lot was because I didn't have skills in eye contact and body language. Those are legitimate skills that I went on to learn in high school, and then I started getting more first places. I had to be taught in a physical way what body language and eye contact are.

I really appreciated the teachers in high school who would accommodate me but who had high expectations. They would ask me, "What can I do that would make this better for you?" but they wouldn't let me slide at all academically. There was a math teacher, an old gruff guy. He would accommodate me, but I had to achieve and I had to earn my grade. I always got B's from him but I respected him so much more than some other teachers who gave me easy A's. The same thing happened in college. I always appreciated the teachers who expected the most out of me and worked my hardest in their classes. I also got the most out of them.

I didn't have a lot of friends in junior high school and high school. Some teachers liked me, but I never had any other children who saw me as their best friend, with one exception, who was a fellow isolate with a disability. I had people who respected me for what I did well, especially in my competitive speech. I even mentored some of them. I did get respect from my peers, and I wanted that. But as far as an intimate friendship with any of my peers, I didn't have it.

My family believed that I would always need to be taken care of and struggled with how they would handle that. My uncle expected more of me than anyone else in the family. He was only nine years older than I was, and we became a bonded pair. He would not baby me at all. He was tough on me. The relatives thought he was a mean person but, in fact, he treated me like an equal. He didn't treat me like a disabled child, and that was the difference. It has always been that way between us.

It has always been true for me that it doesn't matter what the bulk of the people think about me. What has mattered are the thoughts of those significant to me. I like to be professional and have the respect of others whom I respect.

An early mentor for me was my junior high speech coach because he saw my talent and he demanded that I fulfill my potential. In high school, it was my psychology teacher who pushed me to achieve. He made me recognize that there were going to be things that were very hard for me to do, but he expected me to do them anyway. He knew I might not be the best at some things, but he wouldn't let me use my disability as an excuse not to learn basic academic skills. He believed I could go to college and helped me get there. He pushed me and I responded. He helped me get into Cal State Long Beach, where I met two women who became my heroes—Norma Gibbs and Kay Goddard. Kay was the assistant dean of student activities. She started by treating me like I was going to be a professional—not a disabled client, but a professional. Disabilities never really came up in our conversations. She knew I was disabled, but we would just talk about things I needed to develop. She was a person whom I really chose to relate to. Norma is disabled; she had TB. Norma believed in me in even a broader sense—spiritually as well as professionally. She is my picture of a lady, but a lady with no pretense of being anything but what she is. She helped me gain a sense that we should really go out and taste life.

Since those times, Anita Baldwin has become a person I really respect. When issues of blindness come up, I turn to Anita because she has a disability similar to mine. June Kailes has become a role model for me too. June has a disability and has been a leader in the disability movement. June and I are, in fact, role models for each other. We have high expectations of each other and never let up on each other. We always try to make each other better. We motivate and set standards for each other. I compare myself to June to make sure I measure up to her and earn her respect.

As people with disabilities, we have made progress. In the old days, if we wanted to affect social policy, we were dead before we got to the door. Now we've got people with disabilities in positions to make decisions. But we have a long way to go. There are some important things to know about policy development. First, policy is developed by individuals, and those individuals have biases that are incorporated in policy. When policy makers have biases about people who have disabilities of some type, whether intellectual, physical, or sensory, those people are discounted.

Biases against people with disabilities are usually based on pity. We are viewed as not being capable. That view is then incorporated into policy, which is put into practice. Then the system teaches the persons who are discounted in the policy that they should behave in the way predicted in the policy. We do this to disabled people but also to welfare recipients and others.

If the bias is that disabled people can't work, then systems are set up with workers whose job it is to keep people on disability benefits and away from work. We end up with a self-fulfilling prophecy from the creation of the policy. So a major task for people with disabilities is to modify the biases of policy makers. Policy makers need to recognize that accommodations must be made for people with disabilities. But they must also make the assumption that no class of people is burdened by the characteristic of incompetence. There may be individuals in that class—disabled, poor, or other—who will not achieve. But within the class, we must, as a matter of policy, make policy with the assumption that incompetence is an individual characteristic, not a class characteristic. Policy must then be developed with incentives from birth to tell people in society, whoever they are, that they are responsible for achieving to their potential. The tools must then be in place to reinforce that message. We need both public and private polices because the government isn't going to fix it all. The message must be sent early to people with disabilities that we are responsible for ourselves. The message must also be sent that other people are responsible for assisting in areas where assistance needs to happen. Finally, we need to accept people's potential, and we need to judge people on what they do with what they are given.

Another side of the issue rests within people. People with disabilities have to step out of the victim role and take on responsibility for our lives. When we are in bad situations or miserable, we need to take the challenge to get out of it. We need support systems to do that, but it is up to us to do it. We talk about "abs" (able-bodied people) and how they have done things to us. But it is up to us to make things change. People can give 25,000 excuses about why they can't do anything to make things better because they are disabled. I say to them that, as a policy maker, I'm only as powerful in my position as the community that backs me. If I don't have that backing, I have no power in my position at all.

I think it's important for people to get in touch with who they are, who they belong to, their power base. Whether it's women who get in touch with themselves or people with disabilities or whoever, I like to see it happen. Their identity is based on the oneness, something they can be part of. To have empowerment, we need to have something to believe in, something to attach ourselves to.

Going through some of the things my disability has made me go through has given me the character to deal with things and achieve what I need to achieve. Having a disability and saying, "I'm not going to let people's opinions or stereotypes hold me down," has created the strength to do what I've done. I can say that if I had a choice between having my disability and having that character or not having the disability and having what I have seen in what are called able-bodied people, I would rather have the disability. It isn't that I'm proud of being blind. It's that I'm pleased that I used what came to me in a constructive way.

What you do with what you get determines whether you succeed or not. Whether it is gender or ethnicity or disability, you get what comes and there's no second chance. We have to use the tools in our toolkits. My disability was a tool, an opportunity from which I could gain, and it was also a barrier from which I could lose. Every day I confront situations where I can make the choice to use the disability as a gainer or a loser; I choose to use it as a gainer.

In offering advice to professionals, first, I think language is important. There's a reason we say "persons with disabilities." People with disabilities are members of the pool of humanity who have a characteristic that affects their lives—some more, some less. Disability affects people's personalities and affects them emotionally, but it is one of a whole range of things that affects their lives. Second, don't discount anyone based on their disability. Don't believe that anyone is incapable of any task because of what you see before you. There may be tasks that some people can't perform at this moment but could do if given the support to develop their potential. Some of our greatest inventions have been made by refusing to limit ourselves by what we see today and envisioning what is possible in the future. A prime example is telecommunication devices for the deaf.

I would say that the first thing people should drop from their vocabulary is the word *can't*. Once that word is incorporated, it stops creativity and the potential for development of things that eventually will benefit all of society. For example, speech-activated computers were developed for various disabled people, but pretty soon lawyers, court reporters, and others began using them. And all because someone decided it was possible to solve a problem.

Another thing I would say is that people with disabilities are capable of thinking and doing what anybody else does—good,

bad, or indifferent. Don't make us angels and don't make us dev-
ils. There are stupid, angry people with disabilities and there are
people who are very capable. Professionals need to understand
that. Do not stereotype us.

DISCUSSION QUESTIONS

1. What are some of the major issues in defining persons who are blind or
   visually impaired? What cautions must be applied when one is looking at
   functional definitions?
2. How might persons who are blind or visually impaired internalize societal
   stereotypes that result in feelings of inadequacy and depression?
3. Explain how some social service agencies providing services to persons
   who are blind or visually impaired might foster oppression rather than
   empowerment. What kinds of things could social service agencies do to
   avoid this?
4. Prepare a list of jobs that many people in the United States commonly
   think a person who is blind or visually impaired could not do. Then discuss what accommodations could help a person who is blind or visually
   impaired accomplish each of the jobs on your list.
5. Discuss both sides of the issue of preferential treatment for persons who
   are blind or visually impaired. Which argument do you think is stronger,
   and why?
6. What are some of the unique issues concerning persons who are deaf-
   blind? As a practitioner, how would you accommodate a person who is
   both blind and deaf?

SUGGESTED READINGS

Alexander, S. (2000). *Do you remember the color blue? The questions children ask
about being blind.* New York: Penguin Books.
Koesder, F. A. (1976). *The unseen minority: A social history of blindness in America.*
New York: David McKay.
Scott, R. (1969). *The making of blind men: A study of adult socialization.* New York:
Russell Sage Foundation.
Stroman, D. F. (1982). *The awakening minorities: The physically handicapped.* Lan-
ham, MD: University Press of America.
tenBroek, J., & Matson, F. W. (1959). *Hope deferred: Public welfare and the blind.*
Berkeley: University of California Press.

REFERENCES

Albrecht, G. (1992). *The disability business: Rehabilitation in America.* Newbury
Park, CA: Sage.

Beers, M. H. (Ed.). (2003). *The Merck manual of medical information* (2nd ed.). New York: Simon & Schuster.

Berkowitz, E. D. (1987). *Disabled policy: American programs for the handicapped.* London: Cambridge University Press.

Dickson, M. B. (1994). *Working effectively with people who are blind or visually impaired.* Ithaca, NY: ILR Program on Employment and Disability, Cornell University.

Goode, D. (1994). *A world with words: The social construction of children born deaf and blind.* Philadelphia: Temple University Press.

Hogan, J. (2005). There's one rule for the rich . . . anyone trying to redistribute wealth in a market economy may be up against a law of nature. *New Scientist, 185,* 6–7. Retrieved September 11, 2006, from Expanded Academic ASAP via Thomson Gale.

Holte, L., Prickett, J. G., Van Dyke, D. C., Olson, R. J., Lubrica, P., Knutson, C. L., et al. (2006). Issues in the evaluation of infants and young children who are suspected of or who are deaf/blind. *Infants & Young Children, 19*(3), 213–227.

Koestler, F. A. (1976). *The unseen minority: A social history of blindness in America.* New York: David McKay.

Large, T. (1993). The effects of attitudes upon the blind: A reexamination. In M. Nagler (Ed.), *Perspectives on disability: Text and readings on disability* (2nd ed., pp. 165–168). Palo Alto, CA: Health Markets Research.

Meeting the needs of the deaf-blind child. (1994). *Future Reflections, 13*(1). Retrieved September 13, 2006, from http://www.nfb.org/Images/nfb/Publications/fr/fr1/94win.htm

National Federation of the Blind. (n.d.). *The courtesy rules of blindness.* Retrieved September 9, 2006, from http://www.nfb.org/nfb/courtesy_rules.asp?SnID = 176 6641712

Newberry, F. (1993). The blind child: Becoming an independent adult. *Future Reflections, 12*(2), 4–11. Retrieved September 12, 2006, from http://www.nfb.org/Images/nfb/Publications/fr/fr1/93sprsum.htm

Number of blind and vision-impaired Americans expected to increase. (2004). *Review of Optometry, 141,* 9. Retrieved September 6, 2006, from Expanded Academic ASAP via Thomson Gale.

Pharr, S. (1988). *Homophobia: A weapon of sexism.* Inverness, CA: Chardon Press.

Prickett, J. G., & Welch, T. R. (1995). Adapting environments to support the inclusion of students who are deaf-blind. In N. G. Haring & L. T. Romer (Eds.), *Welcoming students who are deaf-blind into typical classrooms: Facilitating school participation, learning, and friendship* (pp. 171–193). Baltimore: Paul H. Brookes.

Richert, M. (2002). Surveying our field: Dividing lines and common boundaries. *Re:view in Health, 34,* 3–4. Retrieved September 10, 2006, from Expanded Academic ASAP via Thomson Gale.

Sasse, H. (2006). *Deafblind FAQ.* Retrieved September 11, 2006, from http://www.deafblind.co.uk/deafblnd_faq.html#5

Scott, R. (1969). *The making of blind men: A study of adult socialization.* New York: Russell Sage Foundation.

Shapiro, J. P. (1993). *No pity: People with disabilities forging a new civil rights movement*. New York: Time Books.

Shore, Z. (1993). Free rides for the blind cost us too much. *Future Reflections, 12,* 1. Retrieved September 12, 2006, from http://www.nfb.org/Images/nfb/Publica tions/fr/fr1/93win.htm

Solomon, B. (1976). *Black empowerment: Social work in oppressed communities.* New York: Columbia University Press.

Stroman, D. E. (1982). *The awakening minorities: The physically handicapped.* Lanham, MD: University Press of America.

tenBroek, J. (1993). Pros and cons of preferential treatment of blind persons. *Future Reflections, 12* (1). Retrieved September 12, 2006, from http://www.nfb.org/ Images/nfb/Publications/fr/fr1/93win.htm

tenBroek, J., & Matson, E. W. (1959). *Hope deferred: Public welfare and the blind.* Berkeley: University of California Press.

Thompson, R. P., & Freeman, C. W. (1995). A history of federal support for students with deafblindness. In N. G. Haring & L. T. Romer (Eds.), *Welcoming students who are deaf-blind into typical classrooms: Facilitating school participation, learning, and friendship* (pp. 17–35). Baltimore: Paul H. Brookes.

Thylefors, B., Negrel, A.-D., Pararajasegaram, R., & Dadzie, K. Y. (1995). Global data on blindness. *Bulletin of the World Health Organization, 73* (1), 115–121. Retrieved September 6, 2006, from Expanded Academic ASAP via Thomson Gale.

Tierney, L. M., McPhee, S. J., & Papadakis, M. A. (Eds.). (2006). *Current medical diagnosis and treatment.* New York: Lang Medical Books/McGraw-Hill.

Vaughan, C. E. (1993). Origins of conflicting professional and consumer images of blindness. *Journal of Rehabilitation, 59* (1), 10–15. Retrieved September 6, 2006, from Expanded Academic ASAP via Thomson Gale.

World Health Organization. (2002). Magnitude and causes of visual impairment. Retrieved October 6, 2008, from http://www.who.int/mediacentre/factsheets/ fs282/en/

Winnick, J. P. (Ed.). (2005). *Adapted physical education and support* (4th ed.). Champaign, IL: Human Kinetics.

9

Developmental Disabilities

People First is saying, "Treat people first and everything else is second." Change your low expectations to positive expectations. People's minds are sort of warped about disabilities because they haven't gotten an education. Society's low expectations have said, "If somebody is different than me, let's lock them away." Something's got to change, and I think that change is positive thinking. People First helps people know what they want to do and stand up to people who say, "You can't do that." We can advocate for people. People First can go into the institutions and educate those people to stand up to the staff. We help them get out of institutions.

—Resa Hayes, disability activist, People First of Washington

STUDENT LEARNING OBJECTIVES

1. To understand issues around defining developmental disabilities
2. To understand the many varieties of developmental disabilities
3. To develop a very basic knowledge of the major developmental disabilities likely to be experienced by clients and consumers
4. To understand issues of autonomy regarding persons with developmental disabilities

The National Association of Councils on Developmental Disabilities (n.d.) estimates that approximately 4 million Americans are experiencing developmental disabilities. Five to ten percent of all children have some form of developmental disability (Moeschler & Shevell, 2006). The foundations of most of the various definitions of developmental disabilities can be found in the federal definition of developmental disability. The current revision of the Developmental Disabilities Assistance and Bill of Rights Act of 2000 defines developmental disabilities as disabilities that are severe and chronic in nature. They are caused by mental and/or physical impairment, present themselves before the person becomes twenty-two, have a strong probability of being present for the rest of the person's life, and significantly limit a person's ability to carry on major life activities, including the ability to live independently and earn a living. Developmental disabilities also include disabilities that are believed to require some kind of intervention, care, or treatment for a long duration, if not for life. Children from birth to the age of nine with significant developmental delays or congenital or acquired conditions can be considered developmentally disabled even if they do not meet three or more of these criteria (U.S. Department of Health and Human Services, Administration for Children and Families, n.d.).

For all practical purposes, the federal definition of developmental disability encompasses most disabilities acquired before the age of twenty-two. Accordingly, if the onset is early and the disability is severe enough to interfere with several major life functions, the condition can be defined as a developmental disability. The National Association of Councils on Developmental Disabilities (n.d.) expands a bit on the federal definition by including individuals with a disability that may not be visible but still limits their life functioning.

Many states have taken it upon themselves to narrow the definition of developmental disability. For example, California defines developmental disability as occurring before the age of eighteen. The California definition includes specific categories of disabilities that are eligible for services, including mental retardation, epilepsy, cerebral palsy, autism, and any disability requiring services similar to those required for mental retardation. These categorical definitions carry a danger of excluding individuals who do not fit predetermined diagnostic categories but share similar functional characteristics and needs. California laws define substantial disability along the federal guidelines (State Council on Developmental Disabilities, n.d.).

No matter which of these definitions we use, several problems occur with any definition of developmental disability that includes intellectual disability. First, as Ansello (1992) points out, although service benefits are linked to classification as developmentally disabled, groups such as people who are blind, who have cerebral palsy, and who are deaf resist being identified as developmentally disabled. A primary reason appears to be the connection of the term *developmental disability* with mental retardation. Categorization as mentally retarded carries with it a significant social stigma. Much of the early legislative and service provisions concerned with developmental disability centered on persons who were diagnosed as mentally retarded. Mental retardation is specifically named in many state definitions of developmental disability, including that of California. Persons who are intellectually disabled have such a low status in our society that few, including many professionals, want to be associated with this group (Hall, Ford, Moss, & Dineen, 1986).

Second, implied by some writers (Smith, 1994) and experienced by many involved in the independent living movement is a kind of dualism: nondisabled reformers use the words of independent living, but the resulting policy and programs leave this ideal far behind. In examining the civil rights quest for persons with developmental disabilities, Shapiro (1993) found extensive parental involvement. Despite great legislative and service provision success, it is still parents doing for their children. This paternalistic value has been translated to some degree into service providers' mentality. Many professionals have an underlying resistance to allowing persons with developmental disabilities to take control of their own lives (Dudley, 1987). This paternalism is repulsive to other groups of persons with disabilities with an independent living perspective, and they in no way seek to be connected with this value of dependence.

Most problems with an inclusive definition of developmental disability have to do with stigma and economics. But a broad definition of developmental disability, cemented in a social context, allows the incorporation of the breadth and complexity of these particular types of disabilities. It also fits within the values of the independent living movement—that persons with different disabilities have more characteristics in common than differences.

Much of the literature and several legal statutes agree that intellectual disability (mental retardation), Down syndrome, autism, epilepsy, and cerebral palsy fall under the category of developmental disability. Since we have explored cerebral palsy under mobility disability, we will concentrate here on intellectual disabilities, Down syndrome, autism, and epilepsy.

INTELLECTUAL DISABILITY (MENTAL RETARDATION)

Evans (1991) traces the evolution of the definition of mental retardation. Intelligence quotient testing started in Paris as a way to determine which students required special education, and an IQ score of two standard deviations below the mean is still one of the major criteria used to determine mental retardation. However, efforts have been made to replace this simplistic diagnostic method. The American Association on Mental Deficiency (which later became the American Association on Mental Retardation and is now the American Association on Intellectual and Developmental Disabilities) first created an adaptive functioning method of classification in response to the limitations of IQ testing. The association used four categories of classification of mental retardation: mild, moderate, severe, and profound. According to this classification system, people who had mild mental retardation could achieve employment on a semi-skilled or unskilled level. They functioned independently, owned their own homes and cars, and generally had families. People who had moderate mental retardation might achieve self-maintenance in unskilled or semi-skilled work, sometimes under accommodated work environments, including sheltered conditions and supported employment. They generally lived with their families or in group home situations. People who had severe mental retardation might help in their own maintenance but generally required supervision in work and living environ-ments. People who had profound mental retardation had limited motor and speech skills. They might achieve limited self-care and needed extensive attendant or nursing care.

In the mid-1990s, the American Association on Mental Retardation revised and simplified its definition of mental retardation as a basic difficulty in learning and performing certain daily, personal, and life skills. Specific limitations included those of a conceptual, practical, and social intelligence nature. According to the association, a person with mental retardation had limitations only in conceptual, practical, and social intelligence. Other areas, such as health and personality, were not included. The one differentiating characteristic of a person with mental retardation was a standard IQ score of 70 to 75 or below, assessed based on a variety of indicators. Based upon these criteria, a person either did or did not have mental retardation. The gradations of mild, moderate, severe, and profound were removed (American Association on Mental Retardation, 1992).

In the first decade of the 2000s, the American Association on Mental Retardation readdressed the definition of mental retardation and changed its name to the American Association on Intellectual and Developmental Dis-abilities (AAIDD). The AAIDD's definition of mental retardation falls squarely within the social model of disability. They define mental retardation as a condition characterized by both intellectual and adaptive limitations. These limitations are manifested in conceptual, social, and adaptive skills. Mental retardation comes about before the age of eighteen. The AAIDD's definition involves five criteria. First, the intellectual and adaptive limitations must exist within the context of the typical environmental system, including age of peers and culture. Second, when a person is diagnosed as having mental retardation, the assessor needs to consider cultural and language dif-ferences as well as community diversity. Third, strengths as well as limita-tions should be taken into account. Fourth, a profile of needed supports must exist. And fifth, it is likely that with the proper supports, life functioning will improve (American Association on Mental Retardation, 2006).

Generally intellectual disabilities do not manifest until preschool. Usu-ally the first characteristic of an intellectual disability emerges as a delay in language development. Many times social development is also atypical because of the language delay. Children with an intellectual disability may learn to dress and feed themselves at a slower rate than a typical child. Some-times, children with an intellectual disability may have behavioral issues, including emotional outbursts, temper tantrums, and/or physically aggres-sive behavioral patterns. In most cases, these characteristics are not endemic to an intellectual disability but are rather a result of environmental frustration and social isolation. Depression may also come about because of social stigma (Beers, 2003).

From the mythology perpetuated by films such as *Forrest Gump,* one might assume that life for persons who are intellectually disabled is truly like "a box of chocolates." If people with intellectual disabilities have supportive families and try hard, they will be financially and socially successful and may even meet or be the president. However, the lives of most people with intellectual disabilities can be ones of misconception, confinement, and stigma.

Dudley (1987) has found that the general public as well as professionals hold several significant misconceptions about persons with intellectual disabilities. The first misconception is that persons with intellectual disabilities have no awareness or understanding of their disability. The reality is that most do and can describe their disability in detail. The second misconception is that persons with intellectual disabilities are passive or indifferent to the pejorative language used to describe them, including the term *mentally retarded.* The reality is that most people with intellectual disabilities do not like the term because of the stigmas attached to it. Furthermore, they do not like the jokes and the negative way they are portrayed in jest. The third misconception is that persons with intellectual disabilities are unaware of the demeaning way they are treated by society in general and professionals in particular. The reality is that most people with intellectual disabilities do not like to be confined in institutions, told what to do with their lives, stared at, joked about, or patronized by professionals.

These misconceptions, if unchallenged and unrecognized by human service professionals, can have dire consequences. Professionals who are unaware that they are guided by these misconceptions may perpetuate them: they may choose to do for consumers rather than help consumers speak and do for themselves. Professionals may bypass consulting consumers in developing plans of action rather than viewing consumer participation in plan development and implementation as crucial. Professionals may feel persons with intellectual disabilities do not have the intellectual capability to know what is best for their lives. In addition, professionals may relinquish a prime opportunity for change and insight by assuming that individuals don't want to talk about their disability. Professionals may actually tear down self-concept with their unwillingness to discuss the disability, reinforcing consumers' fears that their disabilities are too "horrible and undesirable to mention" (Dudley, 1987, p. 81).

One of the authors of this text, as a part of his role as executive director of an independent living center, wrote a grant for a program to develop self-advocacy skills for people experiencing developmental disabilities. The core piece of the program centered on training folks with developmental disabilities to actually train others with similar disabilities in self-advocacy skills. The grant was accepted, with some changes made by a state program designed to provide service provision for people with developmental disabilities. Before the funds were allocated, a delegation from the governmental entity that funded the grant came to visit the author in his office. They wanted to change the peer training component of the program. They wanted the individuals with developmental disabilities to be trained by professionals rather than others with developmental disabilities. The author rejected their request, and the grant was never funded. The belief demonstrated by this governmental entity whose primary mission was providing services for people with developmental disabilities was that people with developmental disabilities are not capable of training or being trained to teach self-advocacy skills to others.

Professionals can help people with intellectual disabilities and their families understand their rights, maximize their potential, and develop resources. For example, DePoy and Werrbach (1996) describe a day program in which persons with intellectual disabilities were responsible for developing rules and programming. Participants were cognizant of their strengths and limitations. They enlisted professional support to assist in enforcing rules and managing problems but maintained great programmatic control. The following two cases provide contrasting examples of the effects that professional attitudes and advice have on lives.

From Evan's birth, it was clear he had developmental disabilities. His family was told by health care providers that Evan should be placed in a state institution for the mentally retarded. Evan, who had an IQ of about 65, spent his life in a state training school with four hundred others with similar disabilities. The staff who cared for Evan concurrently cared for ten to twenty other "patients." Individual attention was rare. Though most were caring and devoted, staff members had little time to help Evan become toilet trained, learn to dress independently, or become independent in other activities of daily living. It was assumed that Evan had little ability to learn. Time for individual nurturing activities such as reading or cuddling was scarce. Evan's social worker maintained contact with Evan's parents, who were encouraged to visit him periodically. She thought Evan was a "sweet boy" but—like Evan's physician, nurses, therapists, and nurse's aides—saw Evan as needing lifelong care and treatment in an institution. When Evan reached adolescence and developed a crush on another patient, contact between the two was discouraged and prevented. When they kissed, their behavior was labeled inappropriate sexual conduct. Evan's girlfriend was sterilized.

Evan died in his early thirties, a result of cardiovascular problems present from birth. Evan had received treatment for his symptoms throughout his life; however, he had not received aggressive treatments that nondisabled children with similar medical problems receive. Although it cannot be stated with certainty, aggressive treatment may have helped Evan live longer. Evan's life was full of caring professionals and caregivers who reinforced his dependence and low functioning. His life consisted of few choices and no opportunities to live outside a large institution.

In contrast, Myra, who had intellectual abilities similar to Evan's, was reared in her family's home. Public health nurses helped educate Myra's parents about her early care needs. A social worker informed the family of early therapeutic and educational opportunities, which they utilized. Myra was enrolled in Head Start and later in public school. By the time Myra began public school, she was independent in toileting, dressing, and grooming herself. Myra was able to attend public schools throughout childhood. She was socially and academically delayed; however, with resource education and one-on-one attention from classroom aides, she developed many more skills than Evan. Myra's parents consulted with an educational psychologist, who helped them negotiate with the school district to ensure they had adequate resources. Myra developed social relationships with classmates and with other children in her neighborhood. She was also involved with school and social groups for children with intellectual disabilities. She had several boyfriends in adolescence. By age twenty, Myra wanted to live away from her family. With the help of the local independent living center, she moved into a supported apartment with a roommate. A social services worker visited to help Myra with finances and other needs. Myra obtained a job bagging groceries, used public transportation independently, and attended social functions for people with intellectual disabilities. She dates and talks about getting married someday.

The lives of Evan and Myra differ dramatically. Professionals in Evan's life assumed he had few abilities and needed constant care and protection. In contrast, professionals in Myra's life helped her family and provided opportunities for Myra to maximize her potential and independence.

Down syndrome

Although some professionals view intellectual disability and Down syndrome as synonymous, because of the many components of Down syndrome that do not affect intellectual development, we deal with it separately. Down syndrome gets its name from Dr. John Langdon-Down, a physician at the London Hospital in the mid-1800s. His place in history stems from his innovative work training children with intellectual disabilities. In his writings, he classified patients according to their facial characteristics. He labeled the characteristics of one such group Mongolism. In the mid-1960s, the Mongolian People's Republic successfully petitioned the World Health Organization to change the name to Down's syndrome (Davies & Hollman, 2001). The National Dissemination Center for Children with Disabilities (2004) estimates that approximately 4,000 children are born with Down syndrome in the United States each year (one in every 800–1,000 live births). The incidence of Down syndrome increases with maternal age at conception, but parents of any age may have a child with Down syndrome.

There are about 250,000 individuals living in the United States with Down syndrome. Although they have differences, people with Down syndrome are more similar than not to individuals without Down syndrome. Although individuals with Down syndrome share several characteristics, they display a vast array of differences. Like the aggregate population, people with Down syndrome exhibit a wide range of personalities, intelligence levels, and styles of human interaction. Individuals with Down syndrome have a high rate of congenital heart defects (35–50 percent). Physical characteristics of persons with Down syndrome include short stature and a small nose with a flat bridge. Additional characteristics include almond-shaped eyes with white Brushfield spots on the irises, a single palmar crease on one or both hands, and small features. Children with Down syndrome look more like members of their families than they do one another.

On standard IQ tests, persons with Down syndrome can score poorly. However, these tests are limited because they do not measure many important areas of intelligence, and persons with Down syndrome often have good memory and insight, and a great deal of creativity and cleverness. The high rate of learning disabilities in persons with Down syndrome sometimes masks their range of abilities and talents.

There are three major types of Down syndrome, of which trisomy 21 is the most common. Trisomy 21 occurs when an individual carries a third twenty-first chromosome rather than the usual pair as a result of the sperm or egg cell failing to divide properly. About 90 percent of people with Down syndrome have trisomy 21. Translocation Down syndrome occurs when the extra twenty-first chromosome breaks off and becomes attached to and exchanges genetic material with another chromosome. Mosaic Down syndrome occurs when only some of the individual's cells have trisomy 21. Incidences of translocation and mosaic Down syndrome are uncommon (Mayo Clinic, 2006).

One of the most prominent pejorative social constructions of Down syndrome centers on the idea that there is no joy to be found in children with this disability. Parent after parent discusses the bias of the medical and social service professionals systems against having children with disabilities, and particularly Down syndrome children. Vicki Noble (1993), in speaking about her son Aaron Eagle, reflects upon this negative bias:

> I worry about the way in which technology has developed a routine amniocentesis, so that any woman can know in advance that she carries a child with Down syndrome and make a supposedly informed choice about whether or not to carry her pregnancy to term. As a feminist, I have no conflicts with a woman's right to choose any form of birth control, an abortion when all else fails. But I'm worried about the seeming consensus that a woman would naturally not want to give birth to a child with "chromosomal damage," in other words, a child like Aaron Eagle. I'm worried about the powerful unspoken agreement in this modern medical approach that wants to eliminate "defectives" from the population. (p. 6)

Hanson (2003) addressed this issue by interviewing families who participated in an early intervention program between 1974 and 1975. The findings go a long way toward breaking down some of the mythology around the process of raising a child with Down syndrome. First, parents found many positive characteristics of children with Down syndrome. They saw their children as a delight and fun. They observed that the children had positive attitudes and personalities. Children were viewed as full participants in the family process. Second, parents found the actual rearing of a child with Down syndrome a positive experience. In fact, many parents in the study experienced their children without Down syndrome as being more difficult to raise because of the looming issues of drug use, teenage sex, and downright obstinate behavior.

Parents interviewed in the study also encountered challenges. Parents experienced the stigma of having a disabled child. The medical complications that can be a part of raising a child with Down syndrome often created both significant economic and psychological drains for the family. In addition, parents worried about the lack of services and support after their child reached the age of twenty-one. Related to the lack of support was parental concern about the lack of independence and development of a social network for their children. Finally, parents addressed their own social isolation resulting from having a disabled child. It is important to understand that most of the problems parents experienced can be traced to the lack of environmental/societal acceptance and support, not the innate characteristics of their children.

AUTISM

The following song expresses the mystery and complexity of autism:

> Damon, the young dreamer, whose only purpose is in dreaming;
> Caught up in a fairy tale, I fear you've been sleeping.
> Trusting is so simple in the child-like way you live.
> Candle burns in silence; light grows ever dim.
> Was your spirit lost and not regained?
> Do you suffer some unknown private pain?
> Damon, can you reveal the secrets your dark eyes are keeping?
> The ghost of the drifter haunts your soul, I fear.
> Is there an unknown voice you alone can hear?
> Living in the past is so much safer, they all say.
> And you have grown secure, accustomed to your ways.
> Will you live in silence, all alone;
> An island in the sea, so far from home?
> Damon, is it true that you exist just for these brief moments?
> Damon, do you believe that we all are children;
> Drifting aimlessly, too busy to even listen?
> My eyes are filled with tears; I do not trust myself to speak.

There's a sadness in your countenance that makes my heart grow weak.
If there were a time to live in chains, will it pass or is it now too late?
Damon, how can you be certain you are not mistaken? (Crevak, 1976)

The song was written by a young therapist, songwriter, and performer to express his disappointment at not being able to reach a young man with autism with whom he regularly worked. The complexity of his client's behavior and thinking perplexed the young social worker. Karande (2006) defines autism as a complex neurodevelopmental disorder that affects social interaction and communication. It can be characterized by repetitive behavior patterns and repetitive interests and activities. The condition is usually evident by the age of three. The *DSM-IV* defines autistic disorder as involving very specific symptoms in the areas of social interaction, communication, and behavior. Commonly referred to today as autism spectrum disorder, it can result in a wide variety of behavioral characteristics. The diagnosis of pervasive developmental disorder not otherwise specified is used when a child displays behaviors similar to those that characterize autistic disorder but does not meet the specific criteria (American Psychiatric Association, 2000).

Studies conducted in the United States, the United Kingdom, various European countries, and Japan estimate that approximately 7 in 10,000 individuals under the age of eighteen experience autism. Generally, males are more likely than females to have autism (about four boys to one girl). Data collected in the mid-2000s indicate that the incidence of autism has almost tripled, probably reflecting improved diagnosis techniques. There are several theories on the cause of autism. Functional brain imaging studies indicate different temporal lobe functioning than observed in a typical brain. Other studies indicate high levels of serotonin in the developing fetus, resulting in neurocircuitry damage. Genetic factors may play a role in some types of autism, as there is a higher incidence rate among siblings. Emerging research indicates that over ten genes contribute to the risk of autism (Karande, 2006).

The Treatment and Education of Autistic and Related Communication-Handicapped Children lists several characteristics of persons with autism (TEACCH, 2006). One characteristic is that they sometimes have difficulty with language development. Language may not develop at all, or if it does, the person uses words or phrases that do not have standard meanings. Sometimes speech is formal and delivered in a monotone manner. For Grandin (1992), a person with autism, the inability to speak as a child was totally frustrating. When her parents or other adults spoke to her, she could understand them but could not respond. Sometimes the only way she could communicate was to scream.

Persons with autism may also have inconsistent patterns of sensory responses (TEACCH, 2006). At times they may not respond at all to sound.

Other times their reaction may be overresponsive. Grandin (1992) states that her hearing was at one extreme or the other. Noises were so loud that she literally had to shut her hearing down. At times her mother thought she was deaf.

The same response swing may occur with pain, heat, cold, or even human touch. Grandin (1995) recounts how she dealt with this—avoidance of human touch. She craved human touch but pulled away from its intensity: "From as far back as I can remember, I always hated to be hugged. I wanted to experience the good feeling of being hugged, but it was just too overwhelming. It was like a great, all-engulfing tidal wave of stimulation, and I reacted like a wild animal. Being touched triggered flight; it flipped my circuit breaker. I was overloaded and would have to escape, often by jerking away suddenly" (p. 62).

In addition, persons with autism may exhibit high levels of intellectual functioning in some areas, and very low levels in other areas. They may have excellent skills in drawing but may not understand composition balance. They may have perfect pitch but not understand rhythm. They may have highly developed computational skills in math but don't understand how to use the skills effectively (TEACCH, 2006). Grandin (1992) discusses this inconsistency in herself. She had perfect pitch and could hum a tune, note for note, that she had heard just once or twice. But she could not master rhythm. Alone, her rhythm was steady. When she tried to clap along with others, however, she had great difficulty.

Finally, persons with autism may exhibit repetitive body movements or repetitive actions. If the routines or repetitions are changed, they may react in a distressed manner (TEACCH, 2006). One of the authors worked with a twelve-year-old boy with autism who, if left alone, would sit on a table cross-legged, methodically tearing a tissue in two, eating half, and stacking the other half neatly to his side. If unsupervised, he would do this continually. When directed toward another task, the youngster would become extremely upset.

Special note needs to be made of a subgroup of autism. Individuals with Asperger syndrome share many of the characteristics of those with autism but have no history of language delay. Their intellectual ability is within the average or above average range. Children with Asperger syndrome appear to have difficulty with the social use of language. This lack of social language use affects their ability to maintain friends and social relationships. These characteristics are generally exhibited when the child reaches the school environment (Block & Groft, 2003; Griswold, Barnhill, Miles, Hagiwara, & Simpson, 2002; Karande, 2006).

Grandin (1992) offers insight for people working with persons with autism. She discusses those who were most helpful to her in helping her achieve her life goals and those who were not. Generally, people who could help her capitalize on her strengths were most helpful: the governess who kept her and her sister busy with structured activities that had narrow choices; the science teacher who helped her translate various fixations into actual scientific problems with great practicality, which eventually led her to her academic career; her mother, who took an active interest in her elementary and high school education; the manager of a local firm who supported her interest in the livestock industry while she was in college and who hired her for her first designing job. Grandin's (1995) indictment of traditional human service professionals is sobering: "As I grew older, the people who were of the greatest assistance were always the more creative, unconventional types. Psychiatrists and psychologists were of little help. They were too busy trying to psychoanalyze me and discover my deep dark psychological problems. One psychiatrist thought if he could find my 'psychic injury,' I would be cured. The high school psychologist wanted to stamp out my fixations on things like doors instead of trying to understand them and use them to stimulate learning" (pp. 98–99).

A most significant skill for anyone in the human service industry working with persons with autism as well as other disabilities is the ability to move away from dogma, ideology, and set ways and to address individuals on their own terms, using their strengths as the beginning points of action.

SEIZURE DISORDERS (EPILEPSY)

Seizure disorder (epilepsy) is a term that defines conditions associated with recurrent seizures. Because of the social stigma tied to the condition, people experiencing this condition generally prefer the term *seizure disorder* rather than *epilepsy*. In addition, many people with seizure disorder resist being classified as persons with developmental disabilities. We place seizure disorder in this chapter because this classification reflects current state and federal definitions. In the United States, the United Kingdom, continental Europe, and Japan, seizure disorder occurs in about 50 per 100,000 people per year (Duncan, Sander, Sisodoya, & Walker, 2006). About 0.5–2.5 percent of the population in the United States has conditions resulting in recurrent seizures. Seizure disorder usually affects children, young adults, and people over the age of sixty-five, although anyone at any age can develop a seizure disorder (Tierney, McPhee, & Papadakis, 2006).

Causes of seizure disorder can be grouped into seven categories. Seizures occurring in infancy and childhood can be caused by congenital issues and perinatal injuries. Metabolic disorders, including withdrawal from drugs and/or alcohol, can result in seizures. Other metabolic disorders such as uremia, hypoglycemia, and hyperglycemia may result in seizures, particularly in young adults. Seizures may develop years after the initial trauma. Tumors and lesions may cause seizure disorder. This is particularly the case in middle and later life. Vascular diseases frequently cause seizures after the age of sixty. Degenerative disorders, including Alzheimer's disease, can cause seizure disorder in later life. Several infectious diseases such as bacterial meningitis and herpes encephalitis can cause seizure disorder, as can AIDS (Tierney et al., 2006).

Seizures are a transient flurry of electrical impulses in the brain that are without order. The result can be anything from a blank stare to convulsions (Valente, 2000). Tierney et al. (2006) discuss classifications of seizures defined by the International League against Epilepsy. Seizures can be classified in two broad categories: partial and generalized. Partial seizures are restricted to only one part of the cerebral cortex. They can be either simple, in which the individual does not lose consciousness, or complex, in which either the individual loses consciousness or consciousness is impaired in some way. Persons experiencing partial seizures of either simple or complex types may have sensory, motor, or autonomic symptoms, such as a tingling feeling, jerking, or sweating. Generalized seizures involve the whole brain, which is suddenly inundated with extra chaotic electrical energy, whereby the entire body can be affected. Generalized seizures have five different forms: the absence (petit mal) seizure, atypical absence seizure, myoclonic seizure, tonic-clonic (grand mal) seizure, and atonic seizure (Tierney et al., 2006). The tonic-clonic, or grand mal, seizure is the most dramatic. Lewis (1993) describes a grand mal seizure: "An individual having a tonic-clonic seizure may suddenly cry out and then fall unconscious. The body stiffens, and then shakes or jerks uncontrollably. Bladder and bowel control may be lost. Breathing is quite shallow—and may even stop briefly during the seizure—but will return to normal when the shaking movements end. When the seizure ends, usually after a minute or two, the person is often confused and tired" (p. 20).

Patlak (1992) connects the drama of a grand mal seizure to the supernatural view of epilepsy. The ancient Greeks thought seizures represented visitation from the gods. During the Renaissance, it was thought that people having seizures were possessed by demons or were themselves demons and that people with seizure disorders received just punishment by being burned at the stake.

The dramatic nature of the seizure can result in stereotypes and discrimination. Saburi, Mapanga, and Mapanga (2006) point out that the quality of life of an individual who has seizure disorder may be negatively affected. Individuals must deal with reduced participation in the community, stigma, and family problems due to the societal stereotypes of seizure disorder. Because of the stigma, people experiencing seizure disorder may have low self-esteem, extreme anxiety, and depression (Raty & Gustafsson, 2006).

Discrimination in finding employment and maintaining employment is a large part of the lives of people experiencing seizure disorder. Persons with seizure disorders have trouble finding jobs and advancing in the jobs they do find (Lewis, 1993). Famulari (1992) found that persons with seizure disorders, on the average, obtain one year less education than people who do not have epilepsy. Males with seizure disorders have much more diffi-culty finding jobs than the general population. Finally, the wages paid to persons with seizure disorders who are employed are almost four dollars per hour less than the wages paid to workers who do not have seizure disorders.

As with other disabilities, the limitations in education and work placed on persons with seizure disorders stem from myths and stereotyping. The reality is that medication, diet, and, in some cases, surgery can be used to control seizures. Sometimes a combination of all three is used. Three-fourths of all persons with epilepsy can control seizures with drug therapy. Drugs used include carbamazepine, clonazepam, phenytoin, valproic acid, pheno-barbital, primidone, and ethosuximide. Sometimes more than one drug is used, but this is rare. Drugs can cause side effects, including drowsiness, confusion, clumsiness, nausea, and learning problems. To eliminate side effects, different drugs may be used and dosages manipulated.

Thomas Young, a friend of one of the authors, is a prime example of how stereotypes of persons with seizure disorders are false. In the mid-1990s, Professor Young was vice president of the California Faculty Associa-tion, the union that represents faculty in the California State University sys-tem. He was a full professor of communication studies at California State University, Stanislaus, as well as the interim affirmative action officer. He was a member of the system-wide academic senate. Professor Young identified himself proudly and openly as a person with seizure disorder. He referred to himself as "a person with a disability" with grace and pride. He took medication such as phenobarbital most of his life to control the seizures. Yet, on occasion, he would experience a seizure.

Professor Young kept an unbelievable calendar. He generally worked hundred-hour weeks. He did not drive. Professor Young was constantly on a plane going somewhere. His life was a constant stream of activity and pressure. Aside from his family duties, his teaching duties, his affirmative action duties, and his academic senate duties, he was the prime negotiator between faculty and the California State University during his tenure. Profes-sor Young's life flies in the face of stereotypical views of persons with disabilities.

When control of seizures cannot be brought about by medication, high-fat diets are sometimes used to control seizures. The high intake of fat pro-duces ketogens, which seem to prevent seizures, particularly in children. However, blood levels must be continually monitored to prevent the keto-gens from raising cholesterol and causing organ damage.

If the seizure activity is limited to a small area of the brain, some persons with seizure disorders can benefit from surgical removal or oblation of the malfunctioning brain cells that cause the seizure. Surgery cannot be used when seizure activity is in the areas of the brain that control speech, lan-guage, hearing, and other major functions. Surgery may also be performed to sever the connections between the left and right brain to prevent the spread of the electrical storm (Patlak, 1992). This procedure, however, is dramatic because it limits the ability of the brain's hemispheres to communicate with each other.

THE RIGHT TO BE ME

The cornerstone of the civil rights movement of people with disabilities has been the concept of self-determination. Self-determination is usually wrested away at every step of development and leaves persons with disabilities stranded and alone, afraid to enter into the game of chance that is life. Without the experience of independently making decisions that have the chance of failing, persons with disabilities are left without a clue about how to gain economic resources and real power within our society. This has been the case particularly among persons with developmental disabilities. Pfeiffer (1993) demonstrates the deep historical roots of society's fear of persons with developmental disabilities. Pfeiffer describes in detail the thoughts of Havelock Ellis, who was a strong advocate for human rights—particularly women's rights—in the 1920s. Ellis represented the thought of the time that the "feebleminded" were at best a burden to society, and at worst a potential threat to the future of human beings. Although Ellis advocated merely sterilization and maintenance, other intellectual leaders of the time advocated total eradication.

Controlling people with developmental disabilities has been the driving force of how people with developmental disabilities are treated not only by aggregate society but also by "knowledgeable" professionals. It is this desire to control that is the focal point of concern for self-advocates. People First is a national self-advocacy organization organized by and for persons with developmental disabilities. There are over 374 chapters and some 10,000 members (Shapiro, 1993). Quite simply, self-advocates are looking for control over their lives and how they are treated. T. J. Monroe, a self-advocate from Tennessee speaking to the President's Committee on Mental Retardation in 1994, said it most succinctly: "I think what we need to do is bring together professionals' knowledge and self-advocates' personal experience. This way, we can build a plan for action that solves the real problems people have. Self-advocates want to become empowered and have a voice in solving the problems they experience. Together with professional and government resources, we can make it work" (qtd. in Smith, 1994, p. 22).

Self-advocates question the basic assumptions made about people with developmental disabilities. The first assumption is that persons with disabilities need extensive protections from the myriad of threats and dangers in society. To this false assumption, we need to direct the following questions: How much protection do they need? Who determines the place and nature of the danger? A second assumption is that persons with disabilities cannot make major life decisions because they cannot deal with the risks and the consequences of the decisions. To this mistaken assumption, we need to ask, How do you experience independence without taking risks? Who benefits from the "protection" from making crucial life decisions? Whose fear is at issue when it comes to decisions about living in an apartment, having a job, having sex, or marrying? The last assumption is that self-advocacy cannot work because parents and professionals provide the direction, organization, and resources. This misconception is the hardest to challenge. Because of the nature of developmental disabilities, the various skills necessary for gaining civil rights are the skills most difficult for persons with disabilities to acquire. Yet there are those in the People First movement who strongly believe that the effectiveness of the movement in gaining real independence for persons with developmental disabilities will be compromised as long as persons without disabilities remain in control (Shapiro, 1993).

Spreading the concept of self-advocacy and independence is difficult for a variety of reasons. First, as is the case with most persons with disabilities, a long history of dependency exists. As was mentioned previously, there has been particular historic oppression of persons with developmental disabilities. Second, both persons with developmental disabilities and their parents find the idea of independence too frightening. Finally, laws and policies still deter self-determination. For example, as late as the 1980s, more than half of the states had laws prohibiting persons with developmental disabilities from marrying (Shapiro, 1993).

The nature of developmental disability, particularly when it is intellectually related, challenges the social welfare service provision industry. Human service professionals must remove themselves from the long historic trend of doing for persons with disabilities and lay the foundation of independence. This is no easy task. Teaching self-empowerment is at times work producing and time consuming. Agencies are wanting more for less. The idea of facilitating self-empowerment may produce resistance on the part of the agency, parents and other family members, and professionals. It is far easier to control and dictate. Nevertheless, aside from the long-term benefits empowerment produces for the person with a developmental disability, facilitating independence allows us as a society to experience the richness and joy that the diversity of disability can produce (Schwier, 1994).

SUMMARY

For all practical purposes, the federal definition of developmental disability encompasses most disabilities acquired before the age of twenty-two. According to the federal definition, if the onset is early and the disability is severe enough to interfere with several major life functions, the condition can be defined as a developmental disability. Whereas others offer more succinct definitions, several problems occur with all definitions of developmental disability that include intellectual disability. First, although service benefits are linked to a person's classification as developmentally disabled, groups such as persons who are blind, persons who have cerebral palsy, and deaf people resist being linked with the developmentally disabled banner primarily because of the link between the terms *developmental disability* and *mental retardation*. Many advocates, administrators, and professionals working with people with developmental disabilities frame their work within the independent living philosophy but produce policies and services that reflect paternalism and dependency. Finally, many states, for economic reasons, limit the definition of developmental disability. Although some may not agree, we have placed intellectual disability (mental retardation), Down syndrome, autism, epilepsy, and cerebral palsy under the category of developmental disability.

Generally speaking, persons with intellectual disabilities differ in some ways from typical individuals. But for the most part, their personal characteristics and human interaction reflect the personalities and socialization of most individuals living in society.

Down syndrome is a set of characteristics stemming from individuals having forty-seven chromosomes (because of an extra twenty-first chromosome) rather than the usual forty-six. On standard IQ tests, persons with Down syndrome can score poorly. However, these tests are limited because they do not measure many important areas of intelligence, and persons with Down syndrome often have good memory, insight, creativity, and cleverness. The high rate of learning disabilities in persons with Down syndrome sometimes masks their range of abilities and talents.

Autism is a condition that affects a person's ability to communicate with and relate to others, understand language, and play. The condition is usually evident by the age of three. Persons with autism sometimes have difficulty with language development and inconsistent patterns of sensory responses. They may exhibit high levels of intellectual functioning in some areas and very low levels in other areas. Persons with autism may also exhibit repetitive body movements or repetitive actions.

Seizure disorder (epilepsy) is a term that defines conditions associated with recurrent seizures. Seizures are a transient flurry of electrical impulses in the brain that are without order. The result can be anything from a blank stare to convulsions. The dramatic nature of the seizure can result in stereotypes and discrimination. Persons with seizure disorders have trouble finding jobs and advancing in the jobs they do find.

Controlling people with developmental disabilities has been the predominant approach used not only by the aggregate society but also by the "knowledgeable" professional. The heart of practice with persons with developmental disabilities lies in helping them gain independence and self-determination.

PERSONAL NARRATIVE: RESA HAYES

Resa Hayes is a disability activist from Spokane, Washington. She works for People First, an organization run by people who have developmental disabilities. As part of her job, she lectures about herself and about disabilities to parents of developmentally disabled people, professionals, students, and others.

I was born in 1960 at Deaconess Hospital in Spokane, Washington. My home was in Davenport, Washington, where I lived on a wheat ranch. I have two brothers and one sister. Their names are John, who is the oldest; Elizabeth, who is the second; and Richard, the third; and I am the youngest. My mom noticed that at six months my arms were slightly stiff. When it was hard to keep my balance while sitting on the floor, my parents took me to a specialist in Spokane. He said that I had cerebral palsy (CP). He demonstrated the way that I would probably walk—he did this several times. Because of the way he did it, my parents were so shocked by his rude and insulting manner that they just wanted to take me and run away from the terrible suggestions of this doctor.

I'd like to tell you about decisions and choices. A decision is the act or process of making a judgment, a determination, or reaching a conclusion. A choice is the option of having the power or right to choose—having the freedom of choice. A choice could be good or bad, constructive or destructive. Some of the early choices my parents made were the product of guessing what would be best for me. We had advice from doctors, which helped some, but a lot of the choices they made came from trial and error. The decision they made to send me to the CP school when I was eight years old is one they still talk about and wonder if it was the right decision.

It was really difficult growing up. I grew up in the 1960s, and people didn't have the information they have today. So we had to talk to doctors who did different things to me. The Shriner's Hospital helped a lot because I had surgeries done there and therapies and things like that. The professionals said I've got CP. Nobody said that I was mentally retarded, and if I heard that, I would punch their noses in because I don't like that word.

I don't think my parents knew what I could do, the potential I had. My mom sheltered me quite a lot. She protected me because I was different and she didn't know how the world was going to treat me. My parents worked with me like they would with any of the other kids to get me to do what I could do for myself. My brothers and sisters treated me no differently. They chased me around with the vacuum cleaner, sucking my hair up with it.

I went to a CP school for eight years, and I was protected from "normal" children. We all had different abilities. We used to tease each other and call each other names, but we didn't think of it like, "He's spastic." We didn't think about having CP much, but they didn't prepare us for the outside world and the cruelty of the people when we got into mainstream schools.

My school was good, but to be sent away from my family was very hard on me. My folks took me home every weekend, and that helped a lot. My parents struggled to find me a good boarding home to live in. My first place had none of the family feeling of home. I cried every Monday night (after I came back from visiting my parents) for the first two years I was in that boarding house, and this broke my family's heart. Today I am pleased to know that there are more regulations to monitor the care of children now, because I was not properly cared for then.

The choice to come home and go to high school in Davenport, a small rural farming community, was a good one. In high school, when I came back to Davenport after eight years of living in Spokane, I had about two hours a day in special education classes, and then my other classes were regular. It was an uneasy time for a few weeks until the kids got used to me. People were mean to me; I remember they used to pinch me and stuff. They used to push my books off my desk in front of the classroom. They used to put toothpaste on my pictures. They used to jam my walker so I couldn't open it. They would put the sign "Kick me" on my back. I laughed, but I didn't like what they did to me. I didn't have the guts like I do today to tell them to knock it off. I made a choice to be the girls' volleyball manager for four years. I was included in nearly all my class activities. That time was the beginning of when I felt accepted on the part of my peers. I was sixteen when I went into high school in Davenport, and I was twenty-one when I graduated. I got along better with my younger classmates than my older classmates. They understood me better than the upperclassmen. At my graduation, I led my class in the procession to our graduation ceremonies. I was so proud.

I think starting kids out in the regular school system would be best, better than special schools. They could have teacher's aides go into the classroom with them. But they should not be ostracized from the regular class. I didn't have anybody to help me, but my mom did a lot of writing and test taking for me. She was kind of like my right hand when I was in regular school.

I had two brothers and one sister who went to high school ahead of me. I wanted to be just like them because when I came home from the CP school every weekend I could see what they were doing. My whole dream was to go to high school like them. When I got into regular high school, I was meeting that dream. But getting the grades was a big standard too. I wanted to make my dad and mom proud of me. They were proud of me, but in their own way. They didn't expect me to do what my brothers and sisters did, because they knew I had a learning disability. When I got C's and D's and didn't qualify for the honor roll, I used to lie in bed and cry myself to sleep because it hurt so bad. I guess my dad and mom were just as proud of me as everybody else in the family, but sometimes I wanted to have that academic recognition like all of us do.

After graduation I made a choice to move back to Spokane; since it was my choice, I thought to myself, "Free at last." I arrived in Spokane with the vision of finding a job and having more opportunities. When I first got there, I was presented with several adult family homes to check into and decide where I wanted to live. The home I picked offered room and board and supervision. I did swimming and softball throws. I also did Special Olympics. I began volunteering at United Cerebral Palsy, and I continued there for five difficult years. But what I really wanted was a real paying job. The agency that was supposed to help me find a job had me doing things I didn't like, such as volunteering at day care centers. They didn't look within me. They thought I could talk good and my hands could work good but my hands did not work as well as the average person's hands. I had to always volunteer because the agencies weren't really meeting my needs by helping me find a job. This experience told me that people said I had choices, but I really didn't, and I had to rely on the decisions of others even when I was quite capable of making my own individual choices. This happens to us a lot.

My mom was scared for me when I moved back to Spokane. She didn't think that I could use the bus system. Well, once again I showed everyone.

I live in my own apartment now. I'm still living my full vision even though I have some help with daily living tasks. I'm really, really thankful for assisted living because without assisted living, I would have to work even harder to do my daily tasks. I have two people that come in twice or three times a week to help me out with daily living tasks and take me to doctor's appointments and grocery shopping. They help me in the community and help me with my personal finances. Without that help, I don't know what I would do.

I found a job several years ago working for People First. People First is a nonprofit organization for people with developmental disabilities. We have a motto, which says, "We are people first and our disabilities are second." We don't like using the word *disability*. We like to use *different abilities,* because we are different and we all have abilities. My self-image really grew when I got involved in People First. I was the state president for two years.

When I started with People First, we were working on the Department of Education grant. We went into schools to teach developmentally disabled students about self-determination skills. It was a three-year project. Now I go out to create and support People First chapters in the state.

People First is saying, "Treat people first and everything else is second." Change your low expectations to positive expectations. People's minds are sort of warped about disabilities because they haven't gotten an education. Society's low expectations have said, "If somebody is different than me, let's lock them away." Something's got to change, and I think that change is positive thinking. People First helps people know what they want to do and stand up to people who say, "You can't do that." We can advocate for people. People First can go into the institutions and educate those people to stand up to the staff. We help them get out of institutions.

There is a Disability culture. When I was back in the CP school, we had a Disability culture in the school. We were safe in the culture we were in. We used to joke and call each other some names because we were safe. In society today, we don't feel safe. People point their fingers at us. But you know something? We found out at a Spokane Transit Authority meeting there was a culture that stuck us together like glue. It was really culturfied. We had lots of disabled people there: old people, young people, people of color. We were voicing our opinions about public transportation and together we felt safe. When they said, "You can't clap," we just clapped louder. Talk about culture—that was a cultural experience for me.

As for role models, I remember my home economics teacher in high school. She treated me like everybody else. I liked the way she acted, the way she ran her class. I would also have to say the Incredible Hulk was a role model. He was deaf but that didn't stop him from acting. It didn't stop him from turning green when he got mad. I often wanted to have him move my bedroom furniture around.

I see other people with disabilities just like I am. When people without disabilities see me, it's shocking for them. They are not accepting and lack education about people with disabilities. I have seen people with disabilities ostracized. People label us. But you don't label people; you label jars. You say, "This is Resa, she's my friend. She has a lot to say." Treat people the way you want to be treated. Our biggest problem is people's low expectations of us. People are in institutions because of that. We've got to get them help and get them educated and say, "Hey, we're going to do our very best jobs to get you out of there." We should educate ourselves by accepting the person and not the disability.

To people with disabilities and their parents, I say talk to your doctors to let the doctors know that you will not accept anything less for your child. Be gutsy, be determined about getting answers. The more guts you have, the better off you are. Treat your children as normally as you can by letting them fall down, letting them experience the pain, letting them know what's right and wrong. Let them fall down on the floor, fall down with other people, share a little hurt, because we learn from our falls. All I am trying to say to all of you is to look within your hearts and accept the disabilities. Your children are people first; their disabilities are secondary. Know when to let go when your sons and daughters say they want to make choices and decisions for themselves.

In everyone's life there comes a time to think about a relationship. What is a relationship? What do I need out of a relationship? What can I give in a relationship? I am no different from any of you out there today. I have the same heart, I have the same feelings, I have the same aches and pains and the same hopes and dreams that you do. I have suffered disappointment in relationships, as have you. I have been hurt too, but through all of this I have grown. I have used these experiences as true learning experiences, not allowing them to turn into bad habits. It's been a hurtful relationship, but I have grown to understand myself better. I have learned to have high expectations. I haven't found Mr. Right; I am happy with that.

I am proud to be me, but there are days I would love not to have this. I think all people with a disability would like not to have their speaking impairment, or hearing impairment, or visual or other impairment, but I think we are all stronger for it. I do like myself. My disability has made me stronger in my beliefs and in speaking out for other people. It makes me appreciate who I am and what I can do.

To people with disabilities, I say educate yourself, be good to yourself. No matter what, you're a worthwhile person. If people say you aren't a worthwhile person, tell them to get a life!

Discussion questions

1. What are some of the major issues in defining persons with developmental disabilities? How are these issues influenced by the social construct of disability in our society?
2. What are the major misconceptions that practitioners need to address in working with persons with intellectual disabilities?
3. Why are self-advocacy organizations so important, and how will they affect your future work with persons with disabilities?
4. What are some of the specific characteristics of autism, and how would knowledge of these characteristics influence intervention strategies?
5. How can social service agencies and practitioners facilitate the empowerment and independence of persons with developmental disabilities?

Suggested readings

Grandin, T. (1995). *Thinking in pictures and other reports from my life with autism.* New York: Doubleday.

Meyer, L. H., Peck, C. A., & Brown, L. (Eds.). (1991). *Critical issues in the lives of people with severe disabilities.* Baltimore: Paul H. Brookes.

Noble, V. (1993). *Down is up for Aaron Eagle: A mother's spiritual journey with Down syndrome.* San Francisco: Harper.

Shapiro, J. P. (1993). *No pity: People with disabilities forging a new civil rights movement.* New York: Times Books.

References

American Association on Mental Retardation. (1992). *Mental retardation: Definition, classification, and systems of supports* (9th ed.). Washington, DC: Author.

American Association on Mental Retardation. (n.d.). *Welcome to AAIDD.* Retrieved October 30, 2006, from http://www.aamr.org/About_AAMR/new_name.shtml

American Psychiatric Association. (2000). *Diagnostic and statistical manual of mental disorders* (4th ed.). Arlington, VA: Author.

Ansello, E. F. (1992). Seeking common ground between aging and developmental disabilities. *Generations, 16*(1), 9–16.

Beers, M. H. (Ed.). (2003). *The Merck manual of medical information* (2nd ed.). New York: Simon & Schuster.

Block, M. E., & Groft, M. (2003). Children with Asperger syndrome: Implications for general physical education and youth sports. *Journal of Physical Education, Recreation, and Dance, 74*(3), 38–43.

Crevak, M. (1976). *Damon.* Unpublished composition. Pittsburgh, PA.

Davies, M. K., & Hollman, A. (2001). Down syndrome. *Heart, 86,* 130. Retrieved November 2, 2006, from Expanded Academic ASAP via Thomson Gale.

DePoy, E., & Werrbach, G. (1996). Successful living placement for adults with disabilities: Considerations for social work practice. *Social Work in Health Care, 23*(4), 21–34.

Dudley, J. R. (1987). Speaking for themselves: People who are labeled as mentally retarded. *Social Work, 32*(1), 80–82.

Duncan, J. S., Sander, J. W., Sisodoya, S. M., & Walker, M. C. (2006). Adult epilepsy. *The Lancet, 367*(9516), 1087–1100. Retrieved September 25, 2006, from Expanded Academic ASAP via Thomson Gale.

Evans, I. M. (1991). Testing and diagnosis: A review and evaluation. In L. H. Meyer, C. A. Peck, & L. Brown (Eds.), *Critical issues in the lives of people with severe disabilities* (pp. 25–44). Baltimore: Paul H. Brookes.

Famulari, M. (1992). The effects of a disability on labor market performance: The case of epilepsy. *Southern Economic Journal, 58*(4), 1072–1088.

Grandin, T. (1992). An inside view of autism. In E. Schopler & G. B. Mesibov (Eds.), *High-functioning individuals with autism* (pp. 105–126). New York: Plenum Press.

Grandin, T. (1995). *Thinking in pictures and other reports from my life with autism.* New York: Doubleday.

Griswold, D. E., Barnhill, G. D., Miles, B. S., Hagiwara, T., & Simpson, R. L. (2002). Asperger syndrome and academic achievement. *Focus on Autism and Other Developmental Disabilities, 17*(2), 94–102.

Hall, J. A., Ford, L. H., Moss, J. A., & Dineen, J. P. (1986). Practice with mentally retarded adults as an adjunct to vocational training. *Social Work, 31*(2), 125–128.

Hanson, M. J. (2003). Twenty-five years after early intervention: A follow-up of children with Down syndrome and their families. *Infants and Young Children, 16*(4), 354–366.

Karande, S. (2006). Autism: A review for family physicians. *Indian Journal of Medical Sciences, 60*(5), 205–215. Retrieved September 25, 2006, from Expanded Academic ASAP via Thomson Gale.

Lewis, S. (1993). Understanding epilepsy. *Current Health, 20*(4), 19–22.

Mayo Clinic. (2006). *Down syndrome: Causes.* Retrieved November 2, 2006, from http://www.mayoclinic.com/health/down-syndrome/DS00182/DSECTION = 3

Moeschler, J. B., & Shevell, M. (2006). Clinical genetic evaluation of the child with mental retardation or developmental delays. *Pediatrics, 117*(6), 2304–2316. Retrieved September 25, 2006, from Expanded Academic ASAP via Thomson Gale.

National Association of Councils on Developmental Disabilities. (n.d.). *Who we are.* Retrieved October 17, 2006, from http://www.nacdd.org/pages/who_we_are .htm#purpose

National Dissemination Center for Children with Disabilities. (2004). *Down syndrome.* Retrieved November 2, 2006, from http://www.nichcy.org/pubs/factshe/ fs4txt.htm

Noble, V. (1993). *Down is up for Aaron Eagle: A mother's spiritual journey with Down syndrome.* San Francisco: Harper.

Patlak, M. (1992). Controlling epilepsy. *FDA Consumer, 26*(4), 28–32.

Pfeiffer, D. (1993). Overview of the disability movement: History, legislative record, and political implications. *Policy Studies Journal, 21*(4), 724–735.

Raty, L., & Gustafsson, B. (2006). Emotions in relation to healthcare encounters affecting self-esteem. *Journal of Neuroscience Nursing, 38*(1), 42–50.

Saburi, G. L., Mapanga, K. G., & Mapanga, M. B. (2006). Perceived family reactions and quality of life of adults with epilepsy. *Journal of Neuroscience Nursing, 38*(3), 156–165. Retrieved September 25, 2006, from Expanded Academic ASAP via Thomson Gale.

Schwier, K. M. (1994). Storytelling: The power of listening. *Developmental Disabilities Bulletin, 22*(2), 24–37.

Shapiro, J. P. (1993). *No pity: People with disabilities forging a new civil rights movement.* New York: Times Books.

Smith, B. (1994). PCMR conference report. *Children Today, 23*(1), 20–24.

State Council on Developmental Disabilities. (n.d.). *About developmental disabilities.* Retrieved October 30, 2006, from http://www.scdd.ca.gov/about_developmental_disabilities/Default.htm

TEACCH. (2006). *Autism primer: Twenty questions and answers.* Retrieved November 6, 2006, from http://www.teacch.com/info_primer.html

Tierney, L. M., McPhee, S. J., & Papadakis, M. A. (Eds.). (2006). *Current medical diagnosis and treatment.* New York: Lang Medical Books/McGraw-Hill.

U.S. Department of Health and Human Services, Administration for Children and Families. (n.d.). *Developmental disabilities assistance and bill of rights act of 2000.* Retrieved October 30, 2006, from http://www.acf.hhs.gov/programs/add/ddact/DDA.html

Valente, L. R. (2000). Seizures and epilepsy: Optimizing patient management. *Clinician Review, 10*(3), 79–104.

10

Mental Health Disabilities

I am better off now than I would have been if I had never had
mental illness. . . . The reaction of others is one of the most difficult parts of mental illness. . . . In lots of ways, the way we are
treated is worse than the symptoms themselves.

—Donna Orrin, business owner

STUDENT LEARNING OBJECTIVES

1. To be able to identify and compare the medical, social, and political
   dimensions of mental health and mental health disabilities
2. To understand how the concepts of mental health, mental illness and
   mental health disabilities have developed and evolved over time
3. To understand how our social contexts influence perceptions of mental
   health disabilities
4. To understand the impacts of mental health disability on the lives of people, their loved ones, and communities
5. To appreciate the influence and value of self-advocacy, the self-help
   movement, and partnerships between persons with mental health disabilities, providers of mental health services, and family members

In the first edition of this text, the title of this chapter used the term *psychiatric disabilities,* whereas we have entitled this chapter "Mental Health Disabilities." We have modified language as our views have changed and, arguably,
matured over time. To provide readers a glimpse of our reasons for this
change, we deconstruct mental health language. First, let's consider the term
mental illness, which is currently most commonly used to describe people
with mental health disabilities. While we respect the collective wisdom of
professionals and others who use this term, we believe *illness* is an inadequate and inaccurate descriptor. For example, individuals with depression

In the first edition of this text, Marilyn Wedenoja authored a chapter entitled "Persons
with Psychiatric Disabilities" that covered much of the material we present in this chapter.
While Professor Wedenoja did not contribute to this new edition, we acknowledge her
invaluable contributions to the previous edition and the ongoing influence of her work
on this second edition.

or schizophrenia may seek medical treatment, but we consider it a misnomer to define them as ill or diseased. They seek help from the medical establishment because these are the societal systems that they must navigate to obtain assistance. Similarly, terms such as *psychiatric illness* and *psychiatric disability* define the characteristics and traits medically. The terms *psychiatric illness* and *psychiatric disability* defer to a specific medical specialty that has defined the field (Andreasen, 2001; Caplan, 1995; Walenstein, 1998); however, the characteristics of this group of conditions occur independent of professional specialty. In fact, worldwide, few people with mental health disabilities will ever see a psychiatrist for diagnosis or help.

We use the term *mental health disability* to refer to disabilities that involve mood, emotion, and perception. Those of us who live with mental health disabilities are not sick, nor are we defined by medical specialties or mental illness systems. Though people with mental health disabilities may seek professional help, mental health disabilities exist independently of mental health service systems. In fact, most mental health systems are *not* primarily devoted to maintaining and promoting mental health; rather, these organizations have been developed to treat people and problems associated with mental health disabilities. Terms such as *mental illness, psychiatric disability,* and *mental health disability* are recent constructs. Characteristics and conditions have been grouped together based on contemporary understanding and knowledge, and diagnostic categories of mental illness have grown greatly in recent decades. In much of the world, today's constructs of mental health disabilities are guided by codified manuals such as the tenth edition of the World Health Organization publication *International Statistical Classification of Diseases and Related Health Problems.* The current edition has been used worldwide to identify and objectively classify illness since the early 1990s along with its companion, the 2001 *International Classification of Functioning, Disability and Health.* Other manuals are used by specific countries or regions. For example, the U.S. classification system is based on the 2000 *Diagnostic and Statistical Manual of Mental Disorders (DSM IV-TR),* which is published by the American Psychiatric Association and has been published in more than a dozen languages (Caplan, 1995). In recent years, the World Health Organization and other bodies such as the American Psychiatric Association have collaborated to bring their respective diagnostic manuals in line with one another.

MAJOR MENTAL ILLNESS CLASSIFICATIONS

Diagnostic mental illness manuals today are several hundreds of pages long and contain descriptions and explanations detailing hundreds of conditions. Readers who are interested in these medically based classifications systems are referred to the diagnostic manuals and the plethora of supplemental books that further elaborate on and interpret them. Herein, we provide brief descriptions of four illustrative and commonly diagnosed categories of "mental illness." The National Alliance on Mental Illness (NAMI), the largest U.S. education and advocacy organization for those with mental health disabilities and their families, is the source of these definitions.

Bipolar Disorder

According to NAMI (2006a), "bipolar disorder, or manic depression, is a medical illness that causes extreme shifts in mood, energy, and functioning. These changes may be subtle or dramatic and typically vary greatly over the course of a person's life as well as among individuals. Over 10 million people in America have bipolar disorder, and the illness affects men and women equally."

Medications commonly used to treat bipolar disorder include lithium (Eskalith or Lithobid), divalproex sodium (Depakote), carbamazepine (Tegretol), olanzapine (Zyprexa), risperidone (Risperdal), quetiapine (Seroquel), ziprasidone (Geodon), aripiprazole (Abilify), haloperidol (Haldol), a combination of olanzapine and fluoxetine (Symbyax), quetiapine (Seroquel), and lamotrigine (Lamictal) (NAMI, 2006a).

Depression

NAMI (2006b) defines major depression as "a serious medical illness affecting 15 million American adults, or approximately 5 to 8 percent of the adult population in a given year. Unlike normal emotional experiences of sadness, loss, or passing mood states, major depression is persistent and can significantly interfere with an individual's thoughts, behavior, mood, activity, and physical health. Among all medical illnesses, major depression is the leading cause of disability in the U.S. and many other developed countries. Depression occurs twice as frequently in women as in men, for reasons that are not fully understood." Medications for depression can be divided into classifications and include

- Selective serotonin reuptake inhibitors (SSRIs), including fluoxetine (Prozac), sertraline (Zoloft), paroxetine (Paxil), citalopram (Celexa), escitalopram (Lexapro), and fluvoxamine (Luvox)
- Serotonin and norepinephrine reuptake inhibitors (SNRIs), including venlafaxine (Effexor) and duloxetine (Cymbalta)
- Bupropion (Wellbutrin), which is a norepinephrine-dopamine reuptake inhibitor (NDRI)
- Mirtazapine (Remeron), which targets specific serotonin and norepinephrine receptors in the brain
- Tricyclic antidepressant medications (e.g., amitriptyline [Elavil]) and monoamine oxidase inhibitors (e.g., phenelzine [Nardil]), which were

the first line of antidepressants introduced several decades ago and, because of their side effects, are rarely used today (NAMI, 2006b).

The World Health Organization (n.d.) estimates 121 million people worldwide experience depression.

Schizophrenia

Schizophrenia, as defined by NAMI (2007), "is a serious and challenging medical illness . . . that affects well over 2 million American adults, which is about 1% of the population age 18 and older. Although it is often feared and misunderstood, schizophrenia is a treatable medical condition. Schizophrenia often interferes with a person's ability to think clearly, to distinguish reality from fantasy, to manage emotions, make decisions, and relate to others. The first signs of schizophrenia typically emerge in the teenage years or early twenties, often later for females. Most people with schizophrenia contend with the illness chronically or episodically throughout their lives, and are often stigmatized by lack of public understanding about the disease." Schizophrenia is characterized by three types of symptoms: (1) positive symptoms, such as hallucinations and delusions; (2) negative symptoms such as emotional blunting, flat affect, and anhedonia that are manifest emotionally and socially; and (3) cognitive symptoms such as the inability to prioritize or organize and lack of insight into one's condition.

The following groups of medications are used to treat schizophrenia.

- Typical antipsychotics/neuroleptics. These include chlorpromazine (Thorazine), fluphenazine (Prolixin), haloperidol (Haldol), thiothixene (Navane), trifluoperazine (Stelazine), perphenazine (Trilafon), and thioridazine (Mellaril). These medications were introduced in the 1950s and have significant and potentially dangerous side effects. They are considered to be more effective in treating positive symptoms than negative and cognitive symptoms.

- Atypical antipsychotics/neuroleptics. Introduced in the 1990s, these medications include risperidone (Risperdal), clozapine (Clozaril), olanzapine (Zyprexa), quetiapine (Seroquel), and ziprasidone (Geodon). They also have significant and sometimes potentially fatal side effects. However, overall they seem to carry less risk than the earlier medications *and* they are more effective at treating negative symptoms (NAMI, 2007).

Attention-Deficit/Hyperactivity Disorder

NAMI (2003) characterizes attention-deficit/hyperactivity disorder (ADHD) as "an illness characterized by inattention, hyperactivity, and impulsivity. The most commonly diagnosed behavior disorder in young persons, ADHD affects an estimated 3–5% of school-age children." There are three predominant types of ADHD: inattentive, hyperactive/impulsive, and combined, each with its own set of symptoms. ADHD often persists into adolescence and adulthood and is frequently not diagnosed until later years.

Stimulant medications are the most widely used drugs and include methylphenidate (Ritalin), dextroamphetamine (Dexedrine, Desoxyn), and a combination of amphetamine and dextroamphetamine (Adderall). Other medications include antidepressants; major tranquilizers; the antihypertensive clonidine (Catapres); and atomoxetine (Straterra), a selective norepinephrine reuptake inhibitor (NAMI, 2003).

ADHD has been included in this chapter because it is defined as a mental health disability by leading mental health experts; however, others perceive it as a cognitive disability. Yet others question its very existence (Armstrong, 1995). This lack of consensus illustrates the fluid and evolving nature of the field and provides a cautionary note relative to the acceptance of current definitions as objective realities.

Anxiety Disorders

According to the Anxiety Disorders Association of America (n.d.), anxiety disorders affect approximately 40 million Americans age eighteen and older and are the most common mental disorder in the United States. Anxiety disorders include generalized anxiety disorder, obsessive-compulsive disorder, phobias, panic disorder, posttraumatic stress syndrome, and social anxiety disorder. In the past, benzodiazapene anxiolytics such as lorazepam (Ativan), clonazepam (Klonopin), alprazolam (Xanax), and diazepam (Valium) were commonly prescribed but have fallen into disfavor due to dependence and withdrawal problems. They are now used for acute anxiety. Contemporarily, antidepressants are commonly used long term with periodic use of anxiolytics. Buspirone (BuSpar), a medication that acts by increasing the action of serotonin receptors in the brain and lacks the sedative effects of benzodiazapenes, is also used to treat anxiety.

SOCIAL CONTEXTS OF DEFINING MENTAL HEALTH DISABILITIES

Descriptions of mental health disabilities used by the World Health Organization, the American Psychiatric Association, and NAMI provide a way for people from all over the world, in multiple disciplines and from diverse backgrounds, to classify characteristics and traits into identifiable and generally agreed-upon categories. They are informed by science, technology, and experience. However, we believe it is a mistake to believe the classification systems currently in use are objective realities. Rather, they reflect the combined knowledge, wisdom, and belief systems of professionals with expertise in identifying, understanding, and treating pathology who provide a common framework for everyone else. They are guides that are constantly being modified to reflect new knowledge, altered perceptions, and changing understanding. They have several limitations, some of which are described below.

Professional classification systems reflect extant wisdom that will change over time. For example, fifty years ago, homosexuality was considered a mental disorder; today gay marriage is increasingly being legalized. In the 1980s, multiple personality disorder, now known as dissociative identity disorder, was a common diagnosis, whereas contemporarily, its prevalence and even its existence are being debated.

Classification systems are primarily valuable as descriptors that identify commonalities. They are less accurate when used to explain the causes of mental health disabilities. For example, a generation ago, schizophrenia was explained as resulting from "schizophrenogenic families," while contemporary explanations are based on genetics, brain chemistry, and neuron functioning.

The classification of mental health disabilities as an illness has been essential to the development and maintenance of multiple professions and systems to treat mental illness. Like the medieval church, psychiatry provides the contemporary lens through which mental health and mental health disabilities are viewed and defined. Psychiatry, psychology, social work, and other professions have been instrumental in improving the inhumane treatment and living conditions of people with mental health disabilities that existed in past centuries. Concomitantly, these professions are afforded sanction because of the people they help. Thus, the medical model is an essential component of the symbiotic relationship. People with mental health disabilities rely on professionals for goods and services to function in society, and professionals need people with mental health disabilities to free up the societal resources to justify and sanction their existence.

Mental health disabilities are biosocial in nature. Extant research provides strong evidence for biological explanations. For example, PET scans can reveal differences in brain activity between persons with and without mental health disabilities. However, these differences exist within social contexts and in people's environments. Let's consider one person's different reactions to two chemical atypicalities in her body. In her adolescence, this individual developed type 1 diabetes, which caused her pancreas to cease producing the hormone insulin, thus requiring her to take insulin injections. In her early twenties she developed depression, which she explained as resulting from insufficient serotonin (a neurotransmitter) levels in her brain, for which she took an antidepressant to increase serotonin. She considered the need to inject herself with insulin as an inconvenience necessity; however, she expressed guilt and shame at her use of medication to treat depression. Her feelings were largely mediated by societal attitudes about "mental illness."

Mental health and mental health disabilities are defined in social and cultural contexts that are determined by those who control those contexts. Consider the clinical experience of one of the authors when he was a hospital social worker. He was asked to intervene because the mother of a patient was burning incense and waving her hands over her comatose son to purify him and cleanse his mind and body. The mother was labeled delusional by health care providers, yet some of these same providers believed in providing blessings and healings within their own religious traditions. The author was struck by the observation that one person's spiritual experiences can be another person's delusional activity.

Our observations are not meant to minimize the impact mental health disabilities have on people who experience them and their family members. However, we believe it is important to recognize that our understanding is continually evolving. We reject the medical/illness classification, while acknowledging that mental health disability has real impacts on the lives of those it affects. Some of those impacts produce different ways of experiencing the world and life experiences that benefit the people who experience them, as well as those around them. For example, a colleague of one of the authors was diagnosed by medical professionals as having obsessive-compulsive disorder (OCD). She acknowledges the difficulties of living with OCD, including social ostracization and intrusive thoughts and behaviors. She has counseling and medical treatment, including medications for her OCD. At the same time, she acknowledges that her OCD has led her down personal and professional paths that have enriched her life. For one, she states she would have never met her husband—and never have had the children she has—were it not for her OCD. Thus, when given the hypothetical choice of never having OCD, she insists she would not change her life to live without it.

HISTORICAL ASPECTS OF MENTAL HEALTH DISABILITIES

In previous chapters, we have discussed the history of disability in some detail. In this chapter we provide a more in-depth analysis of the place of mental health disabilities in society. Peculiarities of thought and action have been with humanity since the beginning of recorded history. Millon (2004) chronicles perceptions of the mind and mental health disabilities in multiple cultures throughout the ages. Skull surgeries from past millennia are thought to have been performed to release spirits or demons. Early cave drawings have been interpreted as indicative of the presence of mental disorders. Ancient Greek and Roman societies prescribed herbs and recommended environmental modifications. The Bible tells the story of King David, who went into hiding and "changed his behavior before them, and feigned himself mad . . . and let spittle fall down upon his beard" (I Samuel 21:13) so that the king of Gath would leave him alone. The Koran exhorts believers to show kindness and to help those with limited capabilities and understanding.

Foucault (2006) chronicles the evolution of "madness" in European traditions. Throughout much of the Middle Ages and early in the Renaissance, those considered mad were often removed from the general population and isolated outside cities and towns. It was believed that their madness gave them unique insights and knowledge not readily available to others, but their peculiarities led to their exclusion from the community. Humanist philosophers of the day, such as Erasmus and Montaigne, contended it was "mad" to claim that one could find absolute truth, and that madness was an indicator of the discrepancy between what humans are and what we pretend to be. It was plausible that they possessed a unique sort of knowledge. Two contrasting schools of thought existed simultaneously: Christian thought, which contended that man's reasoning was madness, and secular thought, which considered divine reason madness. This schism gave rise to the connections between reason and sanity, and unreason and madness. Madness was considered the opposite of reason. Consequently, by the seventeenth and eighteenth centuries those who were considered mad were not required to live separately but were locked up and confined to control them. The "insane" were perceived similarly to others who chose deviance, such as blasphemers and prostitutes. Institutionalization was used to punish, not treat. Foucault defines this period as the Great Confinement. Thus, those who were "mad" were treated according to the moral model. While those in power interned those guilty of rejecting nature, others such as members of the burgeoning medical profession perceived madness as worthy of study and, eventually, treatment. By the end of the eighteenth century, the approach to insanity had evolved into the medical model approach. Those judged to be insane were still confined to institutions; however, at least on the surface these lunatic asylums and psychiatric hospitals were constructed to relieve families, protect society, and cure the insane (Khalfa, 2006).

During the nineteenth century, both medical and moral models were evident in society. Institutionalization was still common in the hopes that treatment could bring about amelioration of symptoms or cure. Concomitantly, mental health disabilities brought shame and embarrassment to individuals and families. By the end of the nineteenth century and into the twentieth century, social Darwinism and eugenics had risen to the forefront. Mental health disabilities were among the defects that were considered important to eradicate from society (Wiggam, 1924). In 1911, the U.S. Immigration Commission issued a report strongly discouraging the immigration of those with mental health disabilities. In 1927, the U.S. Supreme Court in *Buck v. Bell* determined that forced sterilization of the "insane" was in the best interest of society and of those sterilized. Writing for the 8–1 majority opinion, Justice Oliver Wendell Holmes wrote: "It would be strange if it could not call upon those who already sap the strength of the State for these lesser sacrifices, often not felt to be such by those concerned, in order to prevent our being swamped with incompetence. It is better for all the world, if instead of waiting to execute degenerate offspring for crime, or to let them starve for their imbecility, society can prevent those who are manifestly unfit from continuing their kind" (*Buck v. Bell,* 1927).

According to the U.S. Holocaust Memorial Museum (n.d.), more than 30,000 people in U.S. mental institutions and prisons were involuntarily sterilized between 1907 and 1939. The museum documents the parallels between the United States and Nazi Germany, including the 1933 German Law for the Prevention of Progeny with Hereditary Diseases, which forced sterilization on 300,000–400,000 people with mental health disabilities such as schizophrenia and bipolar disorder. By 1939, Germany took the next step by instituting the Tiergartenstrasse 4 program, which exterminated between 200,000 and 250,000 disabled people between 1939 and 1945, initially by lethal injection and shooting, then by carbon monoxide, and eventually by gassing. These programs were administered by psychiatrists and other physicians in facilities such as psychiatric hospitals. It was in these "treatment" institutions that the first gas chambers, fully equipped with shower nozzles to distribute lethal gas, were developed; these were later transported to the concentration camps. Standardized questionnaires were used to determine the nature of people's diagnoses, family histories, and functional capabilities and limitations. A red mark was placed on the questionnaires of those who "failed," which designated them for extermination (Lifton, 1986).

The following story provided by the museum is indicative of the Nazis' "mercy" killings.

> Helene Lebel, raised as a Catholic in Vienna, Austria, first showed signs of mental illness when she was nineteen. Her condition worsened until she had to give up her law studies and her job as a legal secretary. In 1936 she was diagnosed as a schizophrenic and was placed in Vienna's Steinhof Psychiatric Hospital. Two years later, Germany annexed Austria. Helene's condition had improved at Steinhof, and her parents were led to believe that she would soon be moved to a hospital in a nearby town. In fact, Helene was transferred to a former prison in Brandenburg, Germany. There she was undressed, subjected to a physical examination, and then led into a "shower room," where she was killed with a deadly gas. (p. 5)

The primary difference between Nazi Germany and other countries was the extreme measures used to apply the philosophy of eugenics.

The advent of modern psychiatry contributed new ideas and theories about mental health disabilities. By the mid-twentieth century, mental health professionals had developed psychoanalytic theories of mental health disabilities. For example, they explained schizophrenia was caused by dysfunctional schizophrenogenic family dynamics that put children in a double-bind leading to mental health disabilities (Bateson, Jackson, Haley, & Weakland, 1956; Bowen, 1960). These theories helped justify treatment approaches such as institutionalization, or the removal of people with mental health disabilities from families for their own protection—and for the protection of society. However, the development of psychotropic medications for conditions such as anxiety, depression, and psychosis brought significant changes to the handling of mental health disabilities. Medication treatment became widespread, and at one point, anxiolytics such as Valium, which became the first billion-dollar drug in history, were widely prescribed and given nicknames such as "mother's little helpers" and "housewives' candy."

By the 1970s and 1980s, deinstitutionalization and community living found favor. Mental health disabilities became defined as multifactorial, having genetic, biological, and social components, while psychodynamic approaches were being questioned and rejected. Community mental health treatment replaced the emphasis on psychiatric institutionalization. Psychotropic medications became widely used and have been refined over recent decades. Contemporarily, many mental health professionals and persons treated with psychotropics swear by their use, while others believe they are widely misused and question their effectiveness (Barber, 2008; Bentley & Walsh, 2001; Walenstein, 1998). While in the twenty-first century, we consider ourselves much more enlightened than past generations, people whom society labels mentally ill still face significant societal obstacles to inclusion in society. Though psychiatric hospitals have a reduced number of beds, and many have closed, resources have not followed people into the community. This has purportedly had deadly consequences (Torrey & Zdanowicz, 1998). Human Rights Watch (2003) issued a report on people with mental health disabilities who are imprisoned in the United States and concluded:

> Somewhere between two and three hundred thousand men and women in U.S. prisons suffer from mental disorders, including such serious illnesses as schizophrenia, bipolar disorder, and major depression. An estimated seventy thousand are psychotic on any given day. Yet across the nation, many prison mental health services are woefully deficient, crippled by understaffing, insufficient facilities, and limited programs. All too often seriously ill prisoners receive little or no meaningful treatment. They are neglected, accused of malingering, treated as disciplinary problems.
>
> Without the necessary care, mentally ill prisoners suffer painful symptoms and their conditions can deteriorate. They are afflicted with delusions and hallucinations, debilitating fears, extreme and uncontrollable mood swings. They huddle silently in their cells, mumble incoherently, or yell incessantly. They refuse to obey orders or lash out without apparent provocation. They beat their heads against cell walls, smear themselves with feces, self-mutilate, and commit suicide.
>
> Prisons were never intended as facilities for the mentally ill, yet that is one of their primary roles today. Many of the men and women who cannot get mental health treatment in the community are swept into the criminal justice system after they commit a crime. *In the United States, there are three times*

more mentally ill people in prisons than in mental health hospitals, and prisoners have rates of mental illness that are two to four times greater than the rates of members of the general public. While there has been extensive documentation of the growing presence of the mentally ill in prison, little has been written about their fate behind bars. (p. 1, emphasis added)

The Human Rights Watch (2003) report quotes Texas judge William Wayne Justice, who, in a 1999 Texas court decision, *Ruiz v. Johnson,* bemoaned as "deplorable and outrageous" the fact that prisons have become repositories for citizens with mental health disabilities, who are confined in conditions that "nurture, rather than abate," their problems. The World Health Organization (2005) reports similar problems with high incarceration rates and lack of treatment in Europe. The U.S. Mentally Ill Offender Treatment and Crime Reduction Act of 2004 purports that 16 percent of adults and 20 percent of youths who are incarcerated have a mental health disability; the $50 million it allocated for the purposes of the act comes to approximately $200 for every incarcerated person with mental health disabilities. Amnesty International (2006) chronicles the executions of scores of prisoners with mental health disabilities, some of whom have been severely impaired, over the last few decades. Several were executed after committing heinous crimes; however, they had received little or no pre-crime help for their problems, although they had often sought services. While public policies for people considered to have mental health disabilities have come a long way since the days of forced sterilization and institutionalization, the resources to help these people live and function in society continue to be limited, resulting in poverty, involvement in the criminal justice system, and life on the margins of society. Federal policies discriminate against people with mental health disabilities who need treatment. For example, Medicaid guidelines prohibit payments for the care of people between the ages of twenty-two and sixty-four years in "institutions for *mental diseases*" (U.S. Department of Health and Human Services) and limit supports for other types of service. However, Medicaid routinely pays for the care of people who use regular medical hospitals for physical diseases and even for psychiatric units that are part of medical hospitals. Insurance companies routinely provide fewer benefits for mental health treatment than for traditional medical treatment. These policies reflect common societal prejudices about atypical behaviors and thoughts that have been characterized by labels such as madness and insanity.

LANGUAGE, MEANING, AND MENTAL HEALTH DISABILITY

Disability language, including mental health disability language, will most likely continue to evolve in the years ahead. We reiterate here the importance of respecting and using the language individuals prefer. Language referring to mental health disability may also vary by context. Some people with mental health disabilities use language based on their settings. For example, when one seeks health care for problems associated with mental health disability, person-first language (e.g., "person with depression," "person with schizophrenia," "person with mental illness") may be acceptable and preferred. However, in nonmedical contexts, disability-first language may be preferred. Mental health disability can complicate people's lives and the lives of their loved ones. However, living with a mental health disability can also provide insights and life experiences that directly result from the disability and would not occur otherwise. In this context, people may identify as disabled men or women. Disability identity often evolves over time. For more than forty years, one of the authors lived with the internalized ableism and shame of mental health disabilities. However, over the last decade, that shame has been replaced, first with acknowledgment, and gradually with a sense of identity and appreciation. The newfound appreciation for this disability has been adopted much more readily by younger generations, who may experience a similar sense of self and live without the shame the author experienced for decades.

As we have discussed, traditional explanations for mental health disabilities are rooted in the moral model of disability and based on individual pathology. As scientific inquiry began to replace moral and religious thought, the explanations for these characteristics evolved to define them as illness, often a result of bad parenting and biology. Currently, mental health disabilities are primarily characterized as neurobiological dysfunctions that are multifactorial in nature and include a strong genetic component. Advancements in technology give us our best understanding, but we suggest that the explanations for these characteristics are based strongly in culture. These conditions are biosocial in nature, and the meanings of these conditions are socially derived. Western society's three primary religions are all based on the premise that God communicated with prophets and revelators on behalf of all people. Many of these people were rejected by their contemporaries, yet today their words are considered scriptural—as the mind and will of a deity. In Western society today, if one talks with one's deity, one is being religious or spiritual; however, if that deity talks back, one is defined as hallucinating. This observation is *not* made to denigrate people's spiritual beliefs, but to illustrate that the conceptualization of mental health disabilities is culturally mediated and not an objective fact. Thomas Szasz (1997), a psychiatrist and one of the most vocal critics of modern psychiatry, challenges the existence of mental health disabilities or "insanity" and accuses the mental health community of manufacturing and defining mental health disabilities as a means to absolve people of personal responsibility and to exert secular control in a manner similar to religious control mechanisms of past centuries. He states that mental health disability is an idea, not a fact, as are conditions such as diabetes, stating,

Anyone who values the truth ought to think twice before embracing the flood of information about mental illness that carries our government's imprimatur. I am convinced psychiatric explanations and interventions are fatally flawed and that, deep in their hearts, most people think so too. . . . If mental illness is common, can strike anyone, and is just like other illness, as the experts claim, then why do people hardly ever think that they themselves have such an illness? . . . And why, if they themselves are so wonderfully free of mental illness, do they find others so terribly full of it? (p. 5)

In contrast to Szasz, others such as the World Health Organization, NAMI, and the National Institute of Mental Health treat mental health disabilities as a fact. Multiple organizations have been created for people with mental health disabilities. Most conceptualize them as mental illness and/or disease and have been instrumental in advocating their rights and participation in society. NAMI (2006c) describes itself as "a grassroots organization of individuals with serious mental illnesses and their family members whose mission is to eradicate serious mental illnesses and improve the quality of life of persons of all ages who are affected by them." The organization's philosophy is that mental health disabilities are not preventable or curable but are treatable and manageable. It acknowledges its right and responsibility to "forcefully advocate for the rights of persons with serious mental illnesses, even when our views conflict with the views of other disability groups." NAMI identifies mental illness as a brain disorder that has strong genetic components but that is complex and not well understood. It is most concerned with serious and persistent mental health disabilities. While it uses a medical model to explain mental health disabilities, it acknowledges the pervasiveness of discrimination and lack of opportunity in the lives of the people for whom it advocates.

In the United States, the primary governmental organization dealing with mental health is the National Institute of Mental Health (2005), which has a mission to "reduce the burden of mental and behavioral disorders through research on mind, brain, and behavior." Other countries have similar bodies. The World Health Organization (2002) estimates that worldwide, 154 million "suffer" from depression, 25 million have schizophrenia, and more than 100 million have substance use disorders. The World Health Organization estimates that the disease burden of "mental and neurological disorders will increase from 11 percent to nearly 15 percent by 2020." In the United States, the National Institute of Mental Health provides a plethora of resources and initiatives relative to mental health and "mental disorders." The Web site of the National Institute of Mental Health (n.d.) lists mood disorders (e.g., depression, bipolar disorder), schizophrenia, anxiety disorders (e.g., panic phobias), eating disorders, ADHD, autism, and Alzheimer's disease as primary foci of their efforts. The National Institute of Mental Health estimates that approximately one in four adults in the United States experiences a *DSM* diagnosable mental disorder in any given year. Based on the World Health Organization's Mental Health Survey, Kessler, Berglund, Demler, Jin, Merikangas, and Walters (2005) estimate that 46 percent of Americans will experience a *DSM* diagnosable disorder, and that 27 percent will experience two or more disorders at some time during their lives. Leckliter and Matarazzo (1994) assert that 15 percent of the U.S. population lives with a mental disorder at any given time, and that one-third of adults will experience a mental disorder at some time in their lives. Of those with a mental health disorder, Kessler, Chiu, Demler, and Walters (2005) found that about one in five are "serious" in nature. According to these data, approximately one in fifteen to twenty people experience a severe mental disorder, though the National Institute of Mental Health (2005) believes people with severe and persistent mental health disabilities are underrepresented in these studies. It is the smaller group that the National Institute of Mental Health identifies as carrying the primary burden of illness, and toward whom much attention needs to be directed. For example, approximately one-fourth of homeless people in the United States are thought to have severe and persistent mental health disabilities (National Coalition for the Homeless, 2006).

We should be aware that definitions of mental health disabilities as well as estimates of incidence and prevalence vary widely. In a compilation of articles on mental health published by Greenhaven Press (2007), mental health experts take dramatically different stances on issues such as definitions and prevalence, severity, treatments, and societal responses to health disabilities. Conflicts today exist about issues such as social control versus self-determination, insight versus anosognosia, and treatment versus punishment. Some experts emphasize the individual and personal nature of mental health disabilities, while others focus on the problems of diagnosis and stigma (Harman, 2003; Hatfield & Lefley, 1993; Wood, 2006). Lane (2007) chronicles and questions the need for the dramatic expansion of the number of labels and psychiatric disorders in recent decades. Citing several legal cases involving psychiatric diagnosis and legal competence, Kirk and Kutchins (1992) warn about the "validity of diagnoses in the face of shifting diagnostic systems and ideological conflicts about the proper methods of understanding and treating clinical conditions" (p. 4). Others warn about the pervasive influence of psychiatry in defining the scope of mental health disabilities and parameters of mental health (Barber, 2008; Caplan, 1995; Szasz, 1997; Walenstein, 1998).

Increasingly, people who have been diagnosed with mental health disabilities and other advocates are applying a social model approach to mental health disability. The mission of the Judge David L. Bazelon Center for Mental Health Law (n.d.) "is to protect and advance the rights of adults and children who have mental disabilities. The Center envisions an America where people who have mental illnesses or developmental disabilities exercise their own life choices and have access to the resources that enable them to participate fully in their communities." The Bazelon Center acknowledges the significance of discrimination and the need for disability rights. Groups comprised primarily of "psychiatric survivors," such as MindFreedom International (n.d.), have organized to "unite in a spirit of mutual cooperation for a nonviolent revolution of mental health human rights and choice." Mind-Freedom International "is an independent nonprofit coalition defending human rights and promoting humane alternatives for mental and emotional well being" that sponsors "Mad Pride" events that educate about and advocate civil rights protections. They celebrate a culture of people considered by society to have mental health disabilities. As a tongue-in-cheek critique of the overdiagnosis of health disabilities and psychiatric abuse, MindFreedom International board member Janet Foner (n.d.) offers ten warning signs of severe and persistent normality. Her diagnosis includes tearlessnicity, stiff upper lippity, inappropriate smiling, conformity prone, hyper-inactivity, adjustment prone/adjustment reaction, normal naïveté disorder, severe blinder-itis, and corporate asskissingitis. Barber (2008) laments the "rampant overmedication" of Americans in recent years. He states that in 2006 there were 227 million prescriptions for antidepressants and contends that drug companies first create a market for psychotropic medications then rush in to fill the need—and make billions of dollars in profits.

Even governmental and other formal organizations are increasingly recognizing the civil rights needs and applying the social model relative to mental health disabilities. The United Nations (2007) Convention on the Rights of Persons with Disabilities recognizes the pervasive discrimination worldwide and establishes protocols for civil rights protections. In the United States, the National Council on Disability (NCD) is an independent federal agency established to promote equal opportunity, self-sufficiency, and integration of disabled persons. The National Council on Disability (2000) delivered a report to President Clinton that called

> on the President and Congress to address the problems described in its report, particularly by ensuring that people with psychiatric disabilities themselves are involved in a major way in making the policy changes that will enable them to claim their full citizenship rights. The NCD also calls on the media to address the problems described herein, and to avoid the negative stereotyping that has often typified public discussions of mental illness.
>
> The NCD looks forward to the day when the label of psychiatric disability has no more effect on people's rights than does any other disability label. Until that day, the NCD believes that people with psychiatric disabilities will remain among the most underprivileged and disadvantaged of American citizens.

The NCD executive summary included ten recommendations and conclusions.

1. Laws that allow the use of involuntary treatments such as forced drugging and inpatient and outpatient commitment should be viewed as inherently suspect.

2. People labeled with psychiatric disabilities should have a major role in the direction and control of programs and services designed for their benefit.
3. Mental health treatment should be about healing, not punishment.
4. Federal research and demonstration resources should place a higher priority on the development of culturally appropriate alternatives to the medical and biochemical approaches to treatment of people labeled with psychiatric disabilities.
5. Eligibility for services in the community should never be contingent on participation in treatment programs.
6. Employment and training and vocational rehabilitation programs must account for the wide range of abilities, skills, knowledge, and experience of people labeled with psychiatric disabilities.
7. Federal income support programs like Supplemental Security Income and Social Security Disability Insurance should provide flexible and work-friendly support options.
8. To assure [sic] that parity laws do not make it easier to force people into accepting "treatments" they do not want, it is critical that these laws define parity only in terms of voluntary treatments and services.
9. Government civil rights enforcement agencies and publicly funded advocacy organizations should work more closely together and with adequate funding to implement effectively critical existing laws.
10. Federal, state, and local governments, including education, health care, social services, juvenile justice, and civil rights enforcement agencies, must work together to reduce the placement of children and young adults with disabilities, particularly those labeled seriously emotionally disturbed, in correctional facilities and other segregated settings.

It is important to note that the NCD report consistently refers to people with mental health disabilities with the imprimatur "labeled with psychiatric disabilities" in deference to the common nomenclature. The report seems to reflect a hesitance to embrace the use of psychiatry as a reference and to implicitly acknowledge the lack of consensus relative to the extant nomenclature.

Like organizations such as NCD and MindFreedom, we approach mental health disabilities from the social model perspective. It is important to recognize characteristics and attributes that currently carry labels such as mental illness and psychiatric illness. We acknowledge that these conditions and characteristics affect people's lives, due to a combination of internal and external factors. Concomitantly, we believe that societal discrimination and other reactions account for the most significant problems for people who carry these labels. We reject notions separating mind from body for those who integrate them. Understanding of mental health disabilities has increased dramatically, yet we caution against relying to too great an extent on positivistic thinking or defining extant understandings as factual. An examination of how the meanings of multiple personality disorder and dissociative identity disorder have evolved in recent decades serves as a warning. As a young professional, one of the authors attended workshops sponsored by mental health experts and law enforcement officials on the "hidden epidemic" of multiple personality disorder and dissociative identity disorder secondary to ritualistic satanic child abuse. Subsequent research and lack of evidence have debunked many of the claims that were treated as facts in the 1980s. Another example is the passage by several countries and the states of Oregon and Washington of laws sanctioning physician-assisted suicide and/or voluntary euthanasia for people with terminal illness. In the context of terminal illness, suicide is considered rational; however, non-terminally ill people who wish to die are labeled mentally ill and are subject to involuntary detention. We suggest the reasons so many people reject the idea that they have a mental health disability are (1) the shame and guilt associated with the characterization, and (2) the overdiagnosing and pathologizing of atypicalities. The common labeling of mental health disabilities as illness and disease and the use of adjectives such as *afflicted, suffering*, and *tragedy* to describe life with a "mental illness" furthers this prejudice by medicalizing and pathologizing those deemed to have mental health disabilities.

LIVING WITH A MENTAL HEALTH DISABILITY

Shame and guilt are still associated with mental health disabilities; however, changes are occurring. The Americans with Disabilities Act of 1990 includes people with mental health disabilities among the groups of people with disabilities who are eligible for its civil rights protections. In developed countries, when mental health disability impairs people's ability to work (and they can prove incapacity), they may be eligible for income maintenance programs such as Social Security. In most developed countries, medical benefits are universal. However, in the United States those with mental health disabilities are often discouraged from working out of the fear that they will lose medical benefits and become ineligible for income maintenance if they become incapacitated in the future. It is commonly perceived that people with mental health disabilities are incapable of working; however, discriminatory public policies and ableist societal attitudes lead to marginalization and reinforce the shame and assumptions of incompetence associated with mental health disability.

Important recent developments leading to the reduction of shame and stigma associated with mental health disability include several celebrities' revelations of their own mental health disabilities. For example, actress Patty

Duke acknowledges that she lives with bipolar disorder. Newsperson Mike Wallace, author William Styron, and Olympic athlete Greg Louganis have detailed their experiences with severe depression. The late Lionel Aldridge, a pro-football star and television announcer, went public with his schizophrenia. The Academy Award–winning movie *A Dangerous Mind* chronicles the life and schizophrenia of Nobel Prize laureate John Nash. Tipper Gore, wife of former vice president Al Gore, has acknowledged her depression and, like several others cited above, has become an advocate for others. Historical figures purported to have lived with serious mental health disabilities include Abraham Lincoln, Vincent van Gough, Leo Tolstoy, Isaac Newton, Edgar Allen Poe, and Irving Berlin.

Arguably, scientific advances are having a dramatic influence on the lives of people with mental health disabilities. Neuroscientists argue that technology such as MRIs and PET scans provide insight into the biochemical processes that occur in the brain with mental health disabilities. In addition, pharmacological research and development have greatly expanded drug options for people deemed to have atypical brain function and mental health disabilities. These developments have led to the questioning and the rejection of moral model explanations of mental health disabilities. However, when the moral model that generates stigma and ostracization is replaced by the medical model, according to which the lives of "patients" are controlled by mental health professionals, there may be little net improvement in people's lives.

Though technology is increasingly providing information about the biology of mental health conditions, people's functioning is still defined by our social contexts. An early career experience of one of the authors illustrates. As a young professor, the author unsuccessfully attempted to publish the results of a study comparing the experiences of disabled college educators to those of gays and lesbians, women, and faculty of color. In referring to people with mental health disabilities, one reviewer's succinct comments demonstrated the problems the author had getting the article published: "Reject, reject, reject, do you really think we want those people in our profession?" The author subsequently published the study results in a journal devoted to gay and lesbian issues. In addition, the author learned that keeping personal and family history of depression under wraps was critical to professional success. Below, we provide another example of dramatic differences in how what we label mental health disabilities are perceived and defined.

Mark was a twenty-seven-year-old Native American man with multiple fractures and internal injuries as a result of a motorcycle accident. Mark had been raised on a reservation in the western United States, and this was his first experience with modern medicine. Mark considered himself the recipient of spiritual messages, and members of his family and home community perceived him similarly. When Mark informed hospital staff of the voices that were guiding him, a psychiatric consult was immediately ordered and Mark was ascertained to be delusional.

In Mark's community, he was considered spiritually gifted; in the hospital he was diagnosed with a mental health disability. Though no tests were performed, it is highly likely brain scans would have shown elevated activity in areas consistent with others who are similarly diagnosed. Parenthetically, when Mark's spiritual leader visited him in the hospital, chanting over him and moving his hands over Mark's body to work on his energy fields, health providers labeled the actions superstitious and "Voodoo." However, some of those who criticized him most strongly had religious traditions of church elders laying hands on heads to provide blessings of healing.

In contrast to the medical model, the social model posits that people with mental health disabilities have the right and the responsibility to control their own lives. Whereas the medical model labels them patients to be treated, the social model emphasizes the individuality and uniqueness of each individual and the inherent right to autonomy. They have a right to—and society has a responsibility to provide—an environment that is accessible to people with mental health disabilities. At times, when individuals become compromised in their ability to exercise self-determination, others may need to step in. However, in contrast to the moral and medical models, the social model begins with the assumption of competence. Self-determination is reduced or removed only with reluctance and when the danger of harm to self or others warrants it. For example, consider the case of Donna, a forty-seven-year-old woman diagnosed with schizophrenia. Donna lived in an urban setting but was reluctant to empty her garbage because a mountain lion might attack her. She had auditory hallucinations, and voices would periodically tell her to barricade doors in her apartment. In addition, her living conditions were very cluttered but were not unsafe or filthy. She used the local bus system to shop and go to appointments, but she also isolated herself. Donna's caseworker intervened to move Donna to a congregate care facility, a move that Donna resisted but nonetheless was coerced to make. She liked living on her own, with periodic help, but her caseworker insisted she would be better off around others and with supervision. Though Donna acquiesced, she lost her independence and required hospitalization twice over the next six months. Previously, she had gone three years without hospitalization while relying on outpatient treatment. Had a social model approach been utilized, Donna's self-determination would have been given a higher priority in decision making, as opposed to professionals deciding what was best for her. Organizations like MindFreedom International and other advocacy groups are taking active roles to maximize self-determination and resources for people in situations like Donna's.

Kay Jamison (1995), a psychologist with manic depression, provides a personal account of living with a bipolar condition. She also suggests that mental health disabilities can have positive effects on people's lives, stating,

Occasionally an exhilarating and powerfully creative force, more often a destructive one, manic-depressive illness gives a touch of fire to many of those who experience it. . . . There is strong scientific and biological evidence linking manic-depressive illness and its related temperaments to artistic imagination and expression. Biographies of eminent poets, artists, and composers attest to the strikingly high rate of mood disorders and suicide—as well as institutionalization in asylums and psychiatric hospitals—in these individuals, and recent psychiatric and psychological studies of living artists have further documented the link. (p. 240)

Jamison's belief that mental health disabilities have beneficial and difficult components are shared by others such as Patty Duke (Duke & Hochman, 1997). As one of the authors, who lives with depression, has found, periods of depression can also lead to bursts of productivity, sometimes as a therapeutic mechanism to alleviate that depression. However, the societal implications can be devastating: people are shunned, denied basic human rights, and subjected to discrimination. Employment and housing are difficult to obtain and stigma follows people everywhere (Wedenoja, 1999). Leete (1997) illustrates the stigma and discrimination associated with severe mental health disability:

Life is hard with a diagnosis of schizophrenia. I can talk, but I may not be heard. I can make suggestions, but they may not be taken seriously. I can report my thoughts, but they may be seen as delusions. I can recite experiences, but they may be interpreted as fantasies. To be a patient or even ex-client is to be discounted. Your label is a reality that never leaves you; it gradually shapes an identity that is hard to shed. We must transform public attitudes and current stereotypes. Until we eliminate stigma, we will have prejudice, which will inevitably be expressed as discrimination against persons with mental illness. (p. 102)

The late Howard Gelb, also known as Howie the Harp, was a psychiatric patient, then a homeless psychiatric survivor, who subsequently became an advocate for people with mental health disabilities. Howie strongly advocated a social model that emphasized freedom, stating, "The progressive collective minds of our mental health system have slowly, by degrees, crept toward the realization that what is good for everyone—what Americans have fought and died for—what civil rights movements have struggled for—is also good for mental health consumers. I remember a sign at one of our rallies: 'Freedom is the Best Therapy.' Freedom of choice, independence, self-determination, and empowerment are what's best for us" (qtd. in Carling, 1995, pp. xv–xvi).

The documentary film *The Legacy of the Harp* deals with Howie the Harp's work helping improve the lives of people who have been incarcerated and diagnosed as having mental health disabilities. It chronicles their risks of victimization, imprisonment, and suicide. It acknowledges that medications, professionals, and treatments can have a positive influence but reflects his beliefs that a sense of belonging, productivity, and community is the best treatment for those considered to have severe mental health disabilities. Furthermore, it provides a sense of hope for people diagnosed with severe and persistent mental health disabilities who are considered incurable.

We believe that the primary problems facing the majority of people with mental health disabilities continue to be social and societal in nature. Guilt, shame, and fear are common. For those who can hide their disabilities from the public, doing so can reduce the social costs of this disability, albeit with negative personal consequences, such as lack of understanding and denial of one's identity. Descriptors such as *sufferers, victims, patients, dangerous, incompetent, crazy, insane*, and *mad* perpetuate ableism and an abundance of myths. Improvements are being made but are slow in coming. Below, we provide some ideas to improve the quality of life of people with mental health disabilities.

1. Removing barriers to housing, employment, medical/mental health care, and social integration will significantly reduce the burden of mental health disabilities more efficiently than the creation of more institutions and treatment centers.
2. People with mental health disabilities should be assumed to be competent and the experts on their own lives. They have the right to control their lives, a right that should be compromised only in dire circumstances.
3. To maximize quality of life and contributions to society, resources for people with mental health disabilities should be made available in the form of investments that allow people the opportunity to contribute to society. This approach should replace the current service system approach that provides services, but not an opportunity for or expectation of a return on investment.
4. People diagnosed with severe and persistent mental health disabilities have the same rights to live in society as others. We acknowledge that, at times, people may become unable to care for and make decisions for themselves. There are several steps to prevent and ameliorate these instances:
   o "Psychosis" and "psychotic" events should be treated as temporary and episodic rather than permanent, and self-determination should be promoted to the maximum extent possible.
   o Preventive resources allowing for prompt action that ameliorate and/or prevent severe problems should be plentiful.
   o People with mental health disabilities should be able to create mental health advance directives that allow them to outline the preferred avenues of intervention in the event that they are unable to make decisions for themselves.

○ The use of correction and penal systems as a primary mechanism of control of and care for people with severe mental health disabilities should be discontinued, and adequate access to preventive community resources and supports should be provided.

○ Parity in access to mental health and medical resources should be promoted.

○ Holistic supports that account for the needs of families and loved ones and that balance decisions with the primary responsibility of self-determination of the individual should be made available.

5. Self-control and advocacy organizations that follow the social model and support an independent living philosophy should receive high priority. When effective, organizations and approaches that promote an independent living model should replace traditional medical model–based organizations and approaches.

6. Social policies should be modified to promote people with mental health disabilities as experts, advocates, role models, and service providers.

7. Professionals and professional organizations are important resources, and collaboration between them and disabled persons and organizations should be encouraged.

We reject the prevailing philosophy that mental health disability is a tragedy. People with mental health disabilities are a diverse group of people who also share commonalities. The implications of mental health disabilities range from mild to severe, dramatic to imperceptible, and run the gamut from positive to very negative. Though the literature is replete with books and articles that chronicle the pathologies and problems of this group of disabled persons, we contend that social costs would dramatically decrease in direct proportion to decreased ableism and discrimination, and the development of positive social policies and practices.

A recent experience of one of the authors illustrates. While we were writing this text, the author engaged in a discussion with a man who is a social worker, and his adult daughter, who is a psychologist, both of whom had experienced significant depression during their lives. Minutes before, the daughter had been in a conversation with a colleague who, unaware of the daughter's history, articulated the eugenicist philosophy that it would be "best if the mentally ill do not reproduce." The daughter was shocked by the statement but remained silent. However, when she saw her father, she became tearful and told him of the statement. She then asked him, "Dad, do you ever wish you had not had me? Do you wish that I had not been born?" The father answered, "Never," but was saddened that his loving and capable daughter was still subjected to and vulnerable to ableism that questions her worthiness and right to live.

SUMMARY

Hundreds of millions of people live with mental health disabilities world-wide. In many societies, mental disabilities are viewed as a cause for shame and guilt. In the contemporary United States and Europe, they are considered a medical illness. Whatever the explanation, people with mental health disabilities are at increased risk of discrimination, exclusion, and in some cases incarceration. Their treatment is based on the belief that the problems associated with "mental illness" reside within the individual. In contrast, though we recognize personal implications and problems, we suggest that the primary obstacles faced by individuals with mental health disabilities are located in the societies and communities in which they reside. We suggest that the removal of negative attitudes, discrimination, and societal barriers will dramatically improve their lives.

This chapter applies an alternate approach to mental health disabilities to that commonly provided elsewhere. It does not view people with mental health disabilities as ill or diseased; rather it suggests that they have conditions and characteristics that are defined as disabilities. Readers who want an in-depth discussion of the personal pathologies associated with mental health disability have a plethora of other resources to consult. However, we wish to emphasize the importance of eliminating discrimination and providing people with mental health disabilities with access to societal resources and equal opportunities, which will improve their quality of life and will benefit society far more than treatment approaches that focus on individual pathology, disease, and illness.

PERSONAL NARRATIVE: DONNA ORRIN

Donna Orrin, MSW, lives with bipolar disorder. She has worked as a psychiatric social worker and as the president of her own business, Creative Connections. She provides extensive training to consumers with mental health disabilities and their family members. She also provides training for mental health professionals.

The first eighteen years of my life were not very happy because I always had negative, self-critical thoughts. However, I didn't tell anyone about them. My mom always had an enthusiastic, happy sense about her, and I was always very active.

In high school, I was an honor student. I won an award for being the most active senior of the year. I also won humanitarian awards and was always involved in activities. I would put a smile on my face and act happy and people really thought that I was happy. Yet my attention was always riveted on negative, self-critical thoughts criticizing everything I did as I did it. I never told anyone because I didn't think anybody could help. I had lots of friends, and they didn't know how poorly I was doing. However, when I started feeling really bad, they tended to shy away.

At eighteen, I left home to go to college, and the real trouble began. My depression really progressed. I started skipping classes and didn't get involved in any extracurricular activities at all. I ended up not showing up for exams and getting incompletes. I began to feel suicidal.

My twin brother, Dale, was living in the dorm across the street from my dorm. I would contact him when I was suicidal. I reached out to him and he really helped. My God, what a heavy burden to put on an eighteen-, nineteen-, or twenty-year-old. I feel sorry about how much I relied on him because I didn't realize the impact it had on him. Because of all the problems, I ended up dropping out of college after one or two years.

It was then, in 1972, that my psychotic and manic symptoms started. I heard voices and thought I could talk to people who were more than one hundred years old and to others who were no longer alive. I could see things that weren't there. I don't remember quite clearly what my symptoms were at that point, but my friends and family were concerned and suggested I needed inpatient hospitalization. But I was in denial and I didn't think that what they saw were symptoms. I just thought I was having wonderful experiences.

Let me say here that a real problem with mental illness is how denial is often a symptom. There is nothing we have discovered yet to solve the problem of denial. I was finally convinced to seek help by a professor because he told me to think of hospitalization as going to a "human potential seminar." He said to think of it like I was going to be there for a couple of weeks with a bunch of other people who were there for the same reason. He said I would be kind of isolated and I would have time to work on my human potential growth. So, he drove me to Kingswood Hospital, where they diagnosed me with bipolar disorder with psychotic symptoms. They prescribed lithium. That was the beginning of the recovery path of my mental illness. But the road was a long one. I had over thirty hospitalizations spanning the next twenty years.

After I got out of the hospital, my problems continued. I went to visit Dale, who was then in New York City. I was walking around the streets of Harlem late one night and the police picked me up. I wound up at Bellevue Hospital, where they put me on high doses of medication. When I got out, I went to visit my sister, who doesn't believe in medical treatment. She believes in alternative care, so she took me to her chiropractor, who took me off my medication cold turkey and put me on kelp instead. I went through withdrawal from stopping my medication. It was horrendous; the physical symptoms were really bad.

At that time, one of the biggest problems was isolation. People didn't know a lot. I couldn't talk to anyone about mental illness. My mother was frustrated; she didn't know where she could go for help, and she couldn't talk to any family members or friends about it because nobody was willing to talk to her.

I went to live with my mother, and for eight months, I lay on her couch thinking about nothing but all the mistakes I had made in my life. It felt like there was a two-ton car on top of me, and I didn't have the strength to lift it off my chest. I was paralyzed on the couch. I didn't have the energy to move.

Mom insisted that I go for a short walk with her every day. If she hadn't insisted I go with her, I never would have left the couch. Those short ten-minute walks were very hard on me. I talked with only one friend once a week, and we would just chit-chat. She had no idea what my lifestyle was like, and I wouldn't tell her. I didn't know that I could do anything else. I just didn't think I could do anything.

At that time, I was not involved at all in the community mental health (CMH) system; I didn't even know there was such a thing as CMH. I hardly knew anyone with mental illness. My education about mental illness consisted of the book *One Flew over the Cuckoo's Nest,* which was really bad news. I felt all alone, and I believed there were lots of really bad things wrong with me.

After eight months of lying around, my mom said she was taking me to a therapist. It had never occurred to me that there might be some treatment for this. Because I had never been in therapy before and had never been educated about selecting a therapist, I ended up with a therapist who was not well versed in mental illness.

With my therapist's encouragement, I started doing more. I would bake bread once a week. That was a big deal! Then I started doing volunteer work one day a week, then two days a week. Eventually, I started working part-time twenty hours a week. My therapist encouraged me to do these things. I then began to deal with my issues, concerns, and goals.

Eventually, I went back to school. I went to Oakland University because I could commute there and still live at my mom's house. I took one class, then two. I even started working on a novel under a Michigan Council for the Arts grant, about the six months I spent in a mental hospital. Over time, I got my degree and started working in communications, and I started making more and better friends.

When I had gone a period without hospitalization, I started to ask myself if I really had to be on medication for the rest of my life. So I talked to my therapist, my family, coworkers, and my friends. We decided I would try to go off my medications on a trial basis. Within two weeks, I was in a state mental hospital. My doctor there believed that I wasn't manic but schizophrenic, and she tried a different medication on me. My mother and my therapist would try to talk to her, but she wouldn't even see them. They wanted to encourage her to put me on lithium. Not only did she refuse to change my medications, but she wouldn't even give them the time of day. She put me on a variety of other medications, and I was just wiped out. She kept this up for five-and-a-half months before she finally put me on lithium. Within two weeks, I was out of there.

Believe me, a state hospital is no place to go for a five-and-a-half-month vacation. I was left feeling powerless. At the time, I tried to sign myself out voluntarily, but they initiated quick proceedings to involuntarily commit me. I was very angry, but I'm glad now that they were able to prevent me from leaving. My involuntary commitment was beneficial, though I didn't have the insight to realize it at the time. I just wish I had received appropriate treatment.

This hospitalization made me feel powerless; it felt like they stripped me of my soul. I was put in seclusion eighteen times— talk about powerlessness. I was on a ward of thirty women, and we had three seclusion rooms. The seclusion rooms were always full. I was not a danger to myself or others when they put me in seclusion, I swear to God. I know I needed to be in the hospital, but not under the treatment they gave me.

It is ironic that if you go to a hospital for physical care, you have your own phone and your own room. But if you are in a state hospital for mental illness, you get one phone for thirty women, in the hallway, with no privacy. We had to line up to get a chance to use the phone.

One experience during that hospitalization was especially memorable. I was very close to my twin brother, and I was on the phone with him. One of the attendants said to hang up, that it was time to sleep. I put up a finger to signal to him to give me just one minute and I would say good-bye. Before I knew it, two attendants had forced my arms behind my back and dragged me to the seclusion room, leaving the telephone receiver dangling. I was yelling, "Dale, Dale, Dale!" and I couldn't even say good-bye to him. They put me in seclusion overnight. I could only think, "Oh, no, Dale's going to really worry about what happened to me!" I was worried about my brother. I didn't know why they put me in there, didn't know what I had to do to get out, or even when I would get out. All I could do was take four steps one way, then two steps another way. The room smelled really strongly of urine. There was only a plastic bed to lie on and a really high window to look out. Because of my condition, I was experiencing an altered sense of time, so it seemed like I was there for a million years. It was a terrible experience.

Sometimes they threw people in there and told them to calm down as they closed the door. What a joke! Who would calm down? Yeah, right, as if those rooms would calm anyone down. They called this treatment, to help people with calming down. They had to be kidding. One time I felt so powerless and frustrated, I began head banging in the seclusion room. I was sent to intensive care for ten days. I did enough damage to my eyes that there was no white in them; they were completely red for weeks, and I didn't know if I would ever see the whites of my eyes again. Later, I received intensive treatment for this closed head injury.

Back then, there was no multidisciplinary treatment at the state hospital. I remember my social worker telling me to read the Bible and it would treat me. That's all he ever said to me. That was my social work treatment at the state hospital—not extraordinarily effective. As I was being discharged from the hospital, my social worker said, "Donna, face the facts: you're only going to be a store clerk a few months out of every year, and as you get older you're going to have more and more hospitalizations." That was my mental illness "education."

They used to have workshops for us back then. They consisted of reading the front page of the paper and making belts and ashtrays—I didn't even smoke. I remember a funny story about that. A group of us were talking, and somehow we got on the subject of Vincent van Gogh. Someone said, "Gee, isn't it a shame there weren't hospitals like the hospitals we have today back in van Gogh's time?" Someone else in the group said, "Yeah, just think of all those ashtrays and leather belts he missed out on."

Not all my hospitalizations have been like my state hospital experience. There are a lot of good psychiatric hospitals around. I have been to at least three. They provide a lot more freedom, a lot more respect, and better treatment. They provide therapy, though I must admit it is sometimes hard for therapy to be effective when people are functioning at a really low level. Cognitive theory and therapy are wonderful tools. It is hard to teach people much when they are hospitalized for only a couple of weeks, but cognitive therapy has been wonderful for me. I do think that hospitals educate people about their mental illness better than in the past. Yet they used to have more for people to do on weekends so they wouldn't regress.

From 1972 to 1992, I had about forty hospitalizations, but I have turned things around. I have had no hospitalization in the last five years. A number of things have helped me turn things around. One was electroconvulsive therapy (ECT). It was a last-resort treatment after a suicide attempt. I had taken a hundred aspirin, but they pumped my stomach. I also tried to kill myself when I was on MAO inhibitors (an antidepressant). I ate the foods that are prohibited with MAO inhibitors: wine, cheese, and chocolate. I did other things, too. I was really trying to kill myself, and nothing was working. I had given up hope and everyone else, with the exception of my therapist, had given up hope. I had finally found a good therapist. I became able to overcome traumatic times and negative thoughts, feelings, and actions. I created new, positive beliefs by releasing my distress through a form of cognitive therapy. The therapy was instrumental in my development of the quality of life of my choice.

Without the combination of therapy and ECT, I would probably be dead. At a minimum, I certainly wouldn't have the quality of life I have now. ECT alone would not have done the job, but ECT and therapy were really quite wonderful.

A third intervention was also extremely important. It was a simple intervention but was very difficult to get. When I was discharged from the hospital after having ECT, I was a CMH client. I requested that someone from CMH call me every morning and every evening to remind me to take my medications every day. These reminder calls were extremely valuable.

The fourth reason for my success is that I have learned to recognize and know my individual symptoms. I am celebrating my five-year anniversary, but that doesn't mean I haven't had manic and psychotic symptoms over the last five years; I have. However, I now recognize them immediately and I take appropriate action. I go to a non-stimulating environment. I go to my home; it's my own personal retreat. Then I call up my therapist and let him know. I call him every day until I get better. I make sure I get plenty of sleep and plenty of food and do my best not to think about any psychological issues. With an understanding with my psychiatrist, I increase my Thorazine. In three to four days, I'm back to stability. Those four things—ECT, therapy, medication reminder calls, and self-awareness and self-care—are the reasons why I am celebrating my five-year anniversary without hospitalization.

I want to explain more about my reminder calls. The calls were my idea, but the CMH professionals made it really difficult to get this service. They kept asking me to prove that I needed this assistance. At one point they wanted to give me an IQ test; another time they wanted to give me a memory test. It was after being diagnosed with severe attention deficit disorder without hyperactivity that I understood why I don't remember to take my meds. I can be in the bathroom and think, "I've got to remember to take my meds," but two minutes later I haven't taken my meds and have forgotten that I need to take them. When I think about what I had to go through to get those medication reminder calls, it just infuriates me. I'm a pretty assertive person and, in fact, I was on the CMH board at the time. Yet they said I was trying to be taken care of. That's like saying somebody with a physical disability is asking to be taken care of if she needs a wheelchair. No, a wheelchair is a tool or instrument that enables her to have an independent life. A wheelchair is what she needs to take care of herself and move on in life. My medication calls were my tool and were extremely cost effective: two one-minute phone calls a day compared to two months of hospitalization. It makes me wonder: if getting those calls was that difficult for me, what is it like for other consumers when they ask for the help they know they need?

Not being able to work was very hard on me. I come from a hardworking family. My grandmother told us, "Do for others, do for others." We were trained to do for others, so it was painful for me when I was not able to work. I felt just terrible about myself. Though my family and friends kept saying, "Donna, don't work right now; it's not time," I felt like I ought to be working. Financially, I didn't need to work because I got Social Security Disability and was able to squeak by. At different times I got little jobs. But by listening to myself, I knew when it was time, and that's when I went back to work. I must say employment isn't the be-all and end-all of things; recovery is the most important and comes before employment. People must allow time to recover before becoming employed. Had I been rushed into employment before I recovered, I would not be doing as well as I'm doing now. I tell others with mental illness, "Don't feel guilty if you're not working yet. I know that you must do what is best for you. You can't help somebody else if you are not taking care of yourself."

The reaction of others is one of the most difficult parts of mental illness. When things get bad, people really shy away. I understand that now more than I did in the past because I have a family member with mental illness who doesn't want to go public with it, so I see it from that perspective now. In lots of ways, the way we are treated is worse than the symptoms themselves. We're avoided. We're abandoned and treated in very inhumane ways—I think worse than an alley cat or dog should be treated.

With depression, one of the symptoms is poverty of thought; if you have poverty of thought, you're going to have poverty of communication, and if you have poverty of communication, you don't make such a good friend. It seems that when people are most needy and can't do it alone, others usually aren't willing to reach out to them. Maybe it's because they feel helpless.

I think it's very important for family and friends to know that they may be helping out more than they realize when things seem bad. Family members and friends may not realize how helpful they are because they don't know what's going on with the individual. They don't see the person's internal thoughts and realizations and understand the importance of their bond with the person. I can't think of anything more important than a family member or friend helping someone stay alive. There is hope. I've been there. I've gone through years of doing nothing but getting up in the morning and going to bed at night, but I made it through all that.

It's important for people to know that people with mental illness want to contribute and we want to work. People just don't seem to know that, and it's a shame. When people are not allowed to contribute, they are being denied their humanity and spirituality. They are being denied their self-worth. Sometimes mental illness is like drowning in the ocean. We have to concentrate on getting safely to the beach. But once we survive, please let us help. We want to help. I think it would be great if we had psycho-education workshops for families and individuals and professionals all together; we need to see everyone else's perspective. We have a seemingly impossible mission, and we can accomplish it only if we all work together.

I have gone from people hanging up on me, avoiding me, and abandoning me to getting paid really well just so people can hear what I have to say. It is very rewarding. What I am doing now is really exciting. I'm involved in policy making. I have my own business and do lots of public speaking. I love giving talks; I love engaging the audience. I'll give a talk, and all these people will come up to me afterward and tell me how much they got out of it.

Twenty years with almost forty hospitalizations contrasted with thirty speeches in one year. I like the thirty speeches part better; it's just such a wonderful feeling. I have also developed successful recovery materials and ongoing workshops for consumers. I've written six nationally published articles, and another is going to be published soon. I am helping others avoid the kind of pain that I went through. I am helping family members avoid the pain that my family went through. It is extremely rewarding.

When I was in high school, I was known as an activist and took on many causes, but I can't think of a better cause for me to advance than helping people understand mental illness. I believe I have a talent in writing, and I use it for the most important cause I can imagine.

I am better off now than I would have been if I had never had mental illness. One of the reasons is all the therapy that I've had. Therapy has made a monumental difference in my life. It's made me know myself and helped me be myself. In my work, all I have to do is be myself. One of the best rewards in my life is that my mother now feels it was worth it to go through all the pain that she went through. She knows that every person I help is someone she has helped because I wouldn't be here without her.

In offering advice, one thing I would suggest to professionals working in hospitals is to let friends and family members know that visits mean a great deal to your patients. One of the things that my friends have done is visit me in pairs. I couldn't always communicate that well when I was doing poorly, but when people came to the hospital in pairs, they could talk to each other and I could benefit from their discussions. Suggest that people visit in pairs so they can keep the conversation rolling and provide company for the individual. Those visits are very helpful and prevent isolation.

Professionals need to view us as adults, not children. Don't be condescending; expect the person to be a mature person. Sometimes, and in some ways, communication may need to be very basic in the sense of telling the person, "You need to do this, this, and this." But the fact that you may need to help people in very basic ways doesn't mean that you should treat them like children. Professionals need to know that even when an adult's behavior is childlike, the person is not a child. The person can make some decisions and should be treated as an adult.

I think that teaching people about person-centered planning is important—letting individuals decide what their goals and dreams are and helping them go for it. Imagine what we could do if the system believed in us. What if we didn't have to fight the system? What if the system helped us? What levels would we soar to? A social worker told me I would require more and more hospitalizations as I got older and would not be employable. Fortunately, others believed in me. I now have my master's degree in social work from the University of Michigan and have worked as a psychiatric social worker in both state and private hospitals and have my own business. Instead of having more and more hospitalizations, I have had fewer and fewer.

The system has to believe in us. This includes professionals in health and mental health systems. I'm talking about doctors, social workers, nurses, personal care attendants, and other professionals. I was lucky. I had a therapist who believed in me. If it hadn't been for him, I wouldn't have gotten my MSW degree. If it hadn't been for him, who knows, maybe I would be dead. During my worst times, he was there fighting for me, and he never gave up hope in me.

I think hope is a really major issue. Professionals must instill a sense of hope in people and their families. Always give individuals logical, concrete examples of why they should be hopeful. When I speak to groups of consumers, I ask them, "In your suicidal days, were you able to hang on because you had one, just one, person who believed in you?" I also ask, "How many of you have come farther in your recovery than you thought possible because someone, just one person, had hope for you?" When I ask just those two questions, almost all the hands in the audience go up. They tell me they got through their suicidal times because someone had hope for them. The best advice I can give professionals is to encourage people. Provide a sense of hope. You may be saving someone's life. You may be making a lifelong difference to an individual.

Mental health consumers must be involved in decision making. To improve treatment, we need consumer input. I wrote a book on policy making, and in it I have many opportunities for policy making for consumers, including how to apply policy-making strategies. People think that people with mental illness can't contribute, but we can. I will never forget the first state-level community mental health meeting I attended. I was at the Michigan Association of Community Health Boards conference, where board members and directors voted on an amendment for the mental health code revisions that would include consumer representation in policy making. I was appalled. We had a forty-five-minute debate. The amendment to include consumers squeaked by with a vote of 54–48. I sat there for forty-five minutes and listened as these board members and directors came up to the microphone, one at a time, saying things like, "Consumers are not *competent* to sit on the board." There is fear, anger, hesitation, and discrimination about mental illness. Such attitudes demonstrate the very reason why we need consumers on the board—because if those policy makers and professionals don't know what's possible, if they don't know how much we can recover, and if they don't know our perspective, there is no way they are going to come up with the best policies on our behalf.

DISCUSSION QUESTIONS

1. What are some of the specific types of discrimination experienced by persons with mental health disabilities and their family members?
2. Describe the impact of social stigma on persons with mental health disabilities.
3. How has the meaning of mental health disabilities evolved over the last few centuries? In the last twenty to thirty years?
4. How did eugenics affect the lives and treatment of people with mental health disabilities during the nineteenth and twentieth centuries? What were the similarities and differences between Nazi Germany and the United States during the 1930s and 1940s?
5. Traditionally, individual treatment and therapy have been used as a way to reduce the social costs of mental health disabilities. What societal and social changes would be effective in improving the lives of people with mental health disabilities and reducing the social burdens associated with mental health disabilities?
6. What are the strengths and limitations of professional approaches to mental health disabilities? What are the strengths and limitations of the social model and independent living approach to mental health disability? What are effective ways that the two approaches can be utilized in partnership?
7. Review professional books and/or articles and the adjectives used to describe mental health disabilities and the lives of people with mental health disabilities. How do these adjectives portray life with a mental health disability? How would alternate adjectives convey different messages?
8. A significant controversy involving people with mental health disabilities involves the use of involuntary treatment. Describe conditions under which involuntary interventions are justified, and not justified. Describe systemic changes that could reduce the need for involuntary treatment.

SUGGESTED READINGS

Andreasen, N. C. (2001). *Brave new brain*. New York: Oxford University Press.
Barber, C. (2008). *Comfortably numb: How psychiatry is medicating a nation*. New York: Pantheon Books.

Brzuzy, S. (1997). Deconstructing disability: The impact of definition. *Journal of Poverty, 1*(1), 81–91.

Caplan, P. J. (1995). *They say you're crazy: How the world's most powerful psychiatrists decide who's normal.* Reading, MA: Addison-Wesley.

Deegan, P. (1992). The independent living movement and people with psychiatric disabilities: Taking back control over our own lives. *Psychosocial Rehabilitation Journal, 15*(3), 3–19

Duke, P., & Hochman, G. (1992). *A brilliant madness: Living with manic-depressive illness.* New York: Bantam Books.

Foucault, M. (2006). *History of madness* (J. Murphy & J. Khalfa, trans.). London: Routledge.

Greenhaven Press. (2007). *Mental health: Current controversies.* New York: Author.

Jamison, K. R. (1993). *Touched with fire: Manic depressive illness and the artistic temperament.* New York: Simon & Schuster.

Jamison, K. R. (1995). *An unquiet mind: A memoir of moods and madness.* New York: Alfred A. Knopf.

Lefley, H. P. (1996). *Family caregiving in mental illness.* Thousand Oaks, CA: Sage.

Marsh, D. T., & Dickens, R. M. (1997). *Troubled journey: Coming to terms with the mental illness of a sibling or parent.* New York: Putnam.

Millon, T. (2004). *Masters of the mind: Exploring the story of mental illness from ancient times to the new millennium.* New York: John Wiley & Sons.

Phillips, J., & Morley, J. (Eds.). (2003). *Imagination and its pathologies.* Cambridge, MA: MIT Press.

Szasz, T. (1997). *Insanity: The idea and its consequences.* New York: Syracuse University Press.

Torrey, E. E (1995). *Surviving schizophrenia.* New York: Harper Collins.

Walenstein, E. S. (1998). *Blaming the brain.* New York: Free Press.

Wasow, M. (1995). *The skipping stone: Ripple effects of mental illness in the family.* Palo Alto, CA: Science and Behavior Books.

REFERENCES

Amnesty International. (2006). *USA: The execution of mentally ill prisoners.* Retrieved June 9, 2008, from http://www.amnesty.org/en/library/asset/AMR51/003/2006/en/dom-AMR510032006en.pdf

Andreasen, N. C. (2001). *Brave new brain.* New York: Oxford University Press.

Anxiety Disorders Association of America. (n.d.). *Statistics and facts about anxiety disorders.* Retrieved from http://www.adaa.org/AboutADAA/PressRoom/Stats&Facts.asp

Armstrong, T. (1995). *The myth of the A.D.D. child: 50 ways to improve your child's behavior and attention span without drugs, labels, or coercion.* New York: Penguin Putnam.

Barber, C. (2008). *Comfortably numb: How psychiatry is medicating a nation.* New York: Pantheon Books.

Bateson, G., Jackson, D., Haley, J., & Weakland, J. (1956). Toward a theory of schizophrenia. *Behavioral Science, 1,* 251–264.

Bentley, K. J., & Walsh, J. F. (2001). *The social worker and psychotropic medication* (2nd ed.). Belmont, CA: Brooks/Cole.

Bowen, M. (1960). A family concept of schizophrenia. In D. D. Jackson (Ed.), *The etiology of schizophrenia* (pp. 346–372). New York: Basic Books.

Buck v. Bell. 274 U.S. 200. (1927).

Caplan, P. J. (1995). *They say you're crazy: How the world's most powerful psychiatrists decide who's normal.* Reading, MA. Addison-Wesley.

Carling, R J. (1995). *Return to community: Building support systems for people with psychiatric disabilities.* New York: Guilford Press

Duke, P., & Hochman, G. (1997). *A brilliant madness: Living with manic-depressive illness.* New York: Bantam Books.

Foner, J. (n.d.). *The 10 warning signs of normality.* Retrieved August 18, 2008, from http://www.mindfreedom.org/campaign/madpride/other-info/normality-screening/10-warning-signs-of-normality

Foucault, M. (2006). *History of madness* (J. Murphy & J. Khalfa, trans.). London: Routledge.

Greenhaven Press. (2007). *Mental health: Current controversies.* New York: Author.

Harman, C. E. (2003). *The diagnosis and stigma of schizophrenia.* Brookings, OR: Old Court Press.

Hatfield, A. B., & Lefley, H. P. (1993). *Surviving mental illness: Stress coping, and adaptation.* New York: Guilford Press.

Human Rights Watch. (2003). *Ill-equipped: U.S. prisons and offenders with mental illness.* Retrieved June 9, 2008, from http://www.hrw.org/reports/2003/usa1003/usa1003.pdf

Jamison, K. R. (1995). *An unquiet mind: A memoir of moods and madness.* New York: Alfred A. Knopf.

Judge David L. Bazelon Center for Mental Health Law. (n.d.). *About the Bazelon Center for Mental Health Law.* Retrieved August 18, 2008, from http://www.bazelon.org/about/index.htm

Kessler, R. C., Berglund, P., Demler, O., Jin, R., Merikangas, K. R., & Walters, E. E. (2005). Lifetime prevalence and age-of-onset distributions of *DSM-IV* disorders in the national comorbidity survey replication. *Archives of General Psychiatry, 62*(6), 593–602.

Kessler, R. C., Chiu, W. T., Demler, O., & Walters, E. E. (2005). Prevalence, severity, and comorbidity of 12-month *DSM-IV* disorders in the National Comorbidity Survey Replication. *Archives of General Psychiatry, 62*(6), 617–627.

Khalfa, J. (2006). Introduction. In M. Foucault, *History of madness* (pp. xiii–xx). London: Routledge.

Kirk, S. A., & Kutchins, H. (1992). *The selling of DSM: The rhetoric of science in psychiatry.* Hawthorne, NY: Aldine de Gruyter.

Lane, C. (2007). *Shyness: How normal behavior became a sickness.* New Haven, CT: Yale University Press.

Leckliter, I. N., & Matarazzo, J. D. (1994). Diagnosis and classification. In V. B. Hasselt & M. Herson (Eds.), *Advanced abnormal psychology* (pp. 3–18). New York: Plenum Press.

Leete, E. (1997). How I perceive and manage my illness. In L. Spaniol, C. Gagne, & M. Koehler (Eds.), *Psychological and social aspects of psychiatric disability* (pp. 99–103). Boston: Center for Psychiatric Rehabilitation, Sargent College of Allied Health Professions, Boston University.

Lifton, R. J. (1986). *The Nazi doctors: Medical killing and the psychology of genocide.* New York: Basic Books.

Millon, T. (2004). *Masters of the mind: Exploring the story of mental illness from ancient times to the new millennium.* New York: John Wiley & Sons.

MindFreedom International. (n.d.). *MFI portal.* Retrieved August 18, 2008, from http://mindfreedom.org

NAMI. (2003). *About mental illness: Attention-deficit/hyperactivity disorder.* Retrieved from http://www.nami.org/Template.cfm?Section=By_Illness&template=/ContentManagement/ContentDisplay.cfm&ContentID=22571

NAMI. (2006a). *About mental illness: Bipolar disorder.* Retrieved from http://www.nami.org/Template.cfm?Section=By_Illness&Template=/TaggedPage/TaggedPageDisplay.cfm&TPLID=54&ContentID=23037&lstid=325

NAMI. (2006b). *About mental illness: Major depression.* Retrieved from http://www.nami.org/Template.cfm?Section=By_Illness&Template=/TaggedPage/TaggedPageDisplay.cfm&TPLID=54&ContentID=23039&lstid=326

NAMI. (2006c). *Identity and mission.* Retrieved June 12, 2008, from http://www.nami.org/Content/NavigationMenu/Inform_Yourself/About_Public_Policy/NAMI_Policy_Platform/1_Identity_and_Mission.htm

NAMI. (2007). *About mental illness: Schizophrenia.* Retrieved from http://www.nami.org/Template.cfm?Section=By_Illness&Template=/TaggedPage/TaggedPageDisplay.cfm&TPLID=54&ContentID=23036&lstid=327

National Coalition for the Homeless. (2006, June). *Mental illness and homelessness.* Washington, DC: Author.

National Council on Disability. (2000). *From privileges to rights: People labeled with psychiatric disabilities speak for themselves.* Retrieved June 25, 2008, from http://www.ncd.gov/newsroom/publications/2000/privileges.htm

National Institute of Mental Health. (n.d.). *The numbers count: Mental disorders in America.* Retrieved from http://www.nimh.nih.gov/health/publications/the-numbers-count-mental-disorders-in-america.shtml#Anxiety

National Institute of Mental Health. (2005, June 6). *Mental illness exacts heavy toll, beginning in youth* [Press release]. Retrieved August 18, 2008, from http://www.nimh.nih.gov/science-news/2005/mental-illness-exacts-heavy-toll-beginning-in-youth.shtml

Szasz, T. (1997). *Insanity: The idea and its consequences.* New York: Syracuse University Press.

Torrey, E. F., & Zdanowicz, M. (1998, August 4). Why deinstitutionalization turned deadly. *Wall Street Journal.* Reprinted at http://www.psychlaws.org/General Resources/Article2.htm

United Nations. (2007). *Convention on the rights of persons with disabilities and optional protocol.* Retrieved May 19, 2007, from http://www.un.org/esa/socdev/enable/conventioninfo.htm

U.S. Department of Health and Human Services. (2004). *Title 42—public health. Federal financial participation. Institutionalized individuals.* 42CFR435.1008.

U.S. Holocaust Memorial Museum. (n.d.). *Victims of the Nazi era: 1933–1945* [Brochure]. Washington, DC: Author.

U.S. Immigration Commission. (1911). *Immigration and Insanity: Abstract.* Washington, DC: Governmental Printing Office.

Walenstein, E. S. (1998). *Blaming the brain.* New York: Free Press.

Wedenoja, M. (1999). Psychiatric disabilities. In R. W. Mackelprang & R. O. Salsgiver (Eds.), *Disability: A diversity model approach in human service practice* (pp. 167–190). Pacific Grove, CA: Brooks/Cole.

Wiggam, A. E. (1924). *The fruit of the family tree.* Indianapolis, IN: Bobbs-Merrill.

Wood, E. A. (2006). *There's always help, there's always hope.* Carlsbad, CA: Hay House.

World Health Organization. (2005, January). *Mental health services in Europe: The treatment gap.* Briefing at the WHO European Ministerial Conference on Mental Health, Helsinki, Finland.

World Health Organization. (2002). *Mental health.* Retrieved June 13, 2008, from http://www.who.int/mental_health/en/

World Health Organization. (n.d.). *Depression.* Retrieved from http://www.who.int/mental_health/management/depression/definition/en

11

Cognitive Disabilities

I was in the coma for a couple of weeks, and, waking up, I didn't know my mother. My mother had come to visit me, but I didn't know who she was. I did recognize my father. My parents were divorced and had been living apart for many years, but when I was first waking up, I didn't understand that. I didn't understand anything. When I was taken out of intensive care in a wheelchair, it started to register with me: "Wow, something's happened here." I didn't believe anything had happened until I got out of bed and started using the wheelchair. Then it all started coming together.

—Kevin Shirey, former counselor, Center for
Independent Living, Fresno, California

STUDENT LEARNING OBJECTIVES

1. To understand issues around defining the various cognitive disabilities
2. To understand the many varieties of cognitive disabilities
3. To develop a very basic knowledge of the major cognitive disabilities likely to be experienced by clients and consumers
4. To understand the social consequences of having a cognitive disability
5. To understand the issues concerning the recent questioning of learning disabilities and attention-deficit/hyperactivity disorder

Bruyere, Davis, and Golden (2000) define cognitive disabilities as disabilities that affect an individual's ability to comprehend what he or she sees and hears. Included in cognitive disabilities are impairments that affect the ability to gain information from social cues and what is commonly called body language. Individuals with cognitive disabilities may have difficulty learning new things, generalizing from specifics, and using language for expression in both oral and written form. Sigler and Mackelprang (1993) observe that persons with cognitive disabilities can be impulsive, reacting to situations without fully considering consequences. In addition, persons with cognitive disabilities can have difficulty belonging to groups or finding social acceptance. Cognitive disabilities include learning disabilities, intellectual disabilities, developmental disabilities, traumatic brain injury, autism, and Down syndrome. Developmental disabilities, autism, and Down syndrome may fall into a number of disability categories. Since we have previously looked at developmental disabilities, autism, and Down syndrome under other classifications, this chapter concentrates on learning disabilities, attention-deficit/hyperactivity disorder, and traumatic brain injuries. Please keep in mind again that these classifications are arbitrary at worst, and simply a matter of convenience at best. They are not to be interpreted as written in stone.

LEARNING DISABILITIES

Definitions

Thomas (2000) offers three different definitions of learning disability (LD) based upon the *Diagnostic and Statistical Manual of Mental Disorders* (*DSM-IV*), the law concerning disability, and the social construction of learning disabilities. The *DSM-IV* defines LD as occurring when an individual's achievement on standardized testing falls significantly below expectations for age, schooling, and testing in intelligence. The *DSM-IV* stresses the social and psychological consequence of an LD, including demoralization, low self-esteem, poor school performance, and difficulties adjusting to the work environment. The legal definitions offered by the Rehabilitation Act of 1973 and the Americans with Disabilities Act of 1990 address limitations of major life activities, school activities, and employment experiences. The social definition of disability is in a constant state of change and generally centers on a pejorative judgment of a person's intelligence level, capacity to learn, and capacity to express himself or herself either verbally or in writing.

Sternberg and Grigorenko (2001) cite the federal definition of LD, which defines it as an impairment that affects one or more of the physiological processes involved in understanding and using either spoken or written language. These impairments may manifest themselves in difficulties listening, thinking, speaking, writing, spelling, and/or doing mathematical calculations. The federal definition encompasses the clinical perspective focusing on a difference between capability and actual performance.

The National Joint Committee for Learning Disabilities (n.d.) defines LD clearly and succinctly. An LD is a neurological condition. It appears to be caused by a difference in structure from a typical brain in terms of the way information is processed. An LD has little to do with the intelligence level of the individual. It affects reading, writing, spelling, reasoning, recalling, and organizational ability if the individual is left to accomplish the above kinds of tasks in a conventional manner.

The National Joint Committee for Learning Disabilities (n.d.) concludes that 15 percent of the American population has some form of an LD. The most common manifestation of an LD is difficulty with reading and language skills. LD often runs in families. And learning disabilities are not to be confused with other disabilities such as developmental disabilities, autism, and attention-deficit/hyperactivity disorder. The two key elements of this definition to be remembered are that learning disabilities are the result of neurological structural differences from a typical brain and that they are not a manifestation of another disorder.

Common learning disabilities include the following. Dyslexia is a disability where individuals have difficulty understanding written words. Dysgraphia affects the ability to write within a defined space. Individuals with dyscalculia have difficulty conceptualizing mathematical problems and mathematical processes. Learning disabilities also include auditory and visual processing differences that result in difficulty understanding spoken language although there is not a hearing issue present. Also, nonverbal learning disabilities are certain neurological disorders that create issues in a person's ability to determine spatial relationships and understand organizational sequences (National Joint Committee for Learning Disabilities, n.d.).

As with other disabilities, there are several problems in defining learning disabilities. First, the causes of learning disabilities are often an enigma. Case histories as well as neurological testing commonly fail to find an exact etiology. Second, there are no specifically designated physical and/or behavioral manifestations of learning disabilities. Some individuals with learning disabilities may exhibit impairments or behaviors that are totally different from those of others designated as having an LD. Third, no single impairment or base combination of impairments manifests itself in an individual with an LD. There are many combinations of learning abilities and performance levels that differ from one person to the next (Simpson & Umbach, 1989). These ambiguities in characteristics and evaluation support a popular belief that learning disabilities are not real—that individuals with learning disabilities aren't trying hard enough or are just "dumb." We will return to these issues later.

Before we discuss the characteristics of learning disabilities, we offer the observation that learning disabilities are socially and culturally determined, particularly in industrialized society. Learning disabilities are frequently diagnosed in school settings that demand specific types of learning (e.g., reading, writing, mathematics), often in predetermined ways. The experiences of one of the authors and his family are illustrative. The author's child struggled through two years of college, experiencing increasing frustration relative to grades that did not reflect the extent of learning. Self-image suffered until, in near desperation, this youth sought help in developing learning strategies and was subsequently diagnosed with an LD. Upon implementing alternate nontraditional learning techniques that allowed the student to demonstrate knowledge in a traditional manner, grades improved dramatically, scholarships were awarded, and a doctoral education followed. Subsequently, the author realized that his peculiar learning styles were very similar to his child's; he has an undiagnosed LD. Both the father's and child's learning styles are atypical and thus were often labeled abnormal and considered pathological. For example, in math the author would find answers to questions, but he was penalized by instructors because he found answers in atypical, non-sanctioned ways. These experiences have led the author to wonder about one of his uncles, now deceased, who was considered to be not so bright in school. However, the uncle was revered as a farmer and cattle rancher. People far and wide sought his advice. In the societal context of formalized school education that has existed for a couple of hundred years at most, this man was considered learning disabled, and an average student at best. In an agrarian context, this man was brilliant—a prodigy.

Characteristics

Coles (1987) explains that the first real differentiation of learning disabilities was made by James Hinshelwood, an ophthalmologist living at the turn of the twentieth century in Glasgow, Scotland. Researching what was then called congenital word blindness, he found evidence that some schoolchildren had difficulties reading even though they had good mental abilities. Hinshelwood concluded that the etiology of this condition was in the brain, because he found similar dysfunctional reading abilities in adults with brain lesions. He believed that the problem was confined to the area of the brain dealing with visual memory of words and letters. Hinshelwood sought effective ways of teaching children with this condition. Today, research indicates that the cause is not so concrete. Although there is evidence that some learning disabilities have neurological roots, with others there is no apparent brain dysfunction.

There is some agreement, however, on the characteristics of learning disabilities. Keogh (2005) points out that there are both behavioral and learning components to learning disabilities. Cruickshank (1990) discusses ten identifying characteristics of persons with learning disabilities that are encompassed by these two broad components. The first of these is that persons with learning disabilities may have difficulty discriminating fine differences in auditory, visual, and/or tactile input. For example, persons with learning disabilities exhibiting this characteristic may have difficulty feeling the difference between the sizes of different objects or telling the difference in texture:

> Ever since elementary school, John has had trouble telling the difference between denominations of money. He has difficulty telling the difference between a dime and a quarter. At the same time, he gets twenty-dollar bills confused with fives and ones.

They may have difficulty hearing the difference between two similar-sounding words:

> Susan is having real problems at her first social work position. She has trouble following the instructions of her supervisor. Words like *call* and *saw* sound the same to her. In writing reports, she tends to misuse words like *two, too,* and *to.*

The second characteristic of persons with learning disabilities discussed by Cruickshank (1990) concerns memory. Persons with learning disabilities may have a decreased ability to retain and recall discriminating sounds and forms both in the short term and the long term. These individuals can learn and manipulate concepts but sometimes have difficulty with the specifics that support the concepts:

> Richard has been very successful in his academic career. He graduated with a bachelor of science in education with honors. He did very well in classes dealing with concepts such as intellectual history and philosophy. He did adequately in courses involving math through the use of reasonable accommodation in the form of a calculator. Richard understood most math concepts but had trouble recalling the multiplication tables. As long as he could use a calculator, he did well. Now he is facing the state teaching credential test, which prohibits the use of any calculators during the math portion of the exam.

The third characteristic of persons with learning disabilities involves difficulty in sequencing. Related to the characteristic of limited recall, some persons with learning disabilities have difficulty remembering the correct sequence of steps necessary to complete a task:

> Joe was an expert automobile diagnostician. He could merely listen to an engine and pretty much tell what was going on. When he hooked it up to the electronic diagnostic machine, his findings were always corroborated. Yet Joe was having problems on the job. He could diagnose the problem better than any mechanic in the dealership, but it took him three times the "book time" to replace parts and make repairs. He had difficulty remembering the sequence of removing old parts and replacing them. He had to constantly refer to the repair manual even to do simple jobs.

The fourth characteristic that persons with learning disabilities may frequently experience is difficulty with figure-background relationships and distinguishing which is which. These can be visual, auditory, or tactual in nature. This difficulty has ramifications not only in school performance but in the world of work in terms of reading and listening to directions and training:

> Joyce's boss asked her to go to a conference on establishing a computer network within a company with links to the Internet. The conference was held in a busy hotel downtown, and the only separation between conference rooms was a thin moveable wall. Part of the presentation in the next room involved relatively loud music. No one in her room seemed to be annoyed or distracted, but Joyce found it impossible to focus on what the instructor was saying. Joyce was worried because she was going to take the lead in setting up her company's network and she needed this information.

Persons with learning disabilities also may have difficulties with time and space orientation. They may have difficulty answering the question, "Where am I in time and space?" This fifth characteristic has tremendous ramifications in terms of performance and self-esteem. In school and in work, these individuals may have difficulty with time deadlines and restrictions. They may have problems maneuvering geographically within cities, buildings, and offices.

The sixth characteristic of persons who have learning disabilities involves difficulty bringing closure to either a concept or a physical form:

> When asked by her teacher to draw a circle, Alicia would always come up with something that looked like the letter *U*. When she tried to tell a joke to her classmates, she always left out the punch line.

The seventh characteristic of persons who have learning disabilities put forth by Cruickshank (1990) concerns difficulties integrating input from two or more senses—that is, integrating intersensory information. An individual whose LD involves this characteristic may have difficulty coordinating a task that has, for example, a listening component, a visual component, and a motor skills component:

> Jose was having difficulty in math class. The teacher had students copy a problem from the board. Then the class was supposed to work out the problem and give a verbal response. Jose could not make sense out of what the teacher was saying and writing. He was terrified that she would call on him to show his work.

The eighth characteristic, related to sequencing, centers on difficulties relating perception to motor function. Persons with learning disabilities may have difficulty judging the energy requirements of performing a specific task, which can lead them to take on projects well beyond their capabilities to complete. It can mean that a person with an LD will jump into a motor-related task without considering how to go about completing the task:

> Bill was always eager on Saturday morning to get out in the yard and get some work done. Usually by the late morning, the front and back yards were in chaos. Bill had mowed half the front yard but failed to finish the rest. He had started trimming the shrubs, but before he was able to finish this, he became immersed in fixing a sprinkler head and in the process decided to dig a trench to put in a new sprinkler line. At 11:30 A.M., his wife went to get him for an important phone call, but Bill was nowhere to be found. He had left for the local hardware store to find a part to fix the garden fence.

The ninth characteristic discussed by Cruickshank (1990) involves dissociation. Persons with cognitive disabilities may have difficulty viewing specifics in relation to the whole. This may be visual or conceptual or both. Persons with learning disabilities may have difficulty with pegboard designs or other designs related to tasks, like tying shoelaces. This characteristic may manifest itself in the inability to see the importance of a concept or in missing the concept by focusing on the parts ("not seeing the forest for the trees").

The tenth characteristic of persons with learning disabilities described by Cruickshank (1990) involves attention disturbances. This characteristic shows up as an inability to avoid reacting to stimuli from the environment. Although related to learning disabilities, this condition is currently associated with a separate disorder known as attention-deficit/hyperactivity disorder, which will be discussed next.

Because LD is a relatively "new" disability compared to disabilities such as cerebral palsy, and because, particularly for school systems, the cost for reasonable accommodation can be extensive, LD is surrounded by questions and controversy. Many individuals, including mental health professionals and educational professionals, question the existence of LD. Finlan (1994) puts forth this viewpoint: "There is no such thing as a learning disability. You may think LD exists since more than two million schoolchildren have currently been identified with this federally legislated disability, but LD does not exist any more than there are witches in Salem, monsters in Loch Ness, or abominable snowmen in the Himalayas" (p. 1).

Finlan (1994) bases his conclusion on the following. First, the definition of LD is vague and ambiguous. No one has defined any component of the definition in terms of behavior. Second, the testing process for LD is value biased, and the results are inconclusive. In addition, the tests do not adequately predict school performance with or without special supports and accommodation. Third, the existence of LD is rooted not in science but in politics. Through the efforts of middle-class parents who have banded together as a special interest, their children slide under the protective blanket of disability. Finlan states, "LD, by getting itself included as a handicap, benefited from a major political force, and on the basis of legislation brought about by political activism, LD theory became law without evidence" (p. 24).

Spear-Swerling and Sternberg (1998) believe that the concept of LD should be discarded. They argue that the concept merely offers schools and teachers an excuse for doing an inadequate job of teaching. All children with learning difficulties, whether classified as learning disabled or not, need the same kind of remedial programs in order to achieve reading success.

Finlan (1994) has argued that a diagnosis of LD has negative consequences for the child and the schools. First and perhaps most important, a diagnosis of LD puts the problem on the individual, the child. It blames the victim. Blaming the victim relieves parents and schools of responsibility for the problem. Once this occurs, changing the family structure or the educational structure becomes next to impossible, because the problem really resides with the child. The educational structure need not examine the grading system or the pedagogy of reading or math. It can create a special auxiliary system for the child with the LD and basically leave the rest of the system intact. Second, as a product of the medical model, a diagnosis of LD makes the child abnormal and pathologizes him or her. Labeling children as having LD limits them and establishes lowered performance expectations. Finlan states: "Lowered expectations brought about by labels applied by experts damn these children to lives as second-class citizens as soon as the adults in their lives buy into the labels" (p. 60). Labels become self-fulfilling prophecies.

Wilkinson (2005), a person with a learning disability, supports the viewpoint that a diagnosis of learning disability jeopardizes a person's inclusion in the mainstream of society. Isolating people with LD along with persons with any disability by labeling them is unproductive. Wilkinson argues that the removal of the process of labeling is a necessity in order to ensure the full inclusion of people with disabilities, including learning disabilities.

The topic of LD constantly gets bad press in the United States. The media generally provides a negative depiction of LD. The press equates LD with school disruption and criminal behavior. There is silence when it comes to supporting programs and the benefits for schools and society in general for persons with LD (Antrim, 1997).

These questioning viewpoints are important to our discussion of learning disabilities. This viewpoint reveals a component of ableism. Ableism assumes the superiority of people who are nondisabled and views persons with disabilities who have different physical and mental characteristics as somehow inferior. Along with this assumption is a low expectation of the level of performance and responsibility of persons with disabilities. By assigning a person the label of LD, many in this culture relegate individuals to a lower status, with little or no expectation that they reach for the stars.

On the other hand, a significant amount of caution must be exercised when one is considering the preceding views. First, does LD exist? The fact that a condition covers a wide range of behavioral characteristics that are three-dimensional and dynamic rather than linear does not mean that the condition does not exist. Similarly, our inability to fully understand the etiology or physically demonstrate the presence of a condition does not negate its existence. Various relatively new techniques in brain scanning suggest that there are specific regions of the brain where these conditions find their origin. The efficacy of a combination of medical and psychological testing is beginning to pinpoint causes, resulting in effective treatment (Bigler, Lajiness-O'Neill, & Howes, 1998). The fact that political action has spawned investigation does not negate the legitimacy of the findings. In the course of the history of the United States, many health-related problems and solutions have been brought to the surface by political action. This is particularly true in the area of stopping the spread of infectious diseases such as measles and polio. The same can be said about learning disabilities.

Who benefits from a diagnosis of LD and who does not? MacMaster, Donovan, and MacIntyre (2002) empirically examine the assumption that the label of LD results in a decrease in children's self-esteem due to stigma. They hypothesize that adults assume that the label of learning disabled has a negative impact on children based upon an adult's perspective of the world and difference. MacMaster et al. speculate that children might perceive the issue differently. The results of their research indicate that children's self-esteem actually increases significantly after they are diagnosed with an LD. It appears that before diagnosis, children have a general feeling that something is wrong with them. After diagnosis, the issue becomes more focused and thus more manageable. They understand that they can be helped through intervention and remediation.

Accommodation of learning disabilities within the school structure can be expensive. School administrators find it more and more difficult to maintain traditional programs, not to mention providing auxiliary services for students with disabilities. Schools do not benefit economically in the short run by having students diagnosed with LD. But social service administrators as well as educators need to realize that they exist to serve children. In the long run, if changes within "special" programs can be generalized to the total system, then, in fact, everybody benefits (Zentall, 1993).

Sternberg and Grigorenko (2001) question the efficacy of the popular move to increase the labeling of children with behavioral and learning issues as learning disabled. They come up with some suggestions that reflect the concept of universal access that is part of the social model of disability (see chapter 13). School systems need to support all students who have issues in learning. If children with learning difficulties need more time to take a particular exam in order to do well, what would be the benefit of giving all children extra time? What is the pedagogical rationale for timing a particular test? Comparison of potential performance and actual performance manifested in the use of IQ scores hides the real agenda of helping all children who have low achievement. Interventions must focus on the actual learning problem, not on the identified class of disability. It is a mistake to place a child who is gifted in mathematics but has difficulty reading into the category of learning disabled, for which a whole range of interventions may be used based on a diagnosis. That total range of interventions simply may not be needed. Curricula must account for the vast variety of mechanisms of learning and components of learning. Education should value not only children with superior memories and acute analytical skills, but also the child who has artistic talent and/or practical skills. Related to this concept, it is the obligation of school systems to focus on the strengths of the children in the system. If the above approach were taken, many of the controversies and issues around LD would fade away.

ATTENTION-DEFICIT/HYPERACTIVITY DISORDER

The Centers for Disease Control and Prevention (2005) report that statistics gathered from parents in 2003 indicate that 7.8 percent of school-age children were diagnosed with attention-deficit/hyperactivity disorder. Faraone,

Sergeant, Gillberb, and Biederman (2003) report the worldwide prevalence of ADHD to be approximately 8–12 percent. It is more common in boys than girls and tends to be diagnosed most often in preadolescent children. ADHD's etiology appears to be multifactorial in nature and is linked to several different genes with mixed dominant features. Consequently, ADHD tends to run in families. Recent studies have linked trauma to the brain, damage to the fetus by substance abuse, exposure to lead, and premature birth as other factors in the development of ADHD in children (Wolraich, 2006).

Zentall (1993) outlines several characteristics of students with ADHD in an educational environment, which also manifest in other environments, such as work. What has been traditionally defined as attention deficit is more like a strong pull toward certain kinds of stimuli, accompanied by inattention to other kinds of stimuli. Students with ADHD generally focus their attention on things that are novel, such as new colors or sounds, a change in size, or sudden movement. This can result in several problems. In first learning a task, the person with ADHD does not focus on stimuli that are neutral, bland, detailed, or part of an overall task. Therefore, the person with ADHD may fail to learn vital information:

> Tommy couldn't wait to start taking gym. He had always liked sports, particularly basketball. Today the teacher was going to have them start playing. When Tommy got to class, the teacher began the class by explaining the game, how it should be played, and the rules. Tommy was bored and very fidgety. He had difficulty concentrating on what the teacher was saying. There was a game going on on the other side of the gymnasium, with lots of noise and excitement. When his teacher divided the class into teams to start the game, Tommy was lost. He didn't remember the rules and was removed from the game on the first play for inappropriately touching another student in trying to get the ball away from him.

In the performance part of learning, a second characteristic may be a failure to sustain attention. Persons with ADHD find it difficult to continue attending to stimuli when the novelty wears off. This results in increased error in long-term performance. Zentall (1993) has found that persons with ADHD have difficulty sustaining attention, particularly in repeated tasks. When information is repeated, there appear to be more behavioral problems, such as increased activity and impulsivity, which makes it extremely difficult to develop rote skills.

Impulsivity is a third characteristic outlined by Zentall (1993) that limits achievement in most environments. The inability to withhold verbal or behavioral responses produces many problems. It means that the person with ADHD does not consider the full array of data before making a decision—a skill that is crucial to problem solving. Impulsivity results in difficulty planning, which requires the development of priorities based upon consideration of a wide spectrum of information. Impulsivity makes reading and following directions difficult:

> Kirk loved to build models of fighter planes. But his love mostly resulted in frustration and anger. When he got a new model, he would jump right into building it without reading the directions. The end result never matched what was on the box and usually ended up in the waste can after about fifteen minutes of a flurry of activity.

Impulsivity also makes it difficult to obtain help because of distractions or delays in educational and work environments. Because teachers and supervisors may be dealing with large numbers of students and workers, they are not likely to pick up on individual problems. This results in the person with ADHD not completing tasks correctly.

Impulsiveness has social consequences as well. Sigler and Mackelprang (1993) demonstrate that impulsivity affects social judgment and social behavior. Persons with ADHD who exhibit inappropriate impulsivity in social situations can be subject to social isolation and employment vulnerability:

> David had been working successfully at a local fast-food restaurant for two months. He was doing very well, and both his immediate supervisor and his coworkers liked him. Occasionally, he exhibited an eccentric sense of humor, but nobody really took much notice. One day, the supervisor asked David to join her and a couple of other workers for lunch at the restaurant when the noon crunch was over. They were talking and eating when suddenly David grabbed his throat, held his breath, and fell on the floor. The supervisor thought he was choking and proceeded to do the Heimlich maneuver, when suddenly David started laughing, saying that it was a joke. His supervisor and coworkers were enraged. David's impulsivity damaged his social belonging with his coworkers and placed grave questions in his supervisor's mind about his maturity and ability to be successful at the restaurant.

As with LD, there exists a body of literature that questions whether or not ADHD is a disability. Smelter, Rasch, Fleming, Nazos, and Baranowski (1996) question the existence of attention-deficit/hyperactivity disorder. Their work reinforces the position that there is no agreed-upon etiology and no specific test for the disorder. They believe that this diagnosis is an attempt by some professionals, politicians, and parents to excuse antisocial and inappropriate behavior. According to Smelter et al., the "creation" of ADHD alleviates the guilt of both parents and professionals for a job poorly done and serves as a way for parents to avoid punitive action by the schools and the courts. It also results in a number of negative consequences for children so labeled and for the schools they attend. A diagnosis of ADHD gives children a license to misbehave, with little or no consequence to themselves and without regard for the future ramifications to society: "Doing a 'bad' thing implies responsibility and guilt, as well as the need for some punitive action on the part of one's social peers. But having a 'dysfunction' carries no such social stigma; instead, it evokes sympathy, feelings of compassion, and a genuine desire to help the transgressor" (p. 430).

Smelter et al. (1996) also conclude that a diagnosis of ADHD lowers both parent and teacher expectations for achievement and that children with ADHD conform to limitations established by the diagnosis. Schools cannot afford to make the necessary accommodations for cases of ADHD diagnosis. These accommodations mean additional services provided to persons with a condition that has a wide spectrum of characteristics. In addition, the extra attention required for children diagnosed with ADHD puts extensive burdens on classroom teachers.

O'Meara (2002) interviewed Fred A. Baughman Jr., a retired neurologist, on the subject of the credibility of the diagnosis of ADHD. Baughman views the total phenomenon of ADHD as a fraud perpetuated by educators and mental health professionals. His arguments center on the lack of scientific evidence for ADHD. According to Baughman, most of the studies addressing brain functioning of children with ADHD are significantly flawed because they use individuals already on medication in their sampling. Baumann believes that physicians continue to diagnose ADHD because of peer pressure. And finally, there have been few if any longitudinal studies on the drugs used to control ADHD.

Goldstein (2006) questions the influence of pharmaceutical companies' direct advertising campaigns concerning drugs that control ADHD behaviors at the public and physician levels. Over the last thirty years, there has been a significant shift to an aggressive stance in the marketing of ADHD medications. Goldstein does not question the efficacy of psychotropic medications in dealing with ADHD. But effective treatment of ADHD entails a broader stance involving parent training, a variety of educational strategies, and/or various behavioral modification approaches.

As with the questions raised concerning LD, caution must be applied to the preceding critical views. First, does ADHD exist? An overwhelming body of scientific research validates its existence. In fact, it is the most researched child cognitive disability in recent years (Wolraich, 2006). Like with learning disabilities, the fact that mental health professionals and educators have investigated ADHD, and that it is not visually or tactilely observable, does not mean it is not a legitimate disability.

Who benefits from a diagnosis of ADHD and who does not? ADHD is a troublesome disability. It causes extensive pain on the part of the child, the parents, and the child's school environment. When the cause of a painful condition can be found, and based upon its origin, a plan can be developed to eliminate the pain, a sense of guilt and shame is removed from the person experiencing the condition:

> Dr. Frederick's twelve-year-old boy Sam was diagnosed with both LD and ADHD. His condition manifested itself in the inability to use a pencil to write

and difficulty integrating input from two or more senses. The results were that he was doing poorly in his work at school, and his hyperactivity was disrupting the rest of the class. Even though Dr. Frederick, at his own expense, had Sam tested, the school district refused to accept the diagnosis, and the school's psychologist said that Sam was "normal."

As the year moved forward, Sam was becoming progressively worse. Although Sam was taking medication, he still was not doing well at school. Each day he would come home depressed, go up to his room, and shut the door. Sam believed that he behaved this way in school because he was bad. At times, Sam thought he would be better off dead.

At Sam's next individualized educational program meeting, Dr. Frederick was emphatic about the need for certain changes in Sam's school program, including half a day in a special resource room. On threat of legal action, the school complied with Dr. Frederick's demands. Sam's new teacher was himself diagnosed as having an LD. Sam no longer disrupts the classroom. He uses a computer to write and is doing A work in his "regular" English class. Even more important, Sam is no longer depressed and never thinks about killing himself.

Parents do not seek this diagnosis for their sons or daughters to escape responsibility or to gain services that allow them to maintain their status. They seek answers to help their children. In most cases, the diagnosis of ADHD means changing family routine, which includes curtailing the use of the television, establishing a quiet time, and sometimes setting up a behavioral modification program for the child (Fowler, 2002). It may also mean seeking family counseling and examining how family members relate to one another (Beers, 2003).

As with LD, accommodation of ADHD within the school structure can be expensive. But like accommodations in general for persons with disabilities, most accommodations for ADHD are relatively simple and inexpensive. Generally speaking, work on subject areas that require a high level of sophistication should be done early in the day. It is helpful to break down instructions and assignments rather than presenting them all at once. Bringing variety into the classroom and varying activities holds attention. Placing students with ADHD in areas of the classroom where they will be least distracted can be helpful in holding attention ("Working with the ADHD Student," 2006).

TRAUMATIC BRAIN INJURY

Traumatic brain injury (TBI) is a worldwide phenomenon. The National Center for Injury Prevention and Control (2006) estimates that more than 1.4 million Americans experience traumatic head injuries in a year. TBI of children and young adults is the leading killer and cause of disability in the United States, killing approximately 50,000 each year. Approximately 5.3 million Americans (2 percent of the population of the United States) experience lifelong physical, mental, and emotional changes as a result of TBI.

Causes of TBI include falling (28 percent), motor vehicle accidents including motorcycle accidents (20 percent), and some form of physical assault (30 percent). In India, an estimated 1.5–2 million people experience TBI annually (Gururaj, 2002). In Pakistan, over a four-year period, 260,000 patients were admitted to hospitals for TBI (Raja, Vohra, & Ahmed, 2001), an annual rate of about 40 in 100,000, while in South Australia the estimated incidence of TBI is approximately 322 per 100,000 (Hillier, Hillier, & Metzer, 1997). Even mild TBI may result in long-term changes. However, mild TBI often goes unrecognized because its manifestations are often subtle.

Mild TBI—with or without loss of consciousness—can produce an array of sequelae, including memory loss of events occurring shortly before the injury (retrograde amnesia) and memory difficulties relative to events following the injury (posttraumatic amnesia). People with mild TBI can experience diminished reasoning abilities and reduced frustration tolerance, sometimes long term. A condition called post-concussion syndrome can occur, which causes people to experience changes in cognition and personality after a relatively mild brain injury. Symptoms of post-concussion syndrome often ameliorate within weeks or months of injury.

There are two main types of TBI. Closed TBIs typically result from accidents in which the head strikes, or is struck by, an object with no penetration of the skull. Common causes of closed TBI are motor vehicle accidents, wherein the head strikes, or is struck by, an object such as pavement or a windshield and the brain shakes and scrapes along the inside of the skull. Open TBIs occur when an object, such as a bullet, penetrates the skull and enters the brain. Other brain injuries, such as those caused by insufficient oxygen, poisoning, or infection, can cause changes similar to those that occur with closed TBI. Open TBI usually results in localized injury, whereas closed TBI tends to produce diffuse damage to more than one area of the brain. Damage can occur as a result of direct impact, increased cranial pressure, bruising, blood loss, scraping of the brain along the inside of the skull, oxygen deprivation, chemical reactions, and other causes.

The manifestations of TBI vary widely and depend primarily on the specific areas of the brain that are affected and the severity of injury to those sites. When TBI occurs, function is usually lost immediately or within a few hours (as in cases of slow bleeding or slowly increasing pressure in the brain). Severe damage can produce coma or even death. After the initial crisis and stabilization, spontaneous recovery of function can occur for two years or more. Recovery is rarely immediate. For example, situations in which people suddenly awaken from a coma (as shown frequently on television) are extremely rare. As they recover from severe TBI, people generally go through phases of recovery in which arousal, memory, reasoning, judgment, and impulse control gradually improve. Lifelong improvement can occur with sufficient supports.

The brain stem and frontal and temporal lobes are more prone to traumatic injury than other parts of the brain because they are adjacent to hard, bony structures. The brain stem, located at the base of the brain, is also susceptible to damage from cranial pressure as a result of brain swelling. It is involved primarily in primitive life functions, including arousal and nervous system regulation of other organs. It acts as a switchboard, routing messages to and from the body and higher brain centers. Injury to this area can cause coma or even death if basic life functions such as respiration and cardiovascular function are compromised. The temporal lobes are located at the anterolateral aspects of the brain. They are involved in memory and language. Damage to the temporal lobes can result in behavioral changes as well as language impairment and sensory loss to the face and extremities. The frontal lobes occupy the anterior portion of the cranium. Because of their large size and their position, the frontal lobes are especially susceptible when TBI occurs. They are involved in important cognitive functions such as abstract reasoning, judgment, and voluntary muscle control. Injury to this area usually results in behavioral changes associated with decreased judgment, reduced anger control, and increased impulsiveness.

Cognitive changes are common with TBI. These changes can affect language and communication, information processing, memory, and perceptual skills. Both receptive aphasia (an inability to understand language) and expressive aphasia (an inability to express oneself through language) may result. When perception, memory, and higher reasoning are affected, people experience difficulty reading, writing, or reasoning (such as is required in doing math). People with TBI must often develop new compensatory cognitive skills and coping strategies (Beers, 2003; Brain Injury Association of America, 2006; Pieper, Valadka, & Marsh, 1996; Tierney, McPhee, & Papadakis, 2006).

Physical changes can affect ambulation, balance and coordination, general motor skills, strength, and endurance. Psychological changes can also occur and can affect mood, life perspective, emotions, and the senses (Alexander, 1992).

Finally, it is important to note that some people experience disabilities as a result of TBIs sustained over time that may not be identified as such. People who have experienced long-term domestic violence can encounter the subtle but progressive effects of TBI. This is especially true for young children who have been subjected to shaking, whereby their brains are shaken within their skulls.

PSYCHOSOCIAL CONSEQUENCES OF COGNITIVE DISABILITIES

Kronick (1981) focuses on the social development of persons with LD. Although she finds solutions to the social problems of persons with cognitive disabilities through intervention with the individual, her findings offer insight into the psychosocial consequences of cognitive disabilities. Most of the overt characteristics associated with a cognitive disability bring about a lower status within the major systems of social living. Within the family, if learning and academic achievement are the pillars of family culture, there is danger that a positive self-concept will not develop; at best, the family member with a cognitive disability may have doubts about his or her self-worth. As the child or adolescent compares himself or herself to parents and brothers and sisters, the discrepancy may reinforce a negative self-concept. And if the disability is dealt with poorly through punishment, ridicule, discomfort, shame, or secrecy, the family member with the cognitive disability may feel guilt or shame or inadequacy:

> Roger's family consisted of himself; his mom and dad; and his older brother, Ray. Roger's father was a pharmacist who owned and ran a drugstore in the area of the city where mostly Italian and Irish folks lived. Roger's mother taught science at the local high school. Roger's brother just graduated from college and was accepted to Harvard Medical School. Roger had been diagnosed with a learning disability in junior high school. Although he scored well on IQ tests, he did poorly in school. He was about to graduate, but with barely a C average.
>
> Roger's parents were basically ashamed of him. They never mentioned their younger son to friends. They always talked about Ray. When someone asked about Roger, a frown would appear on his mother's face, and his father simply would not reply. Roger knew he was "damaged goods." Even though people at school said he was really intelligent, Roger knew that he was a failure. On report card days, he would stay in his room, telling his parents he was sick. Roger wished he had never been born.
>
> Within the family, Roger's intelligence and other strengths were never acknowledged. As a result, Roger's poor image of himself and his low self-esteem resulted in severe depression and withdrawal. Eventually, Roger turned to alcohol and drugs.

The educational environment presents many potential psychosocial perils to the student with a cognitive disability. The skills involved with reading, writing, math, listening, working independently and within a group, presenting, and critical thinking are in fact the essence of the educational process. A disability that critically affects the acquisition of these skills can make the student with a cognitive disability susceptible to scorn, ridicule, social isolation, and low status. Lack of academic achievement as well as behavioral characteristics of impulsivity and the need for additional attention can stigmatize people with LD and ADHD in the eyes of both teachers and fellow students. If the student with a cognitive disability has difficulty learning and behaving typically, students and teachers can fail to recognize and reinforce his or her unique learning styles and positive behaviors (Kronick, 1981). Our educational establishment's emphasis on a narrow definition of productivity and success results in a world that can be hostile to persons with cognitive disabilities:

A child might be affable, intelligent, creative, humorous, and cooperative yet become discouraged and depressed over his academic or athletic limitations. If he is unable to limit his feelings of failure to the situation in which he has failed, relate the failure to a component of the situation, and find compensatory ways of handling or avoiding the difficult component, then his depression and anxiety will result in disorganization and hence successive failure in other areas of functioning. Eventually he will feel that he has lost so much ground that he becomes overwhelmed and immobilized by his lack of success. (Kronick, 1981, p. 76)

In light of Kronick's observations, it is not surprising that Naylor, Staskowski, Kenney, and King (1994) find a strong connection between the psychiatric condition of school refusal (failure to attend school, despite the physical ability to do so, as a result of anxiety or depression) and cognitive disability.

Dunham, Roller, and McIntosh (1996) discuss difficulties encountered by persons with cognitive disabilities in higher education. Because of issues of low self-esteem, students with cognitive disabilities tend not to be self-advocates in environments where accommodation is minimal. Because the disability may not manifest itself in overt physical characteristics, students must continually "prove" they have a disability. Faculty and staff may be reluctant to provide reasonable accommodation and may even display hostility toward students with LD. Lack of academic accommodation may negatively affect a student's ability to graduate. In addition, students in college with cognitive disabilities find social acceptance with neither nondisabled nor disabled students, which adds to the social isolation.

Dunham et al. (1996) also explore the ramifications of cognitive disabilities (specifically LD) in the work arena. Persons with cognitive disabilities have a harder time finding and keeping jobs than persons without. Generally, persons with cognitive disabilities who find work have jobs with lower pay and lower status than those without. These are usually unskilled entry-level positions. Typically, persons with cognitive disabilities are underemployed, and many remain at home with their families of origin.

On the job, workers with cognitive disabilities encounter difficulties understanding instructions in technical manuals, writing summaries of completed work, and getting along with fellow workers and supervisors. The pity side of ableism also shows up in the work environment, where supervisors give untruthful positive assessments of the work of persons with cognitive disabilities, often resulting in the eventual failure of the worker:

Karen graduated from a nationally known university with a master's degree in rehabilitation counseling. She has fairly severe reading and writing issues brought about by a head injury sustained in a motorcycle accident when she was nineteen. Now almost thirty, she had made her way through the halls of academia with the help of the disabled student services at both the colleges she attended. In addition, most of her professors provided reasonable accommodation in testing and paper writing.

She had been hired by a local junior college to be a staff member of its mental health center, providing mental health counseling to students, staff, and faculty. Karen loved working with her clients. She was adept at helping them understand their strengths and assisting them in finding their way out of circumstances causing them pain. Unfortunately, she had great difficulty doing her paperwork. Afraid to declare herself a person with a disability (this was before passage of the Americans with Disabilities Act, which allows persons with disabilities in the workplace to ask for reasonable accommodation), she stayed late into the evening and spent her lunch breaks trying to catch up on her paperwork.

Because she spent extra time working, she failed to socialize with the rest of the staff. Fellow workers thought that she was stuck up and trying to look good with her supervisor. Her supervisor, John, was concerned about the poor quality of her paperwork and also by the fact that none of the staff liked Karen. He would overhear people joking about her constantly working. John felt uncomfortable approaching Karen about any of these issues, but he knew she had a learning disability. In fact, every time John had to deal with Karen, he felt angry because she had come with such great references and her performance in college really looked good. At her first sixth-month evaluation, he basically said she was doing well. After a year, however, because of many mistakes in treatment notes and poorly written assessments, Karen was let go.

Bruyere et al. (2000) emphasize that direct and honest communication between the supervisor and the worker with a cognitive disability is crucial in the completion of tasks and to the worker's sense of well-being.

SUMMARY

Cognitive disabilities affect the ability to and ways in which people process and comprehend what they see, hear, and experience. Included in cognitive disabilities are impairments that affect the ability to gain information from social cues. Individuals with cognitive disabilities may have difficulty learning in the manner that others typically do, learning new things, generalizing from specifics, and using language for expression in both oral and written form.

Characteristics of persons with learning disabilities include difficulty discriminating fine differences in auditory, visual, and/or tactual input; decreased ability to retain and recall discriminating sounds and forms in both the short term and the long term; difficulty ordering the correct sequences necessary to complete tasks; difficulty distinguishing between figures and background; difficulties with time and space orientation; difficulty bringing closure to either a concept or a physical form and integrating intersensory information; difficulties relating perception to motor function; difficulty judging the energy requirements of a specific task; difficulty viewing specifics in relationship to the whole; and inability to avoid reacting to stimuli from the environment.

Characteristics of students with ADHD include a strong pull toward certain kinds of stimuli in the educational environment, and inattention to other kinds. Students with ADHD generally focus their attention to things that are novel and find it difficult to continue attending once the novelty has worn off. This results in increased error in long-term performance. Impulsivity is another characteristic that limits achievement in many environments.

More than 1.4 million Americans experience traumatic head injuries in a year. Approximately 5.3 million Americans (2 percent of the population of the United States) experience lifelong physical, mental, and emotional changes because of TBI. Physical changes can affect ambulation, balance and coordination, motor skills, strength, and endurance. Cognitive changes can affect language and communication, information processing, memory, and perceptual skills.

Most of the overt characteristics associated with a cognitive disability bring about a lower status within the major systems of social living. Disabilities that critically affect the acquisition of skills such as reading, math, listening, working independently and within a group, presenting, and critical thinking make students with cognitive disabilities vulnerable to scorn, ridicule, social isolation, and low status.

There is a growing body of literature that questions whether or not certain cognitive disabilities really are disabilities. This is particularly the case with ADHD and LD. Although these voices raise some important issues, ADHD and LD are real disabilities with positive ramifications upon discovery for people with these conditions.

PERSONAL NARRATIVE: KEVIN SHIREY

Kevin Shirey was, at the time of this writing, a forty-one-year-old social work student and independent living counselor.

My primary disability is an acquired traumatic brain injury that I received in April 1986 when I was thirty years old. I also have an alcohol problem that is in remission. Before I became disabled, I used to feel sorry for disabled people. I would feel sorry for them and do what I could to avoid them.

I remember the day I became head injured. I had just finished up a twelve-pack of beer that I had on the back of my motorcycle. I had also just hit up on some drugs, and I went for a ride in the mountains. A truck came at me; it surely seemed like it was in my lane. I wound up trying to avoid the truck, not wanting to go underneath it, so I drove off the side of a hill. I tried to get my bike back up to the road, but the rear wheel hit a root hole and I spun out. Being on the side of a cliff, I was powerless, so my bike and I fell. I hit a tree, and that put me into a coma.

I was in the coma for a couple of weeks, and, waking up, I didn't know my mother. My mother had come to visit me, but I didn't know who she was. I did recognize my father. My parents were divorced and had been living apart for many years, but when I was first waking up, I didn't understand that. I didn't understand anything. When I was taken out of intensive care in a wheelchair, it started to register with me: "Wow, something's happened here." I didn't believe anything had happened until I got out of bed and started using the wheelchair. Then it all started coming together.

Mom was the loving type of mom after the accident. Dad was always a distant type of a person, but after my accident he was really assertive. He talked to the doctors at the hospital, and he actually gave up some work to come into town for me. He applied for Social Security, SSI, and MediCal for me. He did that while I was in the coma. It surprised me he had done that for me.

When I got out of rehabilitation, I tried to go back to my old job. They were still honoring my insurance, but they were going out of business. So I didn't have a job to go back to. I looked for other jobs, but I couldn't get any. Some of my friends, my drinking buddies, made fun of my disability. They would say, "Ha, ha, you'll be back." But it didn't look like I would, and I became locked into depression.

Eventually, I went to the independent living center and met the people there. Sharon was an independent living counselor. Her specialty was chemical dependency–type clients. She started talking to me about school possibilities, so I went back to school. I had Social Security Disability, so I didn't have to go back to work right away. I also needed a place to live, and she directed me to some halfway houses. One accepted me, so I lived there for some time. I was really happy with the independent living experience.

I got into recovery for my alcoholism. My Alcoholics Anonymous meetings are really important to me. AA has been one of my main supports. I also went to some brain injury support group meetings. They referred me to a psychologist, who did an evaluation on me and pretty much told me that I should get some mental health counseling. I went to mental health services, but they just wanted to put me on drugs. I figured that I'm an alcoholic so

I can't be doing these drugs, and that's all mental health wanted to do with me. So I totally quit them.

Sharon at the independent living center really helped a lot. She helped me get into recovery. At Fresno City College, Chuck was the adapted PE instructor. He's good at it, really good. I took a lot of gym classes with Chuck. Also, Richard, who was the director of the independent living center and used a wheelchair, was a role model. It was explained to me that he had multiple sclerosis, which is a constant deterioration process that people go through. I saw that he was in charge of the independent living center, and I knew that he had the education. I didn't believe I could ever get an education, but he helped give me hope. I thought if he could do it, maybe I could try.

Right now I'm a student in a bachelor's program in social work. I'm doing an internship at an independent living center. I make it a point to be there for people with disabilities. Though I like to consider myself pretty much recovered cognitively, I'm still disabled and I can be a better peer counselor with people because of that. The people I work with are people just like me. I appreciate them because they've gone through the things that I went through. Also, because of my chemical dependency, I am in a fellowship with others like me. I know I can't have even one sip of a drink. None of us can. We understand each other.

My past is like a lead weight holding me back. It's real; I have to deal with it. I have to be able to explain things in my past from before my head injury. I've been in prison in three different states, in jail in five states. I've already had my third felony, so the next time I offend I go away for good.

I really appreciate Sharon. She helped me accept the alcoholism tag. She helped me find a house, a place to live where I wasn't left to drink. It got me living with people who were sober and got me sober. Then she pushed for me to go to college. She explained to me how to use my MediCal card, which I didn't know how to use. I appreciate her for getting involved. She was important to me. I hope that other students and professionals, whether they are disabled or not, will participate *with* their clients. They need to guide them and to help them.

Disabled people have got to go through so much red tape to be able to get things done. People in society need to understand that. We need to have the opportunity to function in our homes and in society. Society's views of people with disabilities have affected me; that is why those of us with disabilities need each other and need programs to help us deal with these problems.

DISCUSSION QUESTIONS

1. What are some of the major issues involved in defining learning disabilities?
2. Explain the various characteristics of learning disabilities. Which do you think may have the most social impact?
3. Explain the various characteristics of ADHD. What factors make success in the educational system difficult for persons with ADHD? How would a person with ADHD be accommodated in the workplace?
4. What issues might need to be addressed in work with a person with TBI?
5. Discuss the psychosocial consequences for persons with cognitive disabilities in the family, in school, and at work.
6. Discuss the issues concerning the current questions about LD and ADHD diagnoses for children. What is the relationship between these issues and the problems related to defining these disabilities?

SUGGESTED READINGS

Buchman, D., & Farber, C. (2006). *A special education: One family's journey through the maze of learning disabilities.* Cambridge, MA: Perseus Books.

Coles, G. (1987). *The learning mystique: A critical look at "learning disabilities."* New York: Pantheon Books.

Cruickshank, W. M. (1990). Definition: A major issue in the field of learning disabilities. In M. Nagler (Ed.), *Perspectives on disability: Text and readings on disability* (pp. 389–406). Palo Alto, CA: Health Markets Research.

Finlan, T. G. (1994). *Learning disability: The imaginary disease.* Westport, CT: Bergin & Garvey.

REFERENCES

Alexander, R. (1992). *The traumatically brain injured and the law.* Retrieved October 12, 2006, from http://consumerlawpage.com/article/brain.shtml

Antrim, D. S. (1997). Newspaper coverage of learning disabilities. *Education, 118,* 145–150. Retrieved September 17, 2006, from Expanded Academic ASAP via Thomson Gale.

Beers, M. H. (Ed.). (2003). *The Merck manual of medical information* (2nd ed.). New York: Simon & Schuster.

Bigler, E. D., Lajiness-O'Neill, R., & Howes, N. (1998). Technology in the assessment of learning disability. *Journal of Learning Disabilities, 31*(1), 67–82.

Brain Injury Association of America. (2006). *Types of brain injury.* Retrieved October 9, 2006, from http://www.biausa.org/Pages/types_of_brain_injury.html

Bruyere, S., Davis, S., & Golden, T. P. (2000). *Working effectively with persons who have cognitive disabilities.* Ithaca, NY: ILR Program on Employment and Disability, Cornell University.

Centers for Disease Control and Prevention. (2005, September 20). *Attention-deficit/ hyperactivity disorder (ADHD)*. Retrieved September 22, 2006, from http://www .cdc.gov/ncbddd/adhd/symptom.htm

Coles, G. (1987). *The learning mystique: A critical look at "learning disabilities."* New York: Pantheon Books.

Cruickshank, W. M. (1990). Definition: A major issue in the field of learning disabilities. In M. Nagler (Ed.), *Perspectives on disability: Text and readings on disability* (pp. 389–406). Palo Alto, CA: Health Markets Research.

Dunham, M. D., Roller, J. R., & McIntosh, D. E. (1996). A preliminary comparison of successful and nonsuccessful closure types among adults with specific learning disabilities in the vocational rehabilitation system. *Journal of Rehabilitation, 26*(1), 42–48.

Faraone, S. V., Sergeant, J. S., Gillberb, C., & Biederman, J. (2003). The worldwide prevalence of ADHD: Is it an American condition? *World Psychiatry, 2*(2), 104–113.

Finlan, T. G. (1994). *Learning disability: The imaginary disease.* Westport, CT: Bergin & Garvey.

Fowler, M. (2002). *Attention-deficit/hyperactivity disorder.* Washington, DC: National Dissemination Center for Children with Disabilities. Retrieved October 8, 2008, from http://old.nichcy.org/pubs/factshe/fs14.pdf

Goldstein, S. (2006). The marketing of ADHD (attention-deficit hyperactivity disorder). *Annals of the American Psychotherapy Association, 9,* 32–34. Retrieved September 22, 2006, from Expanded Academic ASAP via Thomson Gale.

Gururaj, G. (2002). Epidemiology of traumatic brain injuries: Indian scenario. *Neurological Research, 24,* 24–28.

Hillier, S., Hiller, J., & Metzer, J. (1997). Epidemiology of traumatic brain injury in South Australia. *Brain Injury, 11*(9), 649–659.

Keogh, B. K. (2005). Revisiting classification and identification. *Learning Disabilities Quarterly, 28,* 100–102.

Kronick, D. (1981). *Social development of learning disabled persons.* San Francisco: Jossey-Bass.

MacMaster, K., Donovan, L. A., & MacIntyre, P. D. (2002). The effects of being diagnosed with learning disability on children's self-esteem. *Child Study Journal, 32*(2), 101–108.

National Center for Injury Prevention and Control. (2006). *What is traumatic brain injury?* Retrieved September 22, 2006, from http://www.cdc.gov/ncipc/tbi/ TBI.htm

National Joint Committee for Learning Disabilities. (n.d.). *What is a learning disability?* Retrieved September 25, 2006, from http://www.ldonline.org/ldbasics/ whatisld

Naylor, M. W., Staskowski, M., Kenney, M. C., & King, C. A. (1994). Language disorders and learning disabilities in school-refusing adolescents. *Journal of the American Academy of Child and Adolescent Psychiatry, 33*(9), 1331–1338.

O'Meara, K. P. (2002, February 18). Baughman dispels the myth of ADHD: He may be a pariah in the mental-health community, but retired neurologist Fred A. Baughman Jr. is a hero to those suffering from the stigma of the ADHD label. *Insight on the News, 18,* 36–39. Retrieved September 22, 2006, from Expanded Academic ASAP via Thomson Gale.

Pieper, D. R., Valadka, A. B., & Marsh, C. (1996). Surgical management of patients with severe head injuries. *AORN Journal, 63*(5), 854–867.

Raja, I., Vohra, A., & Ahmed, M. (2001). Neurotrauma in Pakistan. *World Journal of Surgery, 25*(9), 1230–1237.

Sigler, G., & Mackelprang, R. W. (1993). Cognitive impairment: Psychosocial and sexual implication and strategies for social work intervention. In R. W. Mackelprang & D. Valentine (Eds.), *Sexuality and disabilities: A guide for human service practitioners* (pp. 89–106). Binghamton, NY: Haworth Press.

Simpson, R. G., & Umbach, B. T. (1989). Identifying and providing vocational services for adults with specific learning disabilities. *Journal of Rehabilitation, 55*(3), 49–56.

Smelter, R. W., Rasch, B. W., Fleming, J., Nazos, P., & Baranowski, S. (1996). Is attention deficit disorder becoming a desired diagnosis? *Phi Delta Kappan, 77*(6), 429–433.

Spear-Swerling, L., & Sternberg, R. J. (1998). Curing our "epidemic" of learning disabilities. *Phi Delta Kappan, 79*(5), 39–401. Retrieved September 17, 2006, from Expanded Academic ASAP via Thomson Gale.

Sternberg, R. J., & Grigorenko, E. L. (2001). Learning disabilities, schooling, and society. *Phi Delta Kappan, 83*(4), 335–339. Retrieved September 17, 2006, from Expanded Academic ASAP via Thomson Gale.

Thomas, M. (2000). Albert Einstein and LD: An evaluation of the evidence. *Journal of Learning Disabilities, 33*(2), 149–157.

Tierney, L. M., McPhee, S. J., & Papadakis, M. A. (Eds.). (2006). *Current medical diagnosis and treatment.* New York: Lang Medical Books/McGraw-Hill.

Wilkinson, S. (2005). What's so special about being special? *Learning Disability Practice, 8*(10), 30–31.

Wolraich, M. L. (2006). Attention-deficit/hyperactivity disorder: Can it be recognized and treated in children younger than five years? *Infants & Young Children, 19*(2), 86–93.

Working with the ADHD student. (2006). *Techniques, 81,* 8–10. Retrieved October 9, 2006, from Expanded Academic ASAP via Thomson Gale.

Zentall, S. S. (1993). Research on the educational implications of attention deficit hyperactivity disorder. *Exceptional Children, 60*(2), 143–154.

12

Health-Related Disabilities

It is not *my* inabilities that limit me, but the unwillingness or inability of society to grant me the access I need to participate fully—an access that would give all members of society equal opportunity.

—Danny Teachmann, disability advocate

Student Learning Objectives

1. To be able to identify health-related conditions and illnesses that can lead to disability
2. To be able to differentiate medical diagnoses of chronic illness from life with a disability
3. To understand the impacts of stigma and discrimination on the lives of people with health-related disabilities
4. To understand personal and social factors that influence the quality of life for people with health-related disabilities

When the first edition of this book was published, we felt it was missing a component addressing conditions that are traditionally considered health problems, illnesses, or diseases. These conditions result in impairments that affect people's abilities to function in everyday life and in society. People with health-related disabilities are also handicapped by restrictive social policies and lack of access to resources.

The incidence and prevalence of people who live with chronic conditions leading to health-related disabilities have increased in the last century and will continue to increase in coming decades. These trends are multicausal. Life expectancies worldwide have increased dramatically in the last century, in many areas more than doubling. In addition, conditions that led to death within a short time just a few decades ago can be maintained for decades today. For example, people who developed a neurogenic bladder and the inability to empty the bladder voluntarily used to die from kidney-related problems within months or years. A half century ago, urinary problems, combined with hydrocephalus, led to early deaths for most of the approximately 1 in 1,000 children born with spina bifida worldwide. Over the last generation, because of increased knowledge, children routinely began to grow to adulthood and lead productive lives when bladder care and shunts that drain excess fluid from the brain are available (Bowman, McLone, Grant, Tomita, & Ito, 2001).

The prevalence of chronic health problems has steadily risen in the last century, especially those related to lifestyle, such as cardiac and respiratory illness. For example, in the nineteenth century, when life expectancies were less than forty years, people who smoked rarely died of smoking-related illness; they died too soon. These conditions, which typically arise in the fifth through the seventh decades of life, have become the leading causes of illness and death. According to the World Health Organization (2007e), the three leading causes of death worldwide are cancer, ischemic heart disease, and stroke. Tobacco-attributed deaths worldwide will rise from 5.4 million in 2005 to 6.5 million people, or 10 percent of all deaths, in 2015, and to 8.3 million by 2030. Furthermore, it projects that by the second decade of this century, the fourth-leading cause of death worldwide will be AIDS, and that—assuming antiretroviral therapy coverage reaches 80 percent of the world's population—deaths from AIDS will rise from 2.8 million to 6.5 million worldwide by 2030. Of course, people with conditions such as cancer, heart disease, and HIV disease usually live for years or decades with the physical and social effects of these conditions before succumbing to them.

Conditions such as cancer and respiratory illness produce disabilities in people in all countries and social strata. However, some conditions strike the poor and people in less developed countries in far greater numbers. For example, HIV disease, which found initial footholds in the United States and Europe, is now a pandemic and is especially pervasive in sub-Saharan Africa, where nearly 25 million of the approximately 40 million HIV-infected people worldwide live. In several countries, more than 20 percent of the adult population is infected. Unlike North America and Europe, where people have widespread access, in 2005 only about one in five persons who needed them were receiving antiretroviral drugs worldwide (UNAIDS, 2006). And HIV disease is not the only health problem with disabling effects that disproportionately affect the poorest countries. Let's briefly look at two others: malaria and tuberculosis.

Worldwide, malaria is one of the leading diseases causing health-related disabilities. According to the World Health Organization (2007c), more than 500 million people become severely ill with malaria each year, and there are more than a million malaria-related deaths annually. Caused by the parasite plasmodium and spread from person to person through mosquito bites, it is especially prevalent in sub-Saharan Africa, where some countries spend half of their public health budgets on malaria. The World Health Organization further states that "malaria has lifelong effects through increased poverty, impaired learning and decreased attendance in schools and the workplace."

It disproportionately affects marginalized populations, trapping affected individuals and families in a downward spiral of poverty. Drug-resistant strains are complicating malaria treatment, leaving some with malaria with long-term health problems. The elimination of malaria would increase life spans significantly in the approximately ninety countries in which malaria is endemic (Bawah & Binka, 2005).

Another chronic condition that occurs worldwide is tuberculosis (TB), a bacterial infection that infects the lungs and damages lung tissue, compromising the respiratory system. It can also affect and damage other body systems, causing weight loss, energy loss, and digestive and orthopedic problems. It is spread from person to person in the same manner as the common cold. Though 90 percent of people exposed to the TB bacteria do not develop the disease, there are more than 14 million people living with TB today, and 1.6 million annual deaths. HIV infection dramatically increases the risk of lethal TB infection. In recent decades, antibiotics have been used to cure TB; however, multidrug-resistant TB strains have developed, and in many countries medical treatment is woefully inadequate. It is estimated that the largest number of new TB cases in 2005 occurred in Southeast Asia, which accounted for 34 percent of incident cases globally. However, the estimated incidence rate in sub-Saharan Africa is nearly twice that of Southeast Asia, at nearly 350 cases per 100,000 people (World Health Organization, 2007d).

Suffice it to say that chronic health conditions affect hundreds of millions of persons throughout the world. Some, such as stroke, are stable and nonprogressive. Others, such as heart disease and cystic fibrosis, are progressive; as the conditions progress, they have increasing impact on individuals. Among the most prevalent of progressive conditions are autoimmune conditions, in which the body recognizes its own cells as foreign, thus causing the individual's immune system to progressively attack its own tissues and organs. Infectious health conditions such as HIV are contagious through contact with other people. Malaria is spread by mosquitoes that have bitten an individual with malaria. Many people have misconceptions about infectious conditions; for example, some believe that people who have them are unclean or impure, resulting in stigmas that lead to discrimination and social ostracism.

In this chapter, we select a sampling of health-related conditions that precipitate disability, discussing the physical as well as the social implications of these conditions. In selecting specific health problems, we fully recognize that we are omitting several that deserve attention. Our choices are largely based upon those areas that we believe our readers will have the most interest in.

INFECTIOUS CONDITIONS

In this section, we discuss several infectious conditions throughout history. These conditions have struck fear among the general population and have led to social isolation of those infected with them. For example, lepers were considered unclean and forcibly removed from the population to prevent spread of leprosy. And while today, enlightened societies understand that conditions like leprosy and polio are spread through microorganisms and are not divine punishment or a result of moral failure, stereotypes and stigma surrounding other conditions still exist. Among these is HIV/AIDS. We will, therefore, discuss HIV/AIDS in some detail.

History of Infectious Conditions

Infectious conditions are caused when the body is exposed to and damaged by microorganisms such as viruses, bacteria, fungi, and protozoa. They are contagious when they are transmitted through contact with infected hosts, whether directly or indirectly. People become ill when their immune systems are unable to stop the microorganisms from spreading before they multiply and damage the body. Some infections, such as cold and flu, result in acute mild illness, after which people recover their health and the body develops immunity. At the other end of the spectrum are viruses such as Ebola, which kills between 50 percent and 90 percent of acutely infected people.

Increased understanding of disease processes and advances in health care and technology have greatly changed the face of infectious health-related disabilities in recent history. First, the development of vaccines has led to widespread immunity to numerous illnesses. Since Edward Jenner developed the cowpox vaccine to prevent smallpox in 1796, tens of millions of lives have been spared by vaccines to prevent numerous infectious conditions. Second, an understanding of the link with microorganisms has led to prevention. In 1854, Henry Snow and John Whitehead tracked the source of a London cholera outbreak to a well that was contaminated by a nearby cesspit. This discovery led to great diminution of cholera and provided insights into other infectious diseases. Third, the development and wide-spread use of antibiotics beginning in the mid-twentieth century provided avenues for curing previously incurable conditions. Subsequently, curative and palliative treatments for multiple types of microorganisms have ameliorated much of the infectious disease toll worldwide.

Historically, lethal infectious diseases have decimated populations. Smallpox dates back more than 3,000 years, and in the twentieth century alone, acute smallpox killed an estimated 300 million people before it was eradicated through vaccination (Mackelprang, Mackelprang, & Thirkill, 2005). Outbreaks of bubonic plague or the Black Death, caused by a bacterial infection spread via fleas on rodents, killed approximately 75 percent of the populations of Europe and Asia during the 1300s (Columbia Encyclopedia, 2007b).

Unlike diseases that cause acute illness and either fatality or recovery, some infectious conditions lead to lifelong and often progressive disabilities.

Leprosy results from bacterial infection and has been present for millennia; nearly 20,000 European leper colonies and houses existed in the thirteenth century. Leprosy infects the deep layers of the skin and peripheral nerves, causing sensory loss and paralysis throughout the body, including the face and extremities. Ulceration can occur, and amputation of limbs may be required. More than 90 percent of people exposed to Mycobacterium leprae, the bacteria that cause leprosy, never develop the condition. However, without treatment, those who do contract leprosy develop progressive disability that does not shorten the life span appreciably (Columbia Encyclopedia, 2007a). Lepers have been considered society's pariah throughout history, and leprosy continues to carry stigma in countries like India that have limited public health services and post-infection treatments, and where infected persons do not have access to treatments that are available in countries with adequate resources.

Polio

Poliomyelitis, caused by a viral infection, and most commonly known as polio, is another infectious condition that precipitates long-term disability and has been present in the human population for thousands of years. Sometimes known as infantile paralysis, in the twentieth century it frequently infected older children and adults. The immune systems of most people infected with polio successfully fight off serious illness; however, in less than 1 percent of the people infected, a paralytic case of polio develops. Most commonly, the virus attacks the motor nerves of the spinal cord, affecting mobility but not sensation. During the first half of the twentieth century, polio was endemic throughout the world; however, in 1955 the Salk vaccine was introduced. Over the last half century, polio outbreaks have disappeared in developed countries, and cases worldwide have been greatly reduced. The Global Polio Eradication Initiative (2007) reported 1,997 total cases in 2006, 1,798 of which originated in Nigeria and India. In developed countries, new cases of polio have nearly disappeared; however, people who developed polio prior to the introduction of vaccines live with its long-term effects. In addition, about a quarter of people who develop polio eventually develop post-polio syndrome, a condition characterized by fatigue, weakness, and paralysis (Nathanson & Martin, 1979; Sass, Gottfried, & Sorem, 1996).

Polio is spread through person-to-person contact, and before vaccinations, summer polio outbreaks during the first half of the twentieth century struck fear in people throughout the United States and Europe. In the United States, paralytic polio peaked in the summer of 1952, when more than 21,000 cases and over 3,000 deaths were reported (Atkinson, Hamborsky, McIntyre, & Wolfe, 2007; Mayo Clinic, 2007; Sass et al., 1996).

Polio survivors have had a major impact on disability rights and the development of disability culture. Franklin D. Roosevelt, a polio survivor, was elected president of the United States in 1932, twelve years after contracting polio. He helped pull the United States out of the Great Depression and led the United States through World War II before his death on April 12, 1945, just months before the war ended. The country's citizens were aware of Roosevelt's polio; however, he was masterful in hiding its physical effects from the world. His ability to hide the extent of his physical impairments illustrates the fact that polio did not compromise his ability to lead; however, societal reactions would have. Disability rights founders and leaders Justin Dart, Ed Roberts, and Judy Heumann all survived polio and have been leaders in the fight for the rights of disabled persons. Born into wealth and prominence, Dart (1930–2002) proceeded to make himself into an unlikable "super loser" in a family of "super winners" until he developed polio as a teenager in 1948. Unlike many others, Dart did not consider polio a great tragedy. Referring to the health care providers who helped him during acute infection, Dart stated, "I count the good days in my life from the time I got polio. These beautiful people not only saved my life, they made it worth saving." Dart is widely considered the father of the Americans with Disabilities Act, godfather of the disability rights movement, and a major proponent of civil rights for various cultural groups (Fay & Pelka, 2002). Dart's words, read at his memorial service, demonstrate his commitment to disability rights and to human rights throughout the world.

> Dearly Beloved:
> Listen to the heart of this old soldier. . . . I do not go quietly into the night. . . .
> . . . Let my final actions thunder of love, solidarity, protest—of empowerment. . . .
> I adamantly protest the richest culture in the history of the world which still incarcerates millions of humans with and without disabilities in barbaric institutions, backrooms and worse, windowless cells of oppressive perceptions. . . . I call for solidarity among all who love justice, all who love life, to create a revolution that will empower every single human being to govern his or her life, to govern the society and to be fully productive of life quality for self and for all. . . . I do so love you, my beautiful colleagues in the disability and civil rights movement. . . . Thanks to you, I die in the joy of struggle. Thanks to you, I die in the beautiful belief that the revolution of empowerment will go on. . . .
>
> Justin Dart (Fay & Pelka, 2002)

As we have previously discussed, Ed Roberts and Judy Heumann, both child survivors of polio, were instrumental in starting the independent living movement, promoting the politics of inclusion, and promulgating the doctrine of disability rights first in the United States, then throughout the world. These human rights leaders recognized that social policies that reinforced isolation and discrimination were the true tragedies that limit polio survivors and other people with disabilities.

HIV/AIDS

In 1979 and 1980, sporadic cases of strange, seemingly unconnected illnesses started showing up in San Francisco as well as a few others places like Zaire and Copenhagen. Among these were cases of meningitis caused by Cryptococcus, a yeast; Pneumocystis carinii pneumonia, caused by a fungus; and Kaposi's sarcoma, a cancer of the lymphatic endothelium. What perplexed health workers was not the existence of microorganisms like Cryptococcus and Pneumocystis; they are common in the environment. Rather, it was the virulence of infections that people usually have no difficulty combating. Young and seemingly otherwise healthy people were becoming seriously ill and dying. These events signaled the beginning of the AIDS pandemic that has affected tens of millions in the last four decades.

Compare the initial response to AIDS to that of another infectious organism: Legionella pneumophila, a bacterium named after a July 1976 outbreak in Philadelphia at a convention of Legionnaires, U.S. military veterans. Approximately 220 conventioneers were treated, and thirty-four deaths occurred. An unprecedented investigation followed, and within six months the Legionella bacterium was identified by the U.S. Centers for Disease Control (Shilts, 1987). In contrast, Ronald Reagan first publicly addressed HIV/AIDS in 1987, only after 35,000 Americans had been diagnosed and 21,000 had died. By then, HIV/AIDS had spread to more than one hundred countries and infected more than 50,000 people. The U.S. government's nonresponse to AIDS was directly connected to those who were contracting it: first gay men, and subsequently intravenous drug users. The U.S. surgeon general, C. Everett Koop, has recounted how the president's advisors excluded him from HIV policy planning because they believed infected people deserved to get it. Religious leaders such as Pat Robertson and Jerry Falwell have stated that homosexuals who contract AIDS deserve it and get it because of God's judgments against them (Shilts, 1987; White, 2004). Other governments were not much better in their early response.

By the end of the twentieth century, more than 34 million had been infected with HIV worldwide, half of whom had developed AIDS, and 12 million of whom were already dead. UNAIDS (2006) estimates that at the end of 2005, 38.6 million people were living with HIV, and that 4.1 million new infections and 2.8 million AIDS-related deaths occurred that year. Though the number of new HIV infections is declining, more people than ever before are living with HIV. Nearly 25 million people with HIV live in sub-Saharan Africa.

One can only speculate how HIV/AIDS would look today if the United States and other Western governments had responded in the early years of the epidemic. At the very least, millions of lives would have been saved. Shilts (1987) offers several reasons that the "story of AIDS in America is a drama of national failure, played out against a backdrop of needless death" (xxii):

- Reagan administration officials ignored pleas from scientists, refusing to allocate adequate research funding.

- There was a lack of scientific attention because scientists felt that there was little prestige to be gained from studying a homosexual affliction.

- Researchers were engaging in competition rather than cooperation and collaboration.

- Health officials refused to take tough measures to stop the spread (e.g., closing bathhouses).

- Gay leaders played politics, putting dogma ahead of the preservation of human life out of fear that publicizing the danger of HIV among gay men and forcing the closure of bathhouses would reflect badly on them and on the gay rights movement and would force gay men and women back into the closet.

The introduction of HIV into the population of gay men in the United States and Western Europe came at a time of high vulnerability. The birth of the gay rights movement had taken place scarcely a decade earlier when, in 1969, gay and transgender New Yorkers rebelled against the periodic but routine raids on gay bars by New York City police. Originating at a gay bar, the Stonewall Inn, demonstrations lasted several days and spread to other cities. Within a month, the Gay Liberation Front had been created; the movement soon spread to Canada and several countries in Europe, as well as Australia and New Zealand; and Gay Pride parades became commonplace. Contemporarily Pride parades are held throughout the world in June each year to commemorate Stonewall. With the birth of the international gay rights movement, gay men and women were acknowledged and recognized. Increasingly, they left the closet and acknowledged their identities. Cities like New York, San Francisco, Amsterdam, Paris, and Sydney attracted gays and lesbians, where they found community, acceptance, and openness. However, discrimination from outside these communities was still prevalent. Homosexual acts were still considered criminal. In 1986 the U.S. Supreme Court upheld the prosecution of homosexual acts in the confines of one's own home in *Bowers v. Hardwick*, a decision not overturned until 2003.

The congregation of gay men in urban centers that fostered openness—combined with societal prejudices that separated gay men from society, social policies that did not support long-term committed relationships, lack of governmental response, fear that they would be forced back into the closet, high numbers of casual sexual contacts among gay men, and easily accessible national and international air travel—created an ideal climate for the spread of HIV infection from a few thousand in the early 1980s to tens of millions worldwide contemporarily. In industrialized countries, male-to-male sexual contact is still a major HIV transmission risk a generation into the epidemic. For example, in the United States, male-to-male sexual contact continues to account for more than half of new AIDS diagnoses (Centers for Disease Control and Prevention, 2007).

Let's look at the experience of one man, a close friend of one of the authors, who died of AIDS in the early 1990s.

In 1980, at age eighteen, Will left home in his western state and moved to Los Angeles. As a teen, he never felt like he fit in with his conservative community; experimented with drugs; and, as he told the author, couldn't wait to get out of "Hicksville." When he moved to Southern California, he felt like he had found home; he finally fit in. Closeted, even to himself, in high school, he came out as a gay man to the author about a year after moving. However, he was adamant that his parents and the rest of his family not be informed of his sexual orientation. He had a large circle of friends and lived life in the fast lane, which involved engaging in casual sex with multiple partners. In one 1982 discussion with the author, Will expressed concern that a couple of his friends had recently become ill with a strange gay-related immune deficiency (GRID) or "gay plague." Having had bouts of giardiasis and gonorrhea, he stated he was going to be more careful about his sexual choices but minimized his own risk of developing GRID. In 1985, when Will traveled to visit family and attend a family reunion with Chris, his new "roommate," he told a few family members that his roommate was his new lover and life partner but could not bring himself to tell his parents. He was thrilled about his life, having recently acquired a new job, and about entering a stable relationship. He was also volunteering with a community-based AIDS organization, providing respite care. He expressed concern about AIDS but was convinced that behavioral changes he had tried to stick with since 1982, along with his new monogamous relationship, would minimize his risk. When the author visited Will two years later, Chris had lost much weight and had been admitted to the hospital with Pneumocystis carinii pneumonia (PCP). Chris recovered from his bout with PCP, but his AIDS diagnosis was devastating to the couple. Will had support from his Los Angeles "family," but not his biological family. Even though family members told his parents and brother that Will was gay and they were aware of Chris's AIDS-related illnesses, Will's parents and brother steadfastly refused to acknowledge his sexual orientation and referred to Chris only as his roommate. In addition, when Will took time off from work to help Chris, his employer was made aware of Will's sexual orientation and Chris's AIDS. Will had not previously revealed his sexual orientation to his employer due to his perception that his employer was homophobic. Will experienced a significant attitude change from his employer, and within six months Will was terminated because his job was eliminated. Within eighteen months, Chris died, and by then, Will knew he was HIV positive and had developed symptoms of AIDS-related complex. By 1989, Will had full-blown AIDS. He was experiencing cognitive changes and so moved back to live with his parents. However, even then his parents and brother refused to acknowledge that Will had AIDS or that he was gay. When Will died in 1991, his obituary stated that he died of cancer. His family refused to acknowledge his gay friends; they were excluded from Will's viewing and sat in the back row at the funeral service. To this day, Will's family refuses to acknowledge the cause of his death and his sexual orientation.

Will's experience illustrates the double discrimination of many who experience AIDS as well as both ableism and heterosexism. The social model of disability helps one understand that the problems Will and others experience are as much a result of societal forces as HIV itself. When Will was terminated from his job, he stated, "I know it is because my boss thinks I will get AIDS, and because I am gay." Because of the discrimination surrounding HIV infection, states' reporting laws have treated it differently from any other communicable infection. Until the development and ready availability of new antiretroviral therapies, medications that delay AIDS onset and extend life for decades, in 1996, nearly half of states forbade the collection of epidemiological data on HIV infection. Only AIDS diagnoses were reported. This practice departed dramatically from practices concerning other infectious conditions, which are automatically reported. In states such as Washington, in which HIV reporting was forbidden, the primary argument against reporting was that it would subject people with HIV to pervasive discrimination—discrimination fueled both by homophobia and fear of disability associated with AIDS. With multiple reports of HIV-infected persons being fired, assaulted, and driven from their homes, these fears were justified. HIV reporting is now required in all U.S. states, but unlike with other communicable conditions, many states still forbid the name of the infected individual to be reported, again due to fears of discrimination.

Until the 1990 passage of the Americans with Disabilities Act, there were no U.S. disability rights laws that protected people presumed to have HIV or AIDS. Civil rights laws in other countries followed the implementation of the ADA. Section 12102 defines disability as follows: "The term 'disability' means, with respect to an individual (A) a physical or mental impairment that substantially limits one or more of the major life activities of such individual; (B) a record of such an impairment; or (C) being regarded as having such impairment."

Unfortunately, the ADA was passed too late for Will and thousands of others to benefit from its protections. The phrase "being regarded as having such impairment" is critical for persons with HIV in that persons whom others think might have HIV are protected. The ADA provides protections not only for people living with HIV/AIDS but also for people who lose their jobs and housing and are otherwise discriminated against because someone fears they might have it. Indirectly, ADA also provided protections for gay men by protecting them from discrimination based on the belief that because they are gay, they are likely to have AIDS. The pervasiveness of this problem became obvious to one of the authors around the time he was the guest editor of the journal *Human Services in the Rural Environment* (Mackelprang & Morris, 1989), which was the first time a professional journal devoted an issue to rural HIV/AIDS. The dual discrimination became apparent to the author when he came into contact with two families living with AIDS in the same rural area. The first family received an outpouring of community support when they were diagnosed with AIDS after the husband received a blood transfusion with infected blood. A few weeks later, a man from a nearby community revealed that he had attended a community public health meeting devoted to AIDS. After the meeting, community members who assumed he was gay and HIV infected abducted the man and proceeded to anally rape him with a pole while hurling insults about his presumed sexual orientation and HIV status.

As the AIDS pandemic spread from the United States, Europe, and other industrialized countries, the face of HIV transmission also changed. In industrialized countries, AIDS is still disproportionately represented among men who have sex with men. IV drug users are also at significantly increased risk. However, whereas AIDS began as a "gay plague" in North America and Europe and still affects high numbers of men who have sex with men and IV drug users, worldwide, AIDS is spread primarily through heterosexual contact with infected individuals. A startling trend over the last several years, particularly in the United States, is the disproportionate representation among non-whites. For example, as illustrated in table 12.1, in 2005 the rate among female blacks was almost twenty-three times higher than the rate among whites. The rate of AIDS among black males was eight times higher than among white males. Yet access to prevention and health care services in highly affected communities of color lags behind that in white areas.

Today, in regions such as Africa, where two-thirds of the world's infected population live, HIV is primarily a heterosexually spread condition. The lack of health care providers and medications leads to a far greater mortality rate in these areas (UNAIDS, 2006). Families are being decimated, children orphaned, and societal structures weakened. Before the 1996 introduction of protease inhibitors, a new family of medications that were combined with existing medications for "highly active antiretroviral therapy" in industrialized countries, the life expectancy following infection was ten years or less, whereas today life expectancy is computed in decades. However, this progress is not mirrored in Africa. The decrease in life expectancy and quality shown by the 2004 Human Development Index during the 1990s in thirteen sub-Saharan African countries was due primarily to the HIV/AIDS epidemic and its massive impact on life expectancy (United Nations Development Programme, 2004). Studies blame HIV/AIDS for much of the life expectancy discrepancy between Norway (seventy-nine years) and Zambia (thirty-two years) and Zimbabwe (thirty-three years), which have 16 percent and 25 percent adult HIV infection rates, respectively (British Broadcasting

TABLE 12.1 Estimated numbers of adult and adolescent cases and rates (per 100,000 population) of AIDS in the United States

Race/ethnicity	Males		Females		Total	
	No.	Rate	No.	Rate	No.	Rate
White, not Hispanic	10,027	12.1	1,747	2.0	11,773	6.9
Black, not Hispanic	13,048	95.1	7,093	45.5	20,141	68.7
Hispanic	5,949	36.0	1,714	11.2	7,662	24.0
Asian/Pacific Islander	389	7.2	92	1.6	481	4.3
American Indian/Alaska Native	137	14.3	45	4.4	182	9.3
Total	**29,766**	**24.9**	**10,774**	**8.6**	**40,540**	**16.6**

Source: Centers for Disease Control and Prevention. (2007). *HIV/AIDS surveillance report: Cases of HIV infection and AIDS in the United States and dependent areas, 2005* (Vol. 17). Atlanta, GA: Author.

System, 2004). The moral approach to HIV is strongly supported in many circles. For example, in 2004 Stephen Lewis, the special UN envoy on HIV/ AIDS, bemoaned the U.S. governmental limitations and cuts in HIV prevention funding for condoms in African countries and mandates that prevention programs emphasize abstinence over safer sex. Access to condoms, which are effective in reducing HIV transmission, has been limited because some policy makers believe condoms are necessary only when people engage in "immoral" sex. Today, in many African communities, it is common for thirteen- and fourteen-year-old children to be heads of households; children are raising children because parents and other adults in their communities have died of AIDS (Lewis, 2004; Stephen Lewis Foundation, 2007).

CANCERS

The World Health Organization (2003) reports that in 2000, malignant tumors were responsible for 12 percent of 56 million deaths worldwide. Altogether, in 2000, 11 million people developed cancer, and there were 6.2 million cancer deaths. In some countries, one-fourth of deaths were cancer related. Citing the 2003 World Cancer Report, the World Health Organization projects that by 2020, the annual incidence of new cancers could rise to 15 million. In the United States, the National Cancer Institute (2007b) estimates that the lifetime risk of developing cancer is 41 percent, and the lifetime risk of dying from cancer is about 21 percent. However, the World Health Organization suggests that, with proper action, one-third of cancers can be prevented, and another third cured. The primary reason for the increasing cancer incidence is the pervasiveness of tobacco use, combined with the aging of the population. Tobacco use is the most common preventable health problem behavior; 100 million tobacco-related deaths were reported in the twentieth century. For example, the relative risk of lung cancer is twenty- to thirtyfold greater, bladder and renal cancer five- to sixfold greater, mouth and throat cancer over sixfold greater, and pancreas three- to fourfold greater in tobacco users than non-users. Risks of several other cancers are also higher in smokers. Passive, or secondhand, smoke is responsible for up to a 20 percent increase in lung cancer risk. Reductions in smoking, combined with balanced diets, improved lifestyle choices such as exercise, and early screening and prevention programs, would greatly reduce the morbidity and mortality associated with cancer.

Infections are another cause of cancer, causing nearly one-fourth of cancers in developing countries and one-tenth in developed countries. Leading causes of infection-related cancers are hepatitis B and C (liver cancer), human papillomavirus (cervical and anal-genital cancers), and Helicobacter pylori (stomach cancer). The mortality and morbidity burden is especially heavy in developing countries, in which people have very limited access to vaccines, screening, and early treatment (World Health Organization, 2003).

Box 12.1   Sex, Human Papillomavirus, Cancer, and Vaccinations

HPV vaccination prevents HPV infection, which is responsible for the majority of cancers of the cervix. It is contracted through intimate sexual contact and is avoidable if a woman engages in sex only with one person who has also only had sex with her. HPV is very different from other conditions for which there are vaccinations, such as polio. Given that HPV is contracted primarily through voluntary behavior, what should be the social policies surrounding vaccination? Should it be mandatory like other vaccinations? Should it be voluntary and universally accessible and publicly supported? Should it be voluntary and paid for by individuals/families? What are the moral and public health reasons for your opinions?

Two types of human papillomavirus (HPV), types 16 and 18, are responsible for a high proportion of cervical cancers in infected women. In 2006, a vaccine for HPV was introduced and within a year was available in nearly one hundred countries. However, because this virus is transmitted sexually, there has been significant controversy surrounding vaccination policy. Some entities advocate compulsory vaccination of females, others universal voluntary vaccination. However, there is also much resistance to vaccination based on moral arguments; women who have only one sexual partner who, likewise, has had sex only with her have little or no risk of acquiring HPV. Thus, some argue that HPV vaccination promotes casual or promiscuous sexual behavior. In box 12.1 we ask you to consider appropriate public policies and individual decisions about HPV.

Genetics and heredity are major factors in some cancers. The majority of people who develop cancers have no previously known risk factors. However, genes that are associated with higher cancer risks are increasingly being identified. In some cases, cancers can be traced to mutations in specific genes. For example, mutations of BRCA 1, located on chromosome 17, and BRCA 2, located on chromosome 13, are associated with greatly increased risks of breast cancer. According to the National Cancer Institute (2002), approximately one in eight women will develop breast cancer at some time in her life. However, women who inherit the mutated form of one of these genes are three to seven times more likely to develop breast cancer than women without them. They are also more likely to develop uterine cancer, and their cancers tend to be more aggressive with an earlier onset. Another inherited cancer is familial adenomatous polyposis, a colorectal cancer that occurs when a person inherits a mutated form of the APC gene, which accounts for about 1–2 percent of all colorectal cancers. It develops sporadically among about 75 percent of the people who develop it; that is, about 75 percent have no family history of colorectal cancer. Nearly a quarter of people who develop colorectal cancer have some family history, likely related to multiple genes and/or environmental factors. However, nearly all people who inherit a rare mutation in the APC gene develop colorectal cancer, with a median age of onset at forty years (Frank, 2002).

A cancer diagnosis can strike fear into the hearts of people diagnosed and those close to them. However, the health risks associated with different cancers vary widely. For example, basal cell carcinoma, a skin cancer and one of the most common cancers, rarely metastasizes and is generally easily treatable. In contrast, another cancer of the skin and underlying tissue, malignant melanoma, is much less common but more severe.

The implications of cancer are multifactorial and complex. Personal coping with cancer is influenced by several factors that can be divided into three general categories: cancer-related factors, personal factors, and societal factors. Cancer-related factors include the type of cancer and the body parts and functions it affects. The stage and aggressiveness of cancer are also important. Other factors include the availability of treatments, both in terms of technology and resources to access treatments, as well as the effects of treatments themselves. For example, with surgeries to remove body parts such as testes, ovaries, and breasts, people face not only the loss of body organs but an assault on their sexuality and, sometimes, reproductive capabilities. Treatments such as chemotherapy and radiation therapy may precipitate serious side effects and illness. Sometimes persons with cancer are forced to make decisions about aggressive treatments that may extend the quantity of life at the cost of quality of life. Consider the situations in boxes 12.2, 12.3, and 12.4. Each of these situations involves people who are facing serious and life-threatening cancer scenarios. In contrast, the spouse of one of the authors experienced basal cell carcinoma that required outpatient surgery and no significant life changes.

In addition to cancer-related factors, personal factors are also important in determining how people adjust to and cope with cancer. These factors include (1) intrapersonal coping strategies, personality characteristics, and general health; (2) family and social supports; and (3) time and developmental phase of life. Another personal factor is stressors. Those with stronger supports and coping strategies have significant advantages. Coping strategies can be divided into three general categories: problem focused, emotion focused, and meaning focused. Problem-focused strategies are used to overcome the challenges and specific problems associated with cancer. They are more likely to be used by people who view their cancer as a challenge. Emotion-focused strategies are used when people perceive their cancer as a threat and loss and are used to help regulate emotional stress. People use meaning-focused strategies to figure out the meanings of their cancer and its

---

Box 12.2　Margaret's Family

Margaret was a fifty-five-year-old single female who, after experiencing severe headaches, dizziness, and eventually seizures, was diagnosed with a grade 4 astrocytoma, an aggressive form of brain cancer. Her physician informed her that without surgery, she had three to four months to live; with surgery, her life expectancy would double. She consulted with her adult children, who agreed she should have surgery so that "We can have as much time with you as possible." Surgery was performed; however, following surgery, Margaret experienced severe personality changes, including cognitive deficits, and extreme emotional lability. Her son felt that "Mom died on that operating table." Following surgery, Margaret lived nine more months; however, the personality and cognitive changes she experienced did not improve. The family felt cheated, stating, "If we knew what surgery would do to Mom, we would never have consented." What would you want for yourself in a similar situation? What would you want for a loved one?

---

impact on their lives. People who stay active and involved in coping processes are much more likely to maintain meaning and quality of life, whereas those who become passive and disengaged are less likely to cope well (Ahmad, Musil, Zauszniewski, & Resnick, 2005; Brennan, 2001; Folkman & Greer, 2000; National Cancer Institute, 2007a). It is important to remember that coping with cancer is coping with life. Too often, given the fear cancer generates, we assume that adjusting to serious cancer is preparing for death. Though some cancers are eventually fatal, months, years, and even decades of life are there to be fully lived following a cancer diagnosis.

The third category, societal factors, is often one that is overlooked. Societal factors can include cultural beliefs. Also, social policies that influence access to health care, employment, and monetary resources can greatly influence quality of life. Pearlin and Schooler (1978) emphasize the connection between personal coping and societal factors:

> On the basis of the evidence brought together here we can assert that what people do or fail to do in dealing with their problems can make a difference to their well-being. At the same time, there are important human problems, such as those that we have seen in occupation, that are not responsive to individual coping responses. Coping with these may require interventions by collectivities rather than by individuals. Many of the problems stemming from arrangements deeply rooted in social and economic organization may exert a powerful effect on personal life but be impervious to personal efforts to change them. This perhaps is the reason that much of our coping functions only to help us endure that which we cannot avoid. Such coping at best provides but a thin cushion to

Box 12.3 Paul's Decisions

Paul was a sixty-one-year-old married male who, after two years of symptoms, was "finally dragged by my wife" to see a urologist. A series of tests revealed that Paul had advanced prostate cancer. His physician informed him that without aggressive radiation, chemotherapy, and hormone therapies, he could expect to live one to two years. With treatments, he could lengthen his life expectancy "significantly" and see his nineteen-year-old daughter, a college freshman, graduate from college. Treatments would not cure his cancer, but they would work to put his cancer in remission. Paul chose to undergo all the treatments available to him in spite of side effects that included fatigue, loss of hair from radiation, serious nausea and vomiting from chemotherapy, and loss of sexual function from hormone treatments. However, his prostate cancer went into remission. Four years later, his cancer returned. His physician offered a repeat of treatments but warned Paul that this recurrence would be more resistant to treatment and would likely not result in a full remission as it had before.

What would be your decision in Paul's situation? What would you want if Paul were your father? If Paul were your life partner? How would your answers be influenced if you had full health coverage and no financial worries about treatment? How would your answers be influenced if you were in Paul's situation and treatment would severely diminish life savings for your life partner?

Box 12.4 Elizabeth's Conundrum

Elizabeth, a twenty-six-year-old woman, just received the results of a genetic test that confirmed she inherited a mutated BRCA 1 gene, which greatly increases her chances of developing breast cancer. Her mother died from breast cancer when she was thirty-nine; her thirty-two-year-old sister was recently diagnosed. Two of four maternal aunts have also had breast cancer; one of them died. Elizabeth has been informed that she could have a double mastectomy followed by breast reconstruction to reduce her chances of developing breast cancer.

What would you do in Elizabeth's situation? What would you want if Elizabeth were your daughter? Your life partner?

Box 12.5   To Work or Not to Work: That Is the Question

Allison was a fifty-two-year-old woman with kidney cancer who had worked at her university for five years. Following a nephrectomy, Allison underwent a series of radiation treatments that left her exhausted. Within six months, she had used all her vacation and sick time. Work colleagues offered her "shared sick time," but she knew this would run out within a couple of months. Allison worked as much as she was physically able to, but she was facing long-term complications associated with her cancer. Financially, her employment provided Allison, her life partner, and their two children with health care benefits that were paying not only for Allison's cancer treatment but for other family costs, which were significant. If Allison stopped working, she could apply for Social Security Disability, but that would take six months to receive. More importantly, she would lose her employer's contribution to her health care benefits. Under COBRA, she could pay for insurance out of her own pocket; however, she and her family could not afford the premiums of over $600 a month. In addition to coping with cancer, Allison and her family were faced with the prospect of losing their home, bankruptcy, and cessation of medical treatments. How did societal factors complicate life for Allison and her family?

absorb the impact of imperfect social organization. Coping failures, therefore, do not necessarily reflect the shortcomings of individuals; in a real sense they may represent the failure of social systems in which the individuals are enmeshed. (p. 21)

Baker, Denniston, Smith, and West (2005) find that, in addition to personal and cancer-related factors, societal factors affect adjustment. For example, people with lower incomes report greater coping and adjustment problems. In the 1980s, when one of the authors worked with people living with cancer who used wheelchairs, an ongoing frustration was the lack of physical access to restaurants, movies, and public buildings that existed in the United States prior to the ADA. In essence, societal inaccessibility isolated them and prevented them from participating in society. The experiences shared in boxes 12.5 and 12.6 illustrate the societal factors that have an impact on quality of life for people surviving cancer and their loved ones.

We acknowledge the life-altering and often life-shortening effects cancer has on people's lives. We recall the times when cancer diagnoses were routinely withheld from people, in order to spare them pain and discomfort.

Box 12.6   Edward's Faith

Edward was a forty-five-year-old man with leukemia that was in remission; however, his oncologist had informed Edward and his wife, Corrina, that the leukemia would most likely return. The couple had engaged in open and honest discussions with their five children, ages five to eighteen years. Edward, who was an unpaid clergy member in his religious congregation, shared that he was at peace with his future, "come what may." His faith offered him comfort, and his family relationships were strong. The family was enjoying the reprieve his remission was providing. However, one religiously based social problem weighed on Edward more than any other. When Edward was first diagnosed, he informed members of his large congregation. Subsequently, he received a blessing of healing, prayer circles were held, and several church members expressed their "knowledge" that Edward would be cured of his cancer. Edward and Corrina stated that their friends were not willing to discuss the seriousness of his condition and situation. One friend even told Edward, "Your lack of faith will kill you." Another told Corrina, "If Ed dies, it will be because you do not put your trust in God." Since the congregation was their primary social support, the couple felt isolated and unsupported. In addition, one of Edward's biggest concerns was that when he died, his wife and children would be held in low esteem because of their lack of faith. They felt nourished by their spiritual beliefs but bereft of religious support.

How did Edward's and Corrina's faith influence their interpretations of their situation? In what ways can friends and acquaintances help or complicate people's experiences with serious conditions?

In some countries and cultures, this practice is still advocated. We believe that, for the most part, full knowledge and participation maximize quality and even quantity of life. People living with cancer have lives to live, and societal responses to them have significant influence on their quality of life. Negative and ableist responses to cancer or to its manifestations, and responses fuelled by stereotypes, can dramatically affect life with cancer. Those who treat cancer as a death sentence may do well to reconsider how they frame cancer. Certainly, cancer can shorten life; however, one could also frame birth as a death sentence if one chose to, albeit a death sentence with a much more protracted time frame. While we advocate full access to health care and interventions, we reject the medical model approach, which defines people with cancer primarily as patients, and embrace a social model that respects their full lives.

AUTOIMMUNE CONDITIONS

Autoimmune conditions have become increasingly recognized in recent decades, in part because advances in scientific knowledge and technology have led to greater knowledge relative to the existence, identification, and causes of these conditions. As autoimmune conditions have a propensity for increasing in severity as we age, the aging of the world's populations has led to greater prevalence and severity of autoimmune conditions.

Autoimmune conditions arise when the body's immune system, which typically fights against infections and disease, begins fighting its own tissues. It is believed that the immune system mistakes the body's cells as foreign and threatening and thus attacks and destroys them because substances on the surface of the cells resemble an antigen to which the body has been exposed. Two types of immune cells are known to be involved. B cells produce proteins called antibodies that seek out specific infectious agents or antigens and attach to and neutralize them. T cells attack and destroy cells infected with foreign antigens. Other immune cells such as macrophages are nonspecific; that is, they attack any object or substance that is identified as foreign to the body.

People with autoimmune disorders (ADs) may experience several psychosocial problems. One of these is the fact that medical understanding of autoimmunity is in its infancy. A consequence is that some people with an AD have been labeled malingerers and neurotic. Sometimes they are diagnosed as having somatic disorders. The medical model emphasis on scientifically identifiable phenomena has resulted in people with an AD being marginalized—not because of their AD but because of others' reactions to their AD. Concomitant to the negative perceptions of the medical model, they have been considered morally deficient as well. Consider the case of Laura, who had fibromyalgia, a condition thought to have autoimmune origins. In 1987 Laura, a thirty-five-year-old mother of four children, was experiencing fatigue, muscle and general body aches, and headaches and often felt spacey. When multiple medical tests came back negative, her physician informed Laura's husband that she had hypochondriasis and was somaticizing her problems and recommended psychotherapy and rest from her home responsibilities. It was not until the early 1990s that medical understanding had progressed to the point that fibromyalgia was legitimized as a condition. Unfortunately, the medical model approach resulted in her doctor blaming and labeling Laura rather than acknowledging that medicine may lack the sophistication to identify a legitimate physical problem. In contrast, Laura's daughter, who was diagnosed with fibromyalgia in 2000, was treated with respect, and the symptoms she was experiencing were validated.

Other ADs that have more obvious manifestations, such as type 1 diabetes, are viewed as more legitimate. An advantage of advancements in health care has been that people with ADs have access to treatments and interventions that can improve the quality of life and extend life expectancy. Thus, while the medical model has had very negative impacts on people with ADs in terms of marginalization and making them dependent on others, treatments are having a positive effect. We discuss some of the more common putative ADs below.

Juvenile Rheumatoid Arthritis

Juvenile rheumatoid arthritis (JRA) occurs in youths age sixteen years and younger and can occur as early as six months of age. An estimated 50,000 children in the United States have JRA. Worldwide estimates of JRA vary widely in different countries, with as many as 4 to 1,000 in some urban areas with good community health programs (Arthritis Foundation, 2005; Manners & Bower, 2002). Common manifestations of JRA include joint inflammation, swelling, and pain; limited range of motion; contractures; and sometimes shortened stature. There are three types of JRA. About half of JRA cases involve *pauciarticular JRA*. It affects four or fewer joints, usually the larger joints like the wrists, knees, and ankles, and can also cause inflammation of the eyes. It is most common in girls, with an onset before eight years of age. About 30 percent of people with JRA have *polyarticular JRA*, affecting five or more joints. Smaller joints like those in the hand as well as the larger joints can be affected. It too is more common in girls than boys. Approximately 20 percent of JRA cases involve *systemic JRA,* which affects both the joints and internal organs and affects boys and girls in equal numbers. Chronic fevers and rashes are common cues that aid in initial diagnosis. Internal organs such as the spleen can also become inflamed (Arthritis Foundation, 2005; Kids Health, 2005; Lab Tests Online, 2006). As with other disabilities with onset in childhood, the psychosocial impacts of JRA are as important as the physical changes. Family supports are critical, as are role models, economic resources, and access to adequate technology. Affected youths face changes and loss of physical function that require adjustments. The scope and strength of supports, in combination with personal coping strategies, go far in determining quality of life. Access to educational, recreational, job preparation, and other resources helps youths with JRA lead productive, self-determined lives. Overprotectiveness and lack of opportunity can limit people far more than the physical manifestations of JRA.

Type 1 Diabetes

Type 1 diabetes, commonly known as juvenile onset diabetes, occurs when the insulin-producing cells in the pancreas stop producing insulin, the hormone that allows glucose to enter and fuel the body's cells. According to the Juvenile Diabetes Research Foundation International (2007), type 1 diabetes occurs when the immune system destroys the pancreas's beta cells, which create insulin. Thus, to survive, a person must regularly monitor his or her blood sugar, and insulin must be administered artificially through multiple daily injections. Today, those with the technology and resources inject insulin through insulin pumps that are worn and have a line that runs directly into the abdomen. Type 1 diabetes occurs primarily in children, youths, and sometimes young adults. The International Diabetes Federation (2007) estimates that the prevalence of type 1 diabetes for people age fourteen years and younger worldwide is approximately 2 in 10,000, meaning that about 430,000 experience type 1 diabetes. It estimates that the number of individuals diagnosed with type 1 diabetes is growing at an annual rate of 3 percent.

Monitoring type 1 diabetes forces young people into lifestyle changes at a time that is usually much more carefree for them. Feelings of guilt and responsibility can trouble families. Feelings that arise in response to adjustment to diagnosis can range from relief that symptoms such as chronic thirst and malaise have a cause to feelings of being overwhelmed. A challenge for youths with diabetes is maintaining regular control of blood sugar levels. Serious glucose-insulin imbalance can cause immediate and, in rare instances, potentially fatal crises. However, the long-term effects of diabetes are much more insidious. Even the best-maintained glucose-monitoring program cannot match a fully functioning body system in maintaining glucose-insulin balance. Thus, over years and decades, diabetics become susceptible to nerve and other tissue damage that can eventually lead to problems such as visual problems; weakness, sensory loss, and insufficient blood supply to the extremities, which can result in sores, injury, and even amputation; and kidney damage. Children are still developing the cognitive and emotional abilities that allow them to maintain the diligence that minimizes long-term health damage. Supportive environments, including social, economic, and technological resources, are critical to successfully managing diabetes.

Fortunately, youths with diabetes have role models: famous persons who have lead full and productive lives. Just as importantly, their parents and adult caregivers can also see these people, who lead otherwise typical lives. For decades, the actress Mary Tyler Moore, who contracted type 1 diabetes in the late 1960s, has advocated for diabetics, even serving as chair of the Juvenile Diabetes Research Foundation International (2003). An actress familiar to younger audiences is Halle Berry, an Oscar-winning actress whose sudden and unexpected onset of diabetes left her in a diabetic coma in 1989. Athletes with diabetes include Billy Jean King, one of the most celebrated tennis players in history. Adam Byle, a distance runner, ran 6,521 kilometers across North America in his quest to raise money for diabetes research. Adam Morrison, an NBA player, has been shown on national TV managing his blood glucose levels in the middle of basketball games. World leaders with diabetes include Anwar Sadat of Egypt and Yuri Andropov of the former Soviet Union. Others with diabetes include several Nobel Prize winners, musicians, politicians, artists, and people from all walks of life (dLife, 2007).

Clearly, diabetes can produce a number of life complications and health problems. Just as obviously, people with diabetes live productive, happy, and successful lives. Technological advances in the twentieth century made this possible, the most important being the development of insulin injections in 1922 (dLife, 2006). These advances demonstrate the importance and value of technology in improving the lives of people with diabetes and other disabilities. It is important to remember, however, the dangers of using the medical model to define the lives of diabetics. While diabetics may advocate improved technology and even cures, they are not defined as patients. Diabetics are the authorities on their own bodies and lives, just like non-diabetics. Diabetes leads to unique life experiences that shape people's lives. Thus, the quality of life is greatly determined by the social contexts in which diabetics live.

It is important to note here that our focus has been on type 1 diabetes, which less than 10 percent of the total number of people with diabetes have. Unlike type 1, in which the immune system destroys insulin-producing cells, in type 2 diabetes, the body continues to produce insulin, but, for a variety of reasons, in insufficient quantities. Type 2 diabetics frequently manage their condition through weight control, diet, and/or oral medications. It is much more likely to occur in middle age. Though less severe and of shorter duration, type 2 diabetes can also produce problems similar to type 1.

Multiple Sclerosis

Multiple sclerosis (MS) is an autoimmune condition in which the body's immune system attacks the cells that support and nourish the nervous system. Myelin sheaths that support and insulate neurons in the brain, spinal cord, and peripheral nervous system, and that facilitate electrical impulse conduction, are damaged. As a result, multiple symptoms occur, including sensory and motor loss, vision problems, and cognitive changes.

MS is found all over the world, and its causes are multifactorial. Two primary indicators are race and place of residence. It is much more common in higher latitudes in both the northern and southern hemispheres, with lower prevalence in warmer climates near the equator. MS is two to three times as prevalent in women as in men. The prevalence is much higher in whites than in Asians, Native Americans, Siberians, and Africans. In a meta-analysis of multiple prevalence studies, Rosati (2001) found the highest reported rates of MS in the United Kingdom and especially Scotland, with estimated rates as high as 193 per 100,000. MS rates in Scandinavian countries are also relatively high, with some areas reporting rates as high as 132 per 100,000. However, in some areas of Finland and northern Norway, the prevalence is much lower, with rates in the range of 20–50 per 100,000. Rates in North America are also high, in some areas well above 100 per 100,000; however, below the thirty-seventh parallel the rates are significantly lower. Countries near the equator have relatively low rates. For example, rates in North Africa and Central America are less than 10 per 100,000. In addition to latitude, race is also an important factor in MS risk. For example, it is rare in blacks of African descent and among Japanese, with rates of less than 5 per 100,000. Rates in Siberia, one of the harshest climates in the world, range from 18 to 41 per 100,000. MS is found mostly in people of Russian descent yet is rare in native Siberians.

The onset of MS is usually in young and middle adulthood. There are no definitive diagnostic tests for MS, and diagnosis is made through a combination of physical examination and history and tests. One test, magnetic resonance imaging, sometimes graphically shows white lesions where the central nervous system has been demyelinated. However, it may also show nothing. Often, diagnosis is made in a process of excluding other conditions. Visual problems are frequently one of the first symptoms experienced at onset. Other early indicators include numbness or dizziness, fatigue, problems walking, and pain. Other symptoms include bowel and bladder dysfunction, spasticity, sexual dysfunction, balance and gait problems, and weakness or paralysis, as well as sensory loss in the extremities.

One of the most consistent aspects of MS is its unpredictability. The course of MS can range from minor symptoms followed by remission to fulminating MS, which can precipitate sudden quadriplegia and loss of bowel and bladder control with no remission of symptoms. One typical course is relapsing-remitting MS, in which symptoms are exacerbated for several days to weeks, followed by a lessening of symptoms for extended periods of time. With relapsing-remitting MS, however, there is a gradual decline in functioning as each relapse-remission cycle ends. Another common manifestation is chronic progressive MS, in which an individual experiences gradual loss of function over years and decades. The effects of MS vary dramatically from person to person and also fluctuate significantly over time in the same individual.

Because of its unpredictability and seriousness of symptoms, MS can be very complicated to deal with on emotional and social levels. Prior to learning one has MS, frustrations with not knowing what is happening can be as difficult as the symptoms themselves. In the authors' experiences, sometimes finding out one has MS can actually be a relief because it legitimates one's experiences and allows for the opportunity to deal with a tangible condition. Pollin and Golant (1994) discuss eight fears associated with chronic health-related problems that apply to MS.

1. Loss of control. The progressive nature of MS can lead to gradual loss of strength and physical capabilities. In addition, the unpredictability leaves people wondering what is "around the corner" for them. For example, a friend of one of the authors who had MS planned a romantic week with his spouse in Hawaii, yet his biggest fear was

that his MS could be exacerbated at any time and require him to cancel the vacation.

2. Changed self-image. One's personal sense of self changes with the physical and cognitive changes that arise from MS. As we age and our bodies change, all of us go through changes in self-image; however, MS can dramatically accelerate those changes in unpredictable ways. Life activities such as work and recreation can be changed or lost, and new avenues to find self-worth may need to be found.

3. Dependency. We all depend on others in our lives; however, dependence on others for atypical physical assistance, financial aid, and emotional support that are attendant to MS can be distressing.

4. Stigma. When the manifestations of MS are invisible, such as fatigue or memory problems, people with MS are commonly viewed as malingering or as having hypochondria. Visible symptoms such as ataxia, speech impairments, and mobility impairments can lead to stigmas such as those associated with mobility disabilities, intellectual disabilities, and other disabilities.

5. Abandonment. As physical symptoms increase, the fear of losing loved ones, friends, and social supports increases. In countries in which health care is commonly provided institutionally, people may be especially afraid of being abandoned in places such as nursing facilities.

6. Expressing anger. This fear can be precipitated by the concern that, by expressing anger, individuals may alienate those they are close to and lose their love and support, possibly even being abandoned. They may also fear that becoming angry may be seen as ingratitude.

7. Isolation. Related to several of the fears above, MS can put people lower on the social hierarchy, producing dependence and reducing control over one's social circles and emotional supports. In addition, problems such as job loss and loss of leisure activities can constrict meaningful contacts and relationships.

8. Death. This fear can be precipitated by internal conditions, the problems attendant to the progressive nature of MS. In addition, external factors such as inadequate health care and a lack of resources can put lives at risk. In societies in which ableism and a diminished sense of social value come with disability, people with MS and other disabilities may find their lives are considered expendable.

We believe it is critical for readers to critically assess the internal and external forces that drive the fears attendant to MS, as well as other chronic health problems. We do not minimize the internal changes and losses associated with MS, including the uncertainty caused by its unpredictability. However, many of the fears and concerns are externally derived. Fears of dependency and isolation can be greatly ameliorated by social policies that value rather than marginalize disabled persons. As Mackelprang and Mackelprang (2005) observe, court decisions concerning the end of life in the United States have disregarded the deplorable social and living conditions forced on people with severe physical disabilities. Instead, they have attributed the desire to die exclusively to internal conditions. Humane social policies can significantly ameliorate many of the fears persons with MS face.

Other Selected Autoimmune Conditions

Our discussions of JRA, diabetes, and MS provide examples of the effects autoimmune conditions can have on persons' lives. In this section, we briefly discuss the manifestations of several other conditions. We primarily explain the internal consequences of each, with an understanding that some of the implications of other conditions can be generalized to those listed below. For more extensive discussions of these conditions, readers can refer to Medline Plus, which was created and is maintained by the U.S. National Library of Medicine and National Institutes of Health.

Systemic Lupus Erythematosus

Systemic lupus erythematosus affects nine times as many women as men. Symptoms of systemic lupus erythematosus can be intermittent and vary widely from person to person. Most common are joint pain and arthritis, especially in the joints of the fingers, hands, wrists, and knees. Rashes, headaches, fever, and pericarditis are also common and can be treated with anti-inflammatories and steroid creams. In severe cases, damage to internal organs such as the kidneys, heart, and lungs can occur (Medline Plus, 2006).

Sjogren's Syndrome

Sjogren's is linked to rheumatic conditions and usually occurs in people older than forty years. Ninety percent of those affected are women. The immune system attacks moisture-producing glands such as those that make tears and saliva; thus dry eyes and dry mouth are the most common symptoms. In more severe cases it can also affect the joints, lungs, kidneys, blood vessels, digestive organs, and nerves (Medline Plus, 2008e).

Addison's Syndrome

In Addison's, the immune system attacks cells in the kidneys that produce two hormones, cortisol and aldosterone, both of which are critical to life. Manifestations include weight loss, muscle weakness, fatigue, low blood pressure, and dark patches of skin. It is treated with hormone replacement, without which Addison's can be fatal (Medline Plus, 2008a).

Scleroderma

Scleroderma ("hard skin") is a group of conditions that cause abnormal growth of connective tissue. Localized scleroderma affects only the skin, while systemic scleroderma also affects blood vessels and internal organs as it attacks the connective tissue that support them. Treatments for scleroderma are generally symptomatic (Medline Plus, 2008d).

Thyroid Problems

Two thyroid problems are common. Hashimoto's occurs when the immune system creates an inflammation of the thyroid gland, which frequently results in diminished thyroid function, called hypothyroidism. Its onset is often gradual, progressing over months and years. It is most common in women, with an onset usually in middle age. Grave's is an autoimmune thyroid condition that produces hyperthyroidism. Symptoms may include weight loss, rapid pulse, protruding eyes, feeling too warm, restlessness, insomnia, diarrhea, and irritability (Medline Plus, 2008f).

Psoriasis

Psoriasis is a skin disease that causes itchy or sore patches of thick, red skin with silvery scales, most commonly on the elbows, knees, scalp, back, face, palms and feet. The immune system attacks developing skin cells, causing rapid cell turnover so that immature skin cells rise prematurely to the skin's surface. It varies in severity and is generally treated with skin treatments and light therapy. In serious cases, it can cause widespread skin involvement and progress to the joints, causing psoriatic arthritis (Medline Plus, 2008c).

Crohn's

Crohn's is an AD caused by inflammation of the digestive system. It most commonly affects the lower part of the small intestine but can affect any area from the mouth to the anus. It occurs most often in young adults and can cause abdominal pain, diarrhea, rectal bleeding, weight loss, joint pain, skin problems, and fever. In severe situations, intestinal blockage and malnutrition can occur (Medline Plus, 2008b).

Pediatric Autoimmune Neuropsychiatric Disorders Associated with Streptococci

PANDAS is a relatively newly identified condition that causes children to develop obsessive compulsive disorders and associate tics. Researchers hypothesize that PANDAS is associated with strep infection, after which the body's antibodies mistakenly attack an enzyme in the brain and disrupt communication between neurons (National Institute of Mental Health, 2006).

In summary, autoimmune conditions carry multiple physical, emotional, and social implications. Adequate health care can be crucial in ameliorating problems and improving the quality of life for people with ADs. In addition, social and health policies that promote the full participation of people with ADs in society are critical. For example, work disincentives that discourage employment can be removed. Consider Mark, a twenty-five-year-old college graduate with juvenile onset rheumatoid arthritis. Mark was forced to reject a $30,000/year job because it lacked comprehensive health insurance, which he needed to pay for his ongoing health care needs. If he stayed on Medicaid, SSI, and other government programs, he could continue to live on his own. If he accepted the job offer, he would lose his Medicaid and place his health at great risk because his expenses would consume his salary very rapidly. Consider the example of a family affected by MS in box 12.7, paying particular attention to the internal and external factors affecting their lives.

CARDIOVASCULAR CONDITIONS

The World Health Organization (2007a) describes cardiovascular disease as "disorders of the heart and blood vessels, and comprise coronary heart disease including heart attacks, cerebrovascular disease including strokes, raised blood pressure (hypertension), peripheral artery disease, rheumatic heart disease, congenital heart disease and heart failure." The World Health Organization further explains that tobacco use, physical inactivity, and poor diet are the primary causes of cardiovascular disease, which is the number one cause of death globally. In 2005, an estimated 17.5 million deaths globally, or about 30 percent of all deaths, were caused by cardiovascular disease. Strokes accounted for 5.7 million deaths, and heart attacks accounted for another 7.6 million deaths. Eighty percent of cardiovascular deaths occur in low- and middle-income countries.

While organizations such as the World Health Organization and national health organizations focus on cardiovascular deaths, in this chapter we focus on *living* with cardiovascular conditions (CVCs). The most common cardiovascular conditions are described below:

- Coronary heart disease. Disease of the blood vessels supplying the heart muscle
- Cerebrovascular disease. Disease of the blood vessels supplying the brain
- Peripheral arterial disease. Disease of blood vessels supplying the arms and legs
- Rheumatic heart disease. Damage to the heart muscle and heart valves from rheumatic fever, caused by streptococcal bacteria

Box 12.7 Sheila and Joaquin: Tough Dilemmas

Sheila and Joaquin, the parents of two preteens, were faced with serious problems when Sheila's MS progressed to the point that she required a wheelchair for mobility and she needed help dressing and with personal hygiene. She was forced to leave her job as a marketing manager because she could not spend the required forty hours per week in the office. Joaquin was overwhelmed with physical care requirements for Sheila and for their children, as well as his own job. His insurance was essential for her health care needs, as it allowed her to stay in the home, but it provided no help with personal care. Joaquin's income of $40,000 a year disqualified them for any public assistance programs. Joaquin and Sheila talked about how easy it would be to place Sheila in an extended care nursing facility, where she could qualify for Medicaid, which would pay for her institutionalized care.

Consider the following external factors that complicated the internal problems attendant to Sheila's MS.

- With the use of technology, Sheila could still work—if she did so from home and/or for less than forty hours per week. However, this was not acceptable to her employer.
- Sheila did not have sufficient work history to qualify for employment-related Social Security benefits. Her husband's income and family resources were too great for her to qualify for Supplemental Security Income, a program available to disabled poor people.
- The cost of personal care in the home made it inaccessible to Sheila; however, if she were institutionalized, her physical care needs would be met.

To what extent are this family's problems related to the physical effects of Sheila's MS? How do external factors influence their quality of life? What social policies could eliminate problems the family faces?

- Congenital heart disease. Malformations of heart structure existing at birth
- Deep vein thrombosis and pulmonary embolism. Blood clots in the leg veins, which can dislodge and move to the heart and lungs (World Health Organization, 2007b)

CVCs are related to other health conditions. For example, people with diabetes and obesity are at increased risk. Health-related behaviors such as smoking and poor diet increase risk. In addition, other personal and social variables such as chronic stress, personality styles, and high anxiety levels can lead to and arise from CVCs (Daly, Davidson, Chang, Hancock, Rees, & Thompson, 2002; Krantz, 1998).

The eight fears related to chronic health conditions outlined by Pollin and Golant (1994) also pertain to CVCs. Fear of the loss of control arises from internal factors that arise from physical changes such as decreased stamina, fatigue, and onset of new symptoms, while external factors such as high health care costs, financial burden, and lack of access to resources can pose an additional burden. Losses associated with work, leisure, and recreational changes can lead to a changed self-image. Sexual activities may need to be altered, and individuals with CVCs may feel that their sexual self-worth has been assaulted. Physical dependence in activities of daily living may be required as CVCs progress. In some situations, due to advanced conditions and lack of external resources, individuals may be forced into institutional care. Individuals are often blamed for bringing conditions upon themselves, for example, through smoking. Sometimes, when health conditions are invisible to casual observers, people may be viewed as malingerers or hypochondriacs. In societies where independence and physical vitality are emphasized, people can be devalued because they are considered frail and incapable. Because the proportion of people who acquire CVCs is positively associated with age, people with severe CVCs tend to be older, and spouses and life partners are more likely to have their own physical problems or even die. A significant concern for these folks is the fear that their partners will die, leaving them incapable of managing on their own. In countries like the United States, this may lead to institutionalization in long-term care institutions, which some consider a death knell. The fear of expressing anger is especially relevant for those who require significant assistance from others. Some question whether expressions of anger will lead others to reject them or exact revenge, especially when they rely on these people or agencies for support. Societal attitudes and policies that reflect ableism and ageism can lead to societal separation and seclusion. Similarly, increased risks of losing life partners and other long-term supports and friends can lead to isolation. This is particularly problematic when health problems make it difficult to initiate and maintain new relationships. Finally, as the World Health Organization reports show, CVCs are a leading cause of death. While all of us die eventually, CVCs remind people of their mortality on an ongoing basis and lead to millions of early deaths annually.

Counseling interventions and support for people with chronic CVCs can reduce depression and anxiety and improve home functioning (McLaughlin, Aupont, Bambauer, Stone, Mullan, Colagiovanni, et al., 2005). These interventions may be especially important during the initial phase when people first realize they have a CVC, often through medical diagnosis. Crisis intervention may be needed as well as education about resources. As people adjust to the long-term reality of living with a CVC, sometimes called the chronic phase, ongoing assistance with personal, interpersonal, and social adjustments may be called for. Some individuals experience a gradual diminution of function that eventually leads to death. As they enter what is commonly known as the terminal phase, individual and family interventions may make this transition a valued and meaningful time of life (Pollin & Golant, 1994; Rolland, 1988; Sidell, 1997).

The U.S. Agency for Health Care Research (2007), which is deeply involved in research on people with long-term health problems, has developed five basic coping steps that are applicable to people with CVCs.

1. Take the time you need. Take time to understand and cope with your condition.
2. Get the support you need. Supports come from sources such as loved ones, health care providers, communities, and social institutions.
3. Talk with your doctor. Seek information from health care providers and assert control by letting providers know wishes, desires, and treatments.
4. Seek out information. Information comes not only from health care providers but from multiple other sources. Mentors and other supports can help navigate decisions and chart courses of action. In addition, resources such as the Internet, when navigated with caution, can provide a treasure trove of information.
5. Decide on a treatment plan. Asserting control over the directions and courses of interventions helps individuals maintain command over their lives. Health providers and other professionals do not always know what is best, and there is no need to abrogate one's life control because of a CVC.

Boxes 12.8 and 12.9 tell the stories of people affected by CVCs. As you read these stories, consider how societal beliefs and policies and the assumptions and attitudes of professionals have an impact on the lives of people with CVCs.

SUMMARY

Chronic health conditions are a common cause of disabilities throughout the world and will continue to be so for decades to come. In this chapter, we are not concerned with medical diagnoses, but with their functional sequelae. We fully recognize the importance of health care technology, providers, and treatments in prolonging lives and improving quality of life for individuals with health-related disabilities. Concomitantly, however, we reject the medical model approach to managing life with a health-related disability. We advocate a social model approach, in which people with chronic health conditions have control over their lives and treatment decisions. Social and health providers can play important roles in helping people

---

Box 12.8   Gus and Snow on the Roof

Gus was an eighty-one-year-old male with whom one of the authors worked after he experienced a stroke. Gus had a several-decade history of diabetes that had led to the amputation of a foot and visual loss as a result of retinopathy. He also had coronary artery disease requiring medication for stabilization. As his hospital social worker, the author had counseled Gus and Esther, his seventy-nine-year-old wife, on several issues. Shortly before discharge from the hospital, Gus seemed uncharacteristically stressed, which precipitated a meeting with the couple. In session, Gus, with embarrassment, reluctantly revealed that he was distressed about his sex life. First, would sex precipitate another stroke or other health problems? Second, would Esther still find him desirable? The author was thrilled the next week when Gus responded to his inquiry about how things were going at home with a wink and a big grin. This experience revealed the author's assumption that, because of their age and physical limitations, sex would not be a concern for Gus and Esther. Gus later informed the author that "Just because there is snow on the roof, doesn't mean there isn't fire in the furnace." Subsequent to this experience, the author routinely addressed sexuality with others who were hospitalized for stroke.

---

manage their lives. However, the locus of control remains with individuals. Significant problems associated with health-related disabilities arise from social and societal reactions, not just the health conditions themselves. Consider HIV/AIDS as an example. HIV and AIDS are dramatically more lethal in Africa than in the United States and Europe, where health interventions have increased life expectancies and reduced mother-to-baby HIV transmission. On the other hand, even within the United States there are significant disparities. For example, two neighboring communities in New York, Chelsea and Harlem, have similar seroprevalence rates, but Harlem has a much higher mortality rate, in large measure due to differential access to society's resources (Ciezadlo, 2003).

The medical model approaches chronic health conditions by seeking to ameliorate symptoms and help people cope with psychosocial adjustment problems. Traditional Western medicine separates the mind from the body, dividing sickness into two categories: *disease,* which is concerned with physical dysfunction and treatment, and *illness,* which includes the entire human experience with sickness, including beliefs and culture (Brown, Barrett, & Padilla, 1998). The medical model's disease-oriented approach relies on technology, with less attention to the personal and sociocultural implications of health conditions (Mackelprang & Mackelprang, 2005). The more holistic

Box 12.9   Where to Live? What to Do?

Sharon was sixty-three years old and had emphysema and coronary artery disease and had had multiple heart attacks. She had a forty-year history of smoking one to two packs of cigarettes a day and still smoked about five to ten cigarettes a day. Her husband, Mike, brought her for medical and psychological evaluations because she had been experiencing memory problems and confusion. Tests revealed that she was experiencing signs of moderate dementia due to cerebral oxygen insufficiency and possibly multiple transient ischemic attacks, sometimes known as "mini-strokes." Mike and Sharon had a strong personal relationship, and there was no question that Mike was willing to provide Sharon the minimal supervision and support she required for safety as well as help her with activities of daily living. However, Mike was caught in a dilemma relative to taking care of Sharon. He could not quit his job; financially, he needed to work, yet Sharon could not be left alone for eight or nine hours at a time. They also could not afford to have someone stay with Sharon. Mike's job did not provide medical benefits, Mike made too much for Sharon to qualify for medical assistance, and Sharon was too young for Medicare. Mike was informed that if he admitted his wife of forty-five years to an extended care facility, she could receive Medicaid, which would pay for her care. She would financially qualify because his income would not count against her. Another option was for Mike to divorce Sharon, after which they could continue to live together, an option that repulsed him. On Sharon's part, she was still a delightful person, functioned well with minimal supervision, and was terrified at being institutionalized.

What were the sources of Mike and Sharon's problems? To what extent were their problems a result of Sharon's health problems? To what extent did social policies and community structures contribute to their problems?

approach espoused by the social model addresses chronic health conditions as a part of people's lives. Certainly, they complicate and can affect quality of life. The medical model focuses on internal conditions to explain adjustment problems; the social model attends to social and societal implications and personal life skills. Consider, for example, the case of Warren, whose diabetes led to diabetic retinopathy and progressive visual loss. Warren's physician and social worker were certain he would react primarily with grief and feelings of loss. However, Warren, a deeply spiritual man, sought help from an elder and spiritual advisor from his Native American tribe. Warren was challenged to find life meaning from his vision loss. He viewed his experiences as a journey of discovery. We would not suggest that chronic health problems do not cause problems for those affected. We do, however, suggest that these conditions can lead people on a life path that can offer many positives.

PERSONAL NARRATIVE: DANNY TEACHMANN

Danny Teachmann lived with a disability as a teen then became temporarily able-bodied before acquiring a permanent disability as an adult. He is a disability activist and currently works for the Center for Disability Studies and Universal Access at Eastern Washington University.

I became disabled long before I was ready to admit it. I admitted to becoming disabled at around forty-two years of age, but things started happening at about age thirty-five. According to the medical model, I have multiple sclerosis and spinal stenosis, and these diagnoses have taken control of my life and dictate what I can and cannot do. I see it differently. While I live with these conditions, in fact it is society's barriers that create my limitations. As I have become more active and vocal about society's treatment of disability, I would say some would see my disability as acute Defective Disruptive Societal Disorder.

My first disability experience occurred when I was about fifteen years old and was most likely my first episode of MS. I woke up one morning and was unable to get out of bed. I felt like a wet washrag and was as weak as a kitten. After several trips to the doctors, they decided I had injured my lower back in a football game and that my weakness would only last a short while. However, that short while lasted eleven months. I spent that entire time in a wheelchair and it significantly impacted on my life as an adolescent.

After about two months in the wheelchair, I began thinking I would never get better, started to think my life would not be what I had dreamed, and began to become depressed. My family started to change in how they interacted with me. No one wanted to confront me on any issue or any behavior, and I started to realize I could get away with anything. For example, I remember the time I decided to get some revenge on my brother, who had taken a new tire for my bike. I went out to the garage and took the tube out of the tire and filled his bike tire with sand. Of course, no one thought it was me: I was that poor child in the wheelchair who could not even get out of the house without help from his family. To this day, I look back on that one and have a good laugh. No one saw my abilities; they focused on what they perceived as my inabilities.

My friends also treated me differently. In fact, they stopped coming over to see me or even trying to include me in their activities. Many of my friends even told me that their parents did not want them around me because they were scared, afraid that I had something contagious. I had even heard it said that being associated with me would lead people to be shunned by the normal members of society. This isolation from my friends, school, and normal activities led me to feel I had no worth. I started to question what was in store for me in life when my friends did not want to have anything to do with me and my family wanted to isolate me.

I became increasingly isolated. My friends abandoned me and my family stopped taking me on outings with them. I even remember overhearing my brothers argue about who would be forced to stay home with me for a weekend family excursion. I always wondered why they did not take me with them. I guess they saw my condition as a shame to the family.

The one bright spot of my teen disability experience was when I was placed into the special education class with all the other kids who used wheelchairs or had others forms of disabilities. I made some good friends there. These were not fair-weather friends, and we remained linked even after I had gotten out of the chair and became temporarily able-bodied again. I have never forgotten these friendships.

My time in the special education class had another effect on me. I lost interest in school and dropped out after ninth grade; yes, I am a ninth-grade dropout. Because I needed a wheelchair, the school thought I needed special education, my family isolated me, and my friends had nothing to do with me. It is no wonder I became depressed and lost interest in school. The one bright spot was my disabled friends. At least we had each other.

Once my legs were under me once again, I was looking forward to getting back to my old friends and "normal" schedule of classes. However, my old friends and the school system did not share my desire. My friends still treated me like an outcast; they wanted nothing to do with me. They had cast me into the classification of "handicapped." I was damaged goods and in their eyes would never be normal again. As a reinforcement of this perception of me, the school system would not remove me from special education class. They told me that once I was classified as disabled for more than six months, it became a permanent status for me.

So I left school and began my life as an independent adult—as independent as one can be at sixteen. At seventeen I joined the Navy and ended up on SWIFT boats in Vietnam. After my time in Vietnam, I was filled with a feeling of hate and felt I needed to travel the world and see something other than war and its destruction. So I took two years and began my worldly travels. In these travels I discovered that all the people of the world have two things in common: they want to be loved and they want to love.

My travels finally ended after two years in Boston, though it did not end in the normal sense, for it was a not an ending but a beginning. I had landed in a Greek Orthodox monastery in Boston. For the next five years I was known as Brother George. After five years I found my peace with the world and myself and moved on to experience life in the secular world.

I returned to the Seattle area and met the woman of my dreams; we were married and had three daughters. I had what I thought was a life career as a barber. However, after fifteen years of remission, my MS caught up with me once again and I finally ended up in a wheelchair for life. I had to accept the fact that I was disabled and contend with what it meant to me as a person in a nondisabled society.

I was unable to work as a barber anymore, and all my medical providers were telling me to apply for Social Security Disability, lean back, and enjoy the ride. It was not what I wanted out of life, but it seemed as if I had no choice. So I qualified for SSDI, my wife went back to work, and I tried to take on the role of mom for our girls but it was not easy. My world had been turned upside down. I was having trouble dealing with what has happening to me and I just did not seem to have the wherewithal to be the father I wanted to be for my girls.

A critical time for my wife and me came when we realized our girls did not see themselves as having any need to go to college, the one dream my wife and I had always held for them, even through all our troubles in dealing with my disability. I decided something needed to change.

Knowing that our girls would get more from actions than words, I went to the local community college to see if I could enroll in classes. Remember, I am a ninth-grade dropout. To my surprise, they let me in. Nevertheless, I did not have much confidence in my ability to succeed. About the middle of my first quarter I started speaking with my philosophy professor, who told me he thought I had good writing and critical thinking skills. I thanked him, but I was skeptical about my abilities. However, he took me under his wing and always gave me encouragement at a time I needed that little extra nudge. In fact, it was he who told me not to bother getting the transfer degree and advised me to apply directly to the university. Because of his confidence in me, a disabled ninth-grade dropout, I applied and was accepted.

During my two-and-half years as an undergraduate at Western Washington University, I had the best mentor a person could ask for, my brother. He was the chair of the sociology department and was a big help to my confidence. It was easy for me to determine my undergraduate degree—yes, it is sociology. When I was nearly finished with my BA, I realized that as a person with a disability who had several years with no real work history, I would not have an easy time finding a job. Not only did I need a job, but if I was to work, I needed a job that would allow me to survive while getting off Social Security and Medicare. Therefore, I, the ninth-grade dropout, decided to go on and get a master's degree.

I applied to and was accepted into an MSW program at Eastern Washington University, on the other side of the state. I packed my bags and off I went to see if I was up to the challenge of graduate school. I do not know if I realized it at the time, but I was still trying to convince myself I was capable. I had fallen into the trap of society, one that saw me as less than and not equal. In all my actions, I kept comparing myself to nondisabled persons and questioning whether I measured up. Well, that was about to change, for in the spring of my first year of my masters, I had an instructor who had a fire in his belly about how the disabled are treated in our society; we will call him Professor M. I began to see that it is not *my* inabilities that limit me, but the unwillingness or inability of society to grant me the access I need to participate fully—an access that would give all members of society equal opportunity. He did not realize it, but Professor M became a mentor and hero. He helped me realize I am capable of success and that I have abilities far beyond anything I had ever imagined.

I am embarking on a new career. I am capable and competent. I know my work will be in the area of disability—work aimed at making society accessible for all. I find joy in my work. I appreciate those who have had confidence and who have mentored me. I have become a mentor and role model to others. I am also pleased that two of my three daughters are following their father's example by attending college. There is but one question left: will society give me the opportunity to work and be a contributing member of society? I now know I am capable, but is society capable of accepting a strong, independent, and capable person of disability?

DISCUSSION QUESTIONS

1. What societal factors have led to the changes in the incidence and prevalence of health-related disabilities in the last century?
2. How have polio and survivors of polio influenced the development of the disability rights movement?
3. How have attitudes about homosexuality influenced societal responses to HIV/AIDS and the treatment of persons living with HIV/AIDS?
4. What are the impediments worldwide to prevention and the treatment of people with chronic infectious conditions?
5. Compare and contrast the medical and moral model approaches to chronic illness and health-related conditions.
6. Compare and contrast common attitudes about people who develop cancer related to behaviors such as smoking and lung cancer versus people who develop cancer that is unrelated to any identifiable behavior.
7. What internal and external forces can be used to maximize the quality of life for people with cardiovascular conditions?
8. What are the social justice issues in worldwide responses to infectious and other chronic health conditions?

SUGGESTED READINGS

Brown P. J. (Ed.). (1998). *Understanding and applying medical anthropology.* Mountain View, CA: Mayfield.

Davis, L. (Ed.). (2006). *The disability studies reader* (2nd ed.). New York: Routledge.

Mackelprang, R. W., & Mackelprang, R. D. (2005). Historical and contemporary issues in end-of-life decisions: Implications for social work. *Social Work, 50*(4), 315–324.

Medline Plus. (n.d.). Retrieved November 17, 2008, from http://www.nlm.nih.gov/medlineplus

Nagler, M. (Ed.). (1993). *Perspectives on disability.* Palo Alto, CA: Health Markets Research.

National Cancer Institute. (n.d.). Retrieved November 17, 2008, from http://www.nci.nih.gov

National Institute of Mental Health. (n.d.). Retrieved November 17, 2008, from http://www.nimh.nih

Shilts, R. (1987). *And the band played on: Politics, people, and the AIDS epidemic.* New York: St. Martin's Press.

Stephen Lewis Foundation. (n.d.). Retrieved November 17, 2008, from http://www.stephenlewisfoundation.org

World Health Organization. (2001). *International classification of functioning, disability and health.* Geneva, Switzerland: Author.

World Health Organization. (n.d.). Retrieved November 17, 2008, from http://www.who.int/en

Zola, I. K. (1982). *Missing pieces: A chronicle of living with a disability.* Philadelphia: Temple University Press.

REFERENCES

Ahmad, M. M., Musil, C. M., Zauszniewski, J. A., & Resnick, M. I. (2005). Prostate cancer: Appraisal, coping, and health status. *Journal of Gerontological Nursing, 31*(10), 34–43.

Americans with Disabilities Act of 1990. Pub. L. No. 101–336 (1990).

Arthritis Foundation. (2005). *Juvenile arthritis fact sheet.* Retrieved October 14, 2007, from http://ww2.arthritis.org/conditions/fact_sheets/ja_fact_sheet.asp

Atkinson, W., Hamborsky, J., McIntyre, L., & Wolfe, S. (Eds.). (2007). Poliomyelitis. In *Epidemiology and prevention of vaccine-preventable diseases* (10th ed., pp. 101–114). Washington, DC: Public Health Foundation.

Baker, F., Denniston, M., Smith, M., & West, M. M. (2005). Adult cancer survivors: How are they faring? *Cancer, 104*(11 Suppl.), 2565–2576.

Bawah, A. A., & Binka, F. N. (2005). *How many years of life could be saved if malaria were eliminated from a hyperendemic area of northern Ghana?* (Policy Research Division Working Paper No. 203). New York: Population Council.

Bowman, R. M., McLone, D. G., Grant, J. A., Tomita, T., & Ito, J. A. (2001). Spina bifida outcome: A 25-year prospective. *Pediatric Neurosurgery, 34*(3), 114–120.

Brennan, J. (2001). Adjustment to cancer—coping or personal transition? *Psycho-oncology, 10*(1), 1–18.

British Broadcasting Corporation. (2004, July 15). *Big fall in African life expectancy.* Retrieved September 20, 2007, from http://news.bbc.co.uk/2/hi/in_depth/3894733.stm

Brown, P. J., Barrett, R. L., & Padilla, M. B. (1998). Medical anthropology: An introduction to the fields. In P. J. Brown (Ed.), *Understanding and applying medical anthropology* (pp. 10–19). Mountain View, CA: Mayfield.

Centers for Disease Control and Prevention. (2007). *HIV/AIDS surveillance report: Cases of HIV infection and AIDS in the United States and dependent areas, 2005* (Vol. 17). Atlanta, GA: Author.

Ciezaldo, A. (2003). *Worlds apart: Why are HIVers in New York City's Harlem neighborhood dying at twice the rate of HIVers in the gay enclave of Chelsea?* Retrieved April 23, 2004, from http://www.poz.com/index.cfm?p = article&art_id = 3069

Columbia Encyclopedia. (2007a). *Leprosy* (6th ed.). New York: Columbia University Press. Retrieved September 20, 2007, from http://www.encyclopedia.com/doc/1E1-plague.html

Columbia Encyclopedia. (2007b). *Plague* (6th ed.). New York: Columbia University Press. Retrieved September 20, 2007, from http://www.encyclopedia.com/doc/1E1-plague.html

Daly, J., Davidson, P., Chang, E., Hancock, K., Rees, D., & Thompson, D. R. (2002). Cultural aspects of adjustment to coronary heart disease in Chinese-Australians: A review of the literature. *Journal of Advanced Nursing, 39*(4), 391–399.

dLife. (2006). *Leonard Thompson.* Retrieved October 15, 2007, from http://www.dlife.com/dLife/do/ShowContent/inspiration_expert_advice/famous_people/leonard_thompson.html dLife. (2007). *Inspiration and expert advice: Famous people.* Retrieved October 15, 2007, from http://www.dlife.com/dLife/do/ShowContent/inspiration_expert_advice/famous_people/

Fay, F., & Pelka, F. (2002). Justin Dart's obituary. *Ability Magazine.* Retrieved September 24, 2007, from http://www.abilitymagazine.com/JustinDart_remembered.html

Folkman, S., & Greer, S. (2000). Promoting psychological well-being in the face of serious illness: When theory, research and practice inform each other. *Psychooncology, 9*(1), 11–19.

Frank, S. A. (2002). Inheritance of cancer. *Discovery Medicine, 4*(24), 396–400.

Global Polio Eradication Initiative. (2007). *Wild polio virus weekly update: 19 September 2007.* Retrieved September 24, 2007, from http://www.polioeradication.org/casecount.asp

International Diabetes Federation. (2007). *Diabetes incidence.* Retrieved October 14, 2007, from http://www.eatlas.idf.org/Incidence/

Juvenile Diabetes Research Foundation International. (2003, June 24). *Testimony of Mary Tyler Moore before the Senate Governmental Affairs Committee.* Retrieved October 15, 2007, from http://www.jdrf.org/index.cfm?page_id=101390

Juvenile Diabetes Research Foundation International. (2007). *What is diabetes?* Retrieved October 14, 2007, from http://www.jdrf.org/index.cfm?page_id=101982

Kids Health. (2005). *Juvenile rheumatoid arthritis.* Retrieved October 14, 2007, from http://www.kidshealth.org/parent/medical/arthritis/jra.html

Krantz, D. (1998). Environmental stress and biobehavioral antecedents of coronary heart disease. *Journal of Consulting and Clinical Psychology, 56*(3), 333–341.

Lab Tests Online. (2006). *Juvenile rheumatoid arthritis.* Retrieved October 14, 2007, from http://www.labtestsonline.org/understanding/conditions/jra.html

Lewis, R. (2004, May). *AIDS in Africa.* Paper presented at the Fourth International Conference on Social Work in Health and Mental Health, Quebec, Canada.

Mackelprang, R. W., & Mackelprang, R. D. (2005). Historical and contemporary issues in end-of-life decisions: Implications for social work. *Social Work, 50*(4), 315–324.

Mackelprang, R. W., Mackelprang, R. D., & Thirkill, A. D. (2005). Bioterrorism and smallpox: Policies, practices and implications for social work. *Social Work, 50*(2), 119–127.

Mackelprang, R. W., & Morris, L. C. (Eds.). (1989). AIDS in rural areas [Special issue]. *Human Services in the Rural Environment, 13.*

Manners, P. J., & Bower, C. (2002). Worldwide prevalence of juvenile arthritis: Why does it vary so much? *Journal of Rheumatology, 29*(7), 1520–1530.

Mayo Clinic. (2007). *Infectious disease: Polio.* Retrieved September 24, 2007, from http://www.mayoclinic.com/health/polio/DS00572/DSECTION=1

McLaughlin, T. J., Aupont, O., Bambauer, K. Z., Stone, P., Mullan, M. G., Colagiovanni, J., et al. (2005). Improving psychologic adjustment to chronic illness in cardiac patients: The role of depression and anxiety. *Journal of General Internal Medicine, 20*(12), 1084–1090.

Medline Plus. (2006). *Systemic lupus erthematosus.* Retrieved October 19, 2008, from http://www.nlm.nih.gov/medlineplus/ency/article/000435.htm

Medline Plus. (2008a). *Addison's disease.* Retrieved October 19, 2008, from http://www.nlm.nih.gov/medlineplus/addisonsdisease.html

Medline Plus. (2008b). *Crohn's disease.* Retrieved October 19, 2008, from http://www.nlm.nih.gov/medlineplus/crohnsdisease.html

Medline Plus. (2008c). *Psoriasis.* Retrieved October 19, 2008, from http://www.nlm.nih.gov/medlineplus/psoriasis.html

Medline Plus. (2008d). *Scleroderma.* Retrieved October 19, 2008, from http://www.nlm.nih.gov/medlineplus/scleroderma.html

Medline Plus. (2008e). *Sjogren's syndrome.* Retrieved October 19, 2008, from http://www.nlm.nih.gov/medlineplus/sjogrenssyndrome.html

Medline Plus. (2008f). *Thyroid diseases.* Retrieved October 19, 2008, from http://www.nlm.nih.gov/medlineplus/thyroiddiseases.html

Nathanson, N., & Martin, J. R. (1979). The epidemiology of poliomyelitis: Enigmas surrounding its appearance, epidemicity, and disappearance. *American Journal of Epidemiology, 110*(6), 672–692.

National Cancer Institute. (2002). *Genetic testing for BRCA1 and BRCA2: It's your choice.* Retrieved October 4, 2007, from http://www.nci.nih.gov/cancertopics/factsheet/Risk/BRCA

National Cancer Institute. (2007a). *Normal adjustment and the adjustment disorders.* Retrieved October 4, 2007, from http://www.cancer.gov/cancertopics/pdq/supportivecare/adjustment/HealthProfessional/page2#Reference2.16

National Cancer Institute. (2007b). *SEER cancer statistics review: 1975–2004.* Retrieved October 4, 2007, from http://seer.cancer.gov/csr/1975_2004/sections.html

National Institute of Mental Health. (2006). *How strep triggers obsessive compulsive disorder: New clues.* Retrieved October 19, 2008, from http://www.nimh.nih.gov/science-news/2006/how-strep-triggers-obsessive-compulsive-disorder-new-clues.shtml

Pearlin, L. L., & Schooler, C. (1978). The structure of coping. *Journal of Health and Social Behavior, 19,* 2–21.

Pollin, I., & Golant, S. K. (1994). *Taking charge: Overcoming the challenges of long-term illness.* New York: Crown.

Rolland, J. S. (1988). A conceptual model of chronic and life threatening illness and its impact on families. In C. S. Chilman, E. W. Nunnaly, & F. M. Cox (Eds.), *Chronic illness and disability* (pp. 17–68). Newbury Park, CA: Sage.

Rosati, G. (2001). The prevalence of multiple sclerosis in the world: An update. *Neurological Sciences, 22*(2), 117–139.

Sass, E., Gottfried, G., & Sorem, A. (1996). *Polio's legacy: An oral history.* Lanham, MD: University Press of America.

Shilts, R. (1987). *And the band played on: Politics, people, and the AIDS epidemic.* New York: St. Martin's Press.

Sidell, N. L. (1997). Adult adjustment to chronic illness: A review of the literature. *Health and Social Work, 22*(1), 5–11.

Stephen Lewis Foundation. (2007, July). *Grassroots.* Retrieved September 25, 2007, from http://stephenlewisfoundation.org/grassroots/assets/pdf/2007/0707_slf_grassroots.pdf

UNAIDS. (2006). *2006 Report on the global AIDS epidemic: Executive summary.* Geneva, Switzerland: Author.

United Nations Development Programme. (2004). *Human development report 2004: Cultural liberty in today's diverse world.* Retrieved September 25, 2007, from http://hdr.undp.org/reports/global/2004/?CFID=8711891&CFTOKEN=5d8aabb2a38bd631–3EE282C8–1321–0B50–35921A0EDEC5CB17&jsessionid=e630b49c209120534d47

White, A. (2004, June 8). Reagan's AIDS legacy: Silence equals death. *San Francisco Chronicle.* Retrieved September 24, 2007, from http://sfgate.com/cgi-bin/article.cgi?file=/chronicle/archive/2004/06/08/EDG777163F1.DTL

World Health Organization. (1980). *International classification of impairments, disabilities, and handicaps.* Geneva, Switzerland: Author.

World Health Organization. (2001). *International classification of functioning, disability and health.* Geneva, Switzerland: Author.

World Health Organization. (2003). *Global cancer rates could increase by 50% to 15 million by 2020.* Geneva, Switzerland: Author. Retrieved October 1, 2007, from http://www.who.int/mediacentre/news/releases/2003/pr27/en/

World Health Organization. (2007a). *Cardiovascular diseases.* Retrieved October 18, 2007, from http://www.who.int/cardiovascular_diseases/en/

World Health Organization. (2007b). *Cardiovascular diseases factsheet.* Retrieved October 18, 2007, from http://www.who.int/mediacentre/factsheets/fs317/en/index.html

World Health Organization. (2007c). *Malaria fact sheet.* Retrieved September 17, 2007, from http://www.who.int/mediacentre/factsheets/fs094/en/index.html

World Health Organization. (2007d). *Tuberculosis fact sheet.* Retrieved September 18, 2007, from http://www.who.int/mediacentre/factsheets/fs104/en/

World Health Organization. (2007e). *World health statistics: 2007.* Geneva, Switzerland: Author.

Part III

Human Service Practice Framework

In the United States, human services for persons with disabilities have traditionally centered around the medical model. In the medical model, the assessment process directs practitioners to diagnose the characteristics of persons with disabilities against the context of "normalcy." The elements of the person that are not "within normal limits" are defined as "dysfunctional." Practitioners create intervention plans for persons with disabilities geared to fixing their "broken" or "dysfunctional" parts. They apply a combination of medical, psychological, and training interventions to make persons with disabilities as "normal" or as nondisabled as possible. Essentially, this approach expects practitioners to focus on the individual as the source of the problem. Although appropriate for immediate medical concerns, this perspective in human service practice is very limiting and often reinforces the social oppression experienced by persons with disabilities because it takes away their control.

The following chapters propose alternate practice perspectives to the medical model. We discuss assessment and how assessment guides professional relationships. We discuss models of practice and how practitioners work at micro, meso, and macro levels of intervention. We then provide a guide for professional practice based on respect and a focus on strengths.

In chapter 13, we discuss the assessment process from a strengths perspective. When the human service professional helps individuals examine their needs, the professional helps in assessing strengths as well as limitations. This assessment looks not only at the individual but also at the social and economic environment of the person with a disability. We also introduce the concepts of universal design and access.

Chapter 14 explores a variety of practice models that can be utilized in the process of facilitating the empowerment of a person with a disability.

Like the assessment process, the method of intervention must address change not only in the individual but in the individual's social environment.

Finally, chapter 15 looks at a practice model that we have synthesized from other empowerment models. We address in detail four primary roles that human service professionals play in working with persons with disabilities: counselor, teacher, broker, and political advocate. Using the principles articulated in this chapter, practitioners can develop relationships that promote dignity and self-determination and that maximize people's quality of life.

13

Assessment in Practice

I remember this bullheaded psychologist who gave me a small-print IQ test and told my mother that I was retarded. What he had really tested was my ability to read small print. Even my mother knew that his diagnosis was not correct. After all, why would someone give me a small-print test when he knew I couldn't read small print very well? Because I was very determined to go to regular school, my mother told the resistant school officials, "You'll have to fight with her. She wants to go here." So this bull-headed psychologist then said to my mother, "Well, we'll let her go here so she can learn about failure." So my mother says, "Yeah, OK." She only had an eighth-grade education, but she understood intuitively that I was brighter than they gave me credit for.

—Brenda Premo
Western University of Health Sciences

STUDENT LEARNING OBJECTIVES

1. To understand the implications and limitations of medical/professional-based assessment models that utilize a pathological/dysfunctional frame of reference
2. To develop an understanding of the social model of assessment based on the social-ecological model of human development, with its origins in strengths-based practice and the independent living movement
3. To understand the various layers of the social model of assessment, including the biosocial, psychosocial, and social structural domains
4. To learn to apply the social model of assessment, considering multiple systems sizes in the assessment process

A routine and critical component of human service practice is assessment. Assessment occurs at all system levels, from the individual and personal to the institutional and societal. Hepworth, Rooney, Larsen, Rooney, and Strom-Gottfried (2005) state that assessment provides a foundation for contracting, goal setting, and interventions and that the effectiveness of interventions is contingent on accurate assessments. Effective assessments are multidimensional and purposeful. Assessments can be both process and product oriented. *Product-oriented assessments* are assessments that result in the creation of a report or document. For example, a medical history and physical are required when patients are hospitalized, and mental status examinations and their results concerning emotional and cognitive functioning are documented. *Process-oriented assessments* do not necessarily produce a finished product; they are primarily tools used to guide ongoing relationships to direct activities and plans. Of course, assessments frequently overlap in their nature and purpose.

In this chapter, we discuss the implications of the types of assessments in which human services professionals engage. We start our discussion by illustrating assessments as products. We discuss traditional pathology-based assessments, which are often required to justify the need for professional involvement. We also discuss the processes of assessment. We then discuss the social model of assessment based on the social-ecological perspective.

PROFESSIONAL ASSESSMENTS/EVALUATIONS AS PRODUCTS

Assessments of individuals and families can be divided into three components: information and history, impressions and evaluations, and plans. Information and history comprise the *what* section of an evaluation. What is important to know about the people and situations being evaluated? The second section, the *so what* section, organizes and gives meaning to the history and information. What is the meaning of the information one has received? The third section, the *now what* section, outlines plans. Based on the situation at hand, what should be done and what are the desired outcomes? Figure 13.1 provides a skeletal outline of a tool to develop an assessment product.

The first component focuses on people's histories, background information, and current situations and the reasons that bring them into contact with practitioners. This information can be referred to as the *social history* portion of the assessment. Several elements are relevant to this section. Identifying information includes demographic information such as age, gender, ethnicity, onset and type of disability, and living conditions. It also includes the reasons disabled individuals and their families are using professional services. Family background can include information about the person's family of origin; current relationships with family and significant others; and past, present, and anticipated living situations. Social history can include information on a person's educational and work history, friends and relationships, culture, places of residence, substance use history, and involvement with the legal system. Since persons with disabilities are especially susceptible to financial problems, the history should include information on financial

FIGURE 13.1   Assessment and Evaluation Tool

I. What?

  1. Identifying Information (age, gender, ethnicity, residence, etc.)
      Reason for admission, clinic visit, or agency involvement
      Reason for referral to social work

  2. Family Background
      Family of origin or childhood
      Current relationships
      Adult family and significant others
      Living situation—past, present, and anticipated

  3. Social History
      Educational history
      Work history (including military background)
      Friends—relationships
      Cultural influences
      Places of residence
      Substance use history
      Legal involvement

  4. Financial Status
      Income, expenses, obligations
      Insurance—medical coverage and needs

  5. Psychosocial Situation
      Cognitive status
      Emotional/psychosocial status
      Psychiatric—mental health history
      Family reactions, relationships, support, and adjustments
      Sexuality concerns (e.g., questions, orientation, problems)
      Judgment/planning—behavioral situation
      Other relevant issues

  6. Tools
      Genogram
      Ecomap

II. So What? Impressions

  1. Personal strengths and limitations
  2. Social supports
  3. Resources

III. Now What? Plans

  1. Counseling and direct services—individual and significant others
  2. Social interventions, planning, advocacy
  3. Micro, meso, macro interventions
  4. Anticipated outcomes

---

status. This includes income, expenses, and financial obligations as well as insurance, medical coverage, and costs of medical needs. The person's psychosocial situation may also be important to discuss and may include the person's cognitive and emotional status. Sexuality concerns may be ascertained. Information about the person's history with mental health professionals and the mental health system may be relevant. Family reactions and supports should be considered. Information on the person's relationships within the community may be gathered. Strengths in judgment and planning are also relevant to the person's psychosocial situation. Genograms and eco-maps can be valuable tools for developing comprehensive histories. The information gathered in the social history component of an evaluation varies greatly, depending on each person's circumstances and each person's social and family context. In addition, the settings in which assessments are performed affect the areas highlighted in assessment. For example, the foci of human service assessments in school, hospital, and mental health contexts differ in priority and scope.

In the second section of psychosocial assessments, *evaluation* or *impressions,* the human service practitioner and consumer consider the meaning of the information gathered in the social history. For example, a person who has had strong family relationships is likely to be able to rely on family for continued support. An individual who has had multiple marriages and divorces might expect less family support than one with strong long-term relationships. An individual from a background of poverty will likely have fewer resources available than a person who comes from wealth. The evaluation section should include information about people's strengths and their realized and potential capabilities as well as their needs and limitations. It considers individuals' social supports and their ability to affect people and organizations in their lives. The level and adequacy of personal and environmental resources are also evaluated.

The final section of psychosocial evaluations, the *plan,* is based on the evaluation section. Plans should be explicit and goal directed. In the plan, the person and professional determine desired outputs and outcomes. Outputs may include services that professionals may provide (e.g., counseling, advocacy, referrals) and actions in which consumers may engage. Outcomes focus on the results the consumer and practitioner wish to achieve in their work together. Attention to micro, meso, and macro elements of people's lives is a critical element in effective plans.

Five questions that provide a framework for assessment activities can be asked as practitioners develop human service assessments. First, What is the reason for the assessment? This helps practitioners evaluate people's needs and their reasons for engaging in a relationship with a human service agency and professional. Second, What is the scope of the assessment? Scope is determined by a variety of factors, including people's needs, agency mandates, and social conditions. For example, the reasons for and scope of an employment assessment in a vocational rehabilitation agency differ from those of an assessment performed during the course of family therapy. A third question is, Who receives the information and knowledge gained as a result of the assessment? In an individual and family therapy agency, assessment information is usually kept within the confines of the practitioner and family relationship. However, if family therapy is taking place within a medical and/or psychiatric facility, the information is generally more widely disseminated to other professionals and to third parties. A fourth question is, What are the sources of knowledge that will be needed in order to engage in the assessment? This will determine how information is obtained. Some assessments utilize only one source of information, whereas others utilize multiple sources. Court-ordered assessments for substance abuse offenses may utilize numerous informants as well as court records. On the other hand, assessments for participation in an educational group may rely exclusively on an individual interview. Fifth, What will the assessment be used for? For example, if assessments are being paid for by a third party, especially in managed care settings, a clinical (pathology-based) diagnosed assessment is often necessary to obtain reimbursement (Strom, 1992). Medical and psychiatric settings require pathology-based diagnoses. In contrast, assessments performed in independent living centers focus on consumer definitions of needs and problems.

PATHOLOGY AND ASSESSMENT

Traditional assessment models focus on the presence or absence of pathology (Schuler & Perez, 1991). For example, medical histories and physicals required when patients are admitted to hospitals determine whether findings are "within normal limits" or there is pathology. Strengths are not considered. There are several reasons for the diagnostic, problem-focused emphasis in professional evaluations. Persons seeking professional help do so to receive assistance in treating or solving problems. For example, people see physicians to treat or cure illness. Professional training and sanctioning centered on pathology have traditionally driven models of practice. Medical specialties (e.g., neurosurgery, cardiology, rheumatology) concentrate heavily on treating pathological conditions, and there is relatively little emphasis on preventive and health-maintaining specialties (e.g., family practice, epidemiology). Similarly, mental health training primarily focuses not on maintaining mental health, but on treating mental health disabilities. To justify intervention, a *DSM* diagnosis must be provided. The focus on pathology has been driven, in great measure, by financial interests. Funding is institutionally based in places such as hospitals and nursing facilities, and service providers are paid only after diagnosing and treating pathology.

Certainly, the focus on pathology is essential in many situations (Blotzer & Ruth, 1995). A person taken to an emergency room with multiple injuries from an automobile accident requires immediate assessment and treatment for injuries sustained. Empathy is not particularly a high-priority skill in an emergency or operating room. Similarly, a person experiencing an acute psychotic episode needs immediate protection and treatment. However, an exclusively pathological focus is inadequate in the long term. This is especially true in human services.

By attending primarily to problems, assessment can fail to account for individual strengths. A deficiency focus can lead to the devaluing and, in some cases, dehumanizing of people (Cowger, 1994). For example, in reviewing old patient hospital records, one of the authors repeatedly found the notation "FLK" in the records of children with mental retardation. Upon investigating the meaning, he found that FLK was an acronym for "funny-looking kid" used routinely to refer to patients with mental retardation. FLK was originally used as a type of medical shorthand, because children with intellectual disabilities can have atypical facial and body features. However, the term "FLK" devalues the people it supposedly describes.

The individual pathology focus also fails to recognize the complexity of experiences and relationships (Salsgiver, 1996). This is illustrated in the case of a Native American patient hospitalized in a rehabilitation center with an acute spinal cord injury. Nurses and therapists became increasingly frustrated with his lateness for therapy and his nonparticipation in the general milieu of the center. They attributed his behaviors to denial, resistance, and noncompliance. They failed to realize that he had been raised in a remote community on a reservation. He was overwhelmed, not just with his spinal cord injury, but by his surroundings. The rehabilitation center employed far more people than lived in his community. He had never owned a watch, yet they expected him to follow a tight schedule. He was a night person, yet he was expected to begin his day at 7:00 A.M. There were also language and cultural barriers. However, the staff focused only on "fixing" his behavior so they could provide the therapies they determined he needed. A more holistic assessment would have led professionals to assess ways they could change their expectations of him and modify the environment in such a way to better meet his needs while ensuring that he received the medical and physical attention he needed. For example, times for breakfast and therapies could have been modified to meet the demands of his lifestyle. The staff could have taken the time to get to know the patient and learn about his culture.

MEDICAL AND SOCIAL MODELS OF ASSESSMENT

In the last generation, the adequacy of traditional medical assessments based on pathology has been challenged. For example, Trieschmann (1980) compares two models of assessment and service delivery for persons with spinal cord injuries—the medical model and the learning model. Trieschmann points out that "in the medical model, the behavioral equation for rehabilitation success consists of: B = f (O × p). Behavior (B) is a function of treatments to the organic variables (O) unless [these are] hindered by underlying personality problems (p)" (p. 24). In the medical model, an individual's organic, physical, and medical problems are the primary assessment targets. Personality and psychosocial status are assessed in the context of the obstacles they create for the treating professionals. Strengths are not assessed—only the absence of pathology. The unit of assessment is the individual, problems reside within the individual, and treatment plans center on fixing the individual. In addition, professionals are responsible for assessment and treatment decisions. While this model may be appropriate in crisis situations, such as during a medical or mental health emergency, it has limited benefit in the long term.

Condeluci (1995) discusses the limitations of individual pathology assessments that focus on disabled persons' problems and ignore the social obstacles that prevent them from being productive. Condeluci states: "Today, in the human service world that surrounds disability, a battery of tests and surveys attempts to identify and predict the economic potential of its clients. These tests look at aptitude, interests, skills, education, and deficits. It is mostly the deficits, however, that cast a shadow on the plan that is set up for the individual" (p. 72).

Trieschmann (1980) offers a more progressive model of assessment and intervention—the learning model—and contrasts it to the medical model. She advocates its use in rehabilitation settings, stating, "The behavioral equation for rehabilitation success is: B = f (P × O × E). Behavior [B] is a function of the person [P], the organism [O], and the environment [E]" (p. 26). In Trieschmann's learning model, "person" variables include personality style, coping mechanisms, and internal or external locus of control. Organic variables include age, health, and severity of disability. Environmental variables include family support, finances, and public policies. Assessment broadens to include psychological and environmental well-being. Individuals are still the focus, but assessment is used to help professionals determine how to educate clients to function better. Assessments are performed to identify knowledge and skills that clients need to function as independently as possible. Control still resides primarily with professionals, who act as educators. The learning model attends to internal strengths and social variables. It may be appropriate in the initial stages of disabilities, when persons with disabilities and their families are in need of knowledge and skill development. However, it is inadequate in the long run because the perception of problems and needs as well as the control of services still rest with professionals.

As long as professionals maintain control, people with disabilities are vulnerable to their biases. For example, Condeluci (1995) observes that in the employment arena, people with certain types of disabilities are likely to be stereotyped and that the experts "push people with certain disabilities toward job areas thought to be best with disability groups" (p. 74). For example, people with intellectual disabilities are often pushed into custodial, dish washing, and bus-person jobs, whereas those with brain injuries are traditionally pushed into repetitive work. Assessment tools and interventions such as aptitude tests can be valuable aids in the quest for economic self-sufficiency. However, this model is similar to other models in that it focuses primarily on the individual's deficits and possible interventions to overcome problems.

A social rather than individual approach to disability is the approach that best meets the needs of persons with disabilities. Hahn (1991) labels this approach the "minority group model" and states that social stigma is the major problem facing persons with disabilities, which is best "addressed through civil rights rather than social services. The minority group model also alters the view of the disabled person as defected or deficient. . . . [The] call for improvements in social services is a step in the right direction, but it should be expanded to include civil rights as the major focus for improving the lives of the disabled" (p. 17).

Condeluci (1995) emphasizes the importance of the economic aspects of people's lives. From this perspective, problems lie in the person's inability to earn a living. Professional assessment focuses on problems people have that prevent them from being productive. Condeluci labels this approach an "interdependence paradigm." He contends that interdependence focuses on individual capabilities rather than deficits. Problems reside in systems rather than individuals, and actions are tailored to create environmental supports and consumer empowerment.

There are several elements in approaching assessment from a social perspective. A critical component of the independent living approach is that individuals identify their own needs (Mackelprang & Salsgiver, 1996). The minority group model, the interdependence paradigm, and the independent living approach have many similarities. For ease of use, we call our approach to assessment the social model.

Using Trieschmann's behavioral framework, the social model of assessment might be diagrammed as follows: $B = f(P \times O \times E \times Pe \times C)$. Behavior (B) is a function of the sum of personal attributes (P), organic and biological characteristics (O), and social and environmental factors (E). In addition, we add internal and external definitions of personal characteristics and attributes (Pe) and control over life choices (C). When societal perceptions (Pe) are negative, choices are limited and people develop a tendency to internalize others' messages, such as occurs with internalized ableism. Of course, the social model emphasizes the importance of individuals having choice and responsibility over life decisions.

On the personal (P) level, the social model emphasizes people's strengths and potential. Strengths encompass the knowledge and skills that an individual possesses (Saleebey, 1996). Potential refers to the potential abilities that people can develop with sufficient resources. Persons with disabilities can identify their own strengths, and sometimes professionals can help them identify strengths they may not perceive that they possess. With consumer direction, professionals can also consult to help them develop their potential. This is illustrated in the case of a young couple, both with neuromuscular disabilities, who requested assistance from one of the authors. This couple, both in their early twenties, had met and fallen in love in the nursing facility in which they resided. Their medical records, which focused on their physical limitations, clearly justified their continued stay in the facility. Initially, they came into contact with one of the authors because of their desire to get out of the nursing facility for occasional recreation. With increased community exposure, they began to realize that others with similar capabilities were not forced to live with their parents or in nursing facilities, with others directing their lives. Encouraged to identify their strengths, they began to believe that they could marry and have a sexual relationship if they chose. Both began to realize that their need for physical assistance in daily living activities did not mean they had to give up control over how, what, where, and by whom assistance was provided. Eventually, they each developed their potential and identified their strengths to the point that they left the nursing home to live in their own apartments with attendant care assistance. Their relationship evolved platonically; they maintained their friendship yet began to see themselves as sexual beings. Along the road to independent living, each person began to assess and develop strengths, eschewing traditional pathology-based models of assessment and treatment.

At the organism (O) level, the social model acknowledges that people with disabilities have atypical functioning or characteristics; however, disabled persons are not defined by their impairments (Fine & Asch, 1993). For example, people with mental health disabilities have many other traits, interests, and capabilities. Medical labels such as "schizophrenic" define individuals by their diagnoses. However, acknowledging that a person lives with schizophrenia recognizes that the person has other qualities and traits. People may choose to adopt a disability-first identity, wherein they embrace the totality of the disability as an integral part of themselves, not just the part that needs treatment and intervention. Using impairment as a person's defining characteristic is a natural outgrowth of traditional models that focus on problems and ways to fix problems. In contrast, the social model views the disability as one aspect of people's existence and, possibly, of identity.

In the social model, a critical element of assessment is the environment (E). For example, people who use wheelchairs for mobility face problems, not because they are "confined" to wheelchairs but because of physical barriers that limit their access to full societal participation. The fact that "persons with disabilities tend to make up a disproportionate share of residents at the lower end of the economic scale" (Bryan, 1996, p. 17) has much to do with social policies and institutions that make it extremely difficult for them to be economically self-sufficient. Assessment emphasizes the availability and limitations of social and community resources and looks at ways to enhance opportunities

Another environmental element in the social model of assessment is the reversal of traditional medical model roles. Disabled persons are experts over their lives, while professionals act as consultants. Rather than professionals making decisions based on client information and feedback, consumers identify needs and problems and enlist the help of professionals to meet their needs. Professionals may not always agree with the individual's perceptions, but this approach assumes that people with disabilities have the ability to recognize their individual realities (Condeluci, 1995). Unlike other approaches, the social model does not assume that professional perceptions are superior to those of clients. Rather, it assumes that the consumers of professional services understand their own lives.

The perception element (Pe) of the social model acknowledges that beliefs and values relative to disability dramatically affect the lives and behaviors of disabled persons. Negative societal perceptions lead to institutionalized oppression and devaluation of people with disabilities. Szymanski and Trueba (1994) offer the observation that "the difficulties faced by persons with disabilities are not the result of functional impairments related to the disability, but rather are the result of a castification process embedded in societal institutions for rehabilitation and education that are enforced by well-meaning professionals" (p. 12).

The "castification" that Szymanski and Trueba (1994) refer to is pervasive throughout societal institutions, even those that have been developed to serve persons with disabilities. Traditionally, long-term dependence on health or social services has been assessed as a functional individual problem. For example, in the United States, some disabled people are forced out of the job market by their need to maintain Medicaid benefits that are available only to those who are poor. Social model assessment acknowledges a problem in societal institutions wherein people are forced to choose between low-paying jobs and hazard losing health coverage or being financially dependent so they can maintain access to health care. Another example of this castification occurs in vocational rehabilitation agencies, where pressure to employ people quickly and with limited resources induces counselors to find the easiest sources of employment (e.g., dish washing, custodial work) and to exclude people with severe disabilities by labeling them unemployable. When societal perceptions are pervasively negative, people also internalize the ableism they experience daily. They can begin to accept the negative messages and incorporate them into their identities. In contrast, social model assessment emphasizes societal elements rather than primarily individual concerns.

A major philosophical difference between assessments of people with disabilities based on the traditional medical model and the social model is that the social model assessment begins with perceptions of capability and the assumption that disabled persons are competent and have the right and responsibility to control their lives and to manage the professionals who enter their lives (DeJong, 1979). In contrast, other assessments begin with the assumption that professional assessment is needed to fix individuals' problems. The terminology used is an example of this contrast in assumptions. In the social model, independent living specialists consult with clients, who direct the interventions. In a traditional model, case managers assess and manage cases (i.e., clients, students, or patients). The locus of control resides with the person with the disability in the social model, and with the case manager in the traditional model.

The social model of assessment acknowledges that disabled persons have a right and responsibility to control (C) their lives and resources. Condeluci (1995) contends that "people must be deemed capable to be in control of their lives, and only challenged if family, support people, and advocates are convinced, beyond a shadow of a doubt that they are not" (pp. 102–103). Most professional approaches assume that people with disabilities must prove they are capable before others relinquish control. Unfortunately, those to whom control is relinquished often have conflicts of interest, in that their loss of control also means loss of their role and, possibly, their usefulness. For example, the nursing facility in which the previously cited couple resided had significant disincentives to discharge them—the most important of which was the loss of tens of thousands of dollars in annual revenue.

In the social model, disabled persons determine how and to whom resources are expended. For example, persons with intellectual disabilities in a supported living situation can determine what help they need with finances, but they may use social workers and independent living specialists as consultants to assist them in managing their affairs. Rather than having a home health agency employ attendants on their behalf, individuals with physical disabilities who need physical assistance handle their own financial concerns and employee decisions.

Both traditional and social models recognize that there are situations where people are not able to function independently. Traditional models, however, are inclined to impose professional control over individuals to fix their pathology. The social model, on the other hand, considers the need for assistance to be a part of human existence for all people. No one person is completely independent in today's society. DeJong (1979), in tracing the philosophic roots of the independent living movement, states that the movement "has steered away from destructive individualism. It has encouraged community support and mutual responsibility. The emphasis on self-help and self-reliance has a communal as well as an individual component" (p. 50). People without disabilities use the expertise of others in everything from buying automobiles to purchasing groceries. Likewise, people with disabilities rely on others. People with severe intellectual disabilities may need assistance managing their money or using transportation. For decades, people with hearing disabilities used TTYs to communicate from a distance. Today, text messages, instant messaging, and e-mail are readily available to deaf and hearing people alike, who depend on functioning Internet and/or phone companies. Reliance on others, or what Condeluci (1995) calls "interdependence," is a reality for everyone in society. Problems arise because of limited or absent resources, and people can meet their needs through empowerment and by creating adequate supports. Assessment is a mutual effort that goes beyond solving problems to assessing needs, ascertaining potential and identifying strengths, and finding solutions.

SOCIAL-ECOLOGICAL ASSESSMENT

Effective assessments are contextual; that is, the context in which the assessment occurs determines the nature and extent of the assessment (Miley, O'Melia, & DuBois, 1995). According to Rosenthal (1989), a comprehensive, holistic individual and family assessment includes the biological, psychological/emotional, and social domains. Fee (1994) adds to this the importance of the cultural domain in assessment. Bronfenbrenner (2005) provides a framework for looking at micro, meso, exo, and macro systems and has recently refined his conceptualization to more explicitly include human biology.

In chapter 2, we introduced you to the social-ecological model of human development and behavior. The application of the social-ecological model provides an approach that rejects the pathology-based medical and moral models in favor of what we have been calling the social model of viewing disability. We make this distinction to help readers avoid confusing the social model, which provides an overarching framework, with the social-ecological model, which is one approach to describing and explaining human behavior and which we are applying to human service assessment.

The biosocial, psychosocial, and social structural domains of the social-ecological model encompass the personal elements of traditional human services assessments as well as the social, community, and cultural spheres in which people live. Stated another way, assessments encompass the traditional micro level of the biological, personal, and family elements of the person in the environment; the meso-level influences that are involved in physical and social climates, social systems, organizations, and communities; and the macro-level systems of the environment, societal structures, and cultures in which people reside. Each of the three domains overlaps and is interrelated with the others, as illustrated in figure 2.1 in chapter 2. In addition, influence is reciprocal; not only are people influenced by their environments, but people can help shape their contexts.

Biosocial Domain

The biosocial domain encompasses all of the body's systems. However, biological functioning does not define people. For example, people with spinal cord injuries have paraplegia or quadriplegia—but their medical diagnosis as a paraplegic or quadriplegic does not define them. In a social context, they may identify themselves as belonging to a group of "paras" and "quads," as opposed to "walkies" or the "temporarily able-bodied," or they may choose *not* to identify themselves as part of a disability community. Given opportunities, people with intellectual disabilities that are biologically based are no longer imprisoned in institutions and have strong vibrant communities and organizations such as People First. Biological characteristics have not changed, but their social contexts have.

The social-ecological model assesses biological functioning in the holistic context. Human service workers need to rely on persons with disabilities to identify their levels of biological functioning and the meaning of that functioning in their lives. The focus is on their strengths and capabilities. This can be illustrated using the example of a person with T-12 paraplegia. Traditional assessment focuses on paralysis and lack of sensation in the lower extremities and the genitals, lack of bowel and bladder functioning, sexual dysfunction, and "wheelchair confinement." From this assessment, treatments are developed that are intended to make people closer to "normal." Long leg braces for walking are often prescribed but rarely used. Interventions are developed that focus on helping people deal with their physical losses. In contrast, when assessing biosocial functioning, practitioners seek the meaning of paraplegia to the individual. Together, the individual and professional seek the meaning of paraplegia while assessing strengths and capabilities. Rather than viewing the person as confined to a wheelchair, the professional perceives the person as using a wheelchair for mobility. Sexual function is seen as different, but not as inherently dysfunctional. The gamut of emotional responses are jointly evaluated, with a focus on building strengths, not just fixing pathology.

At the intersection of the biosocial domain and the psychosocial domain is what we call the biopsychological component of human experience. In other words, biology and emotional, psychological status are interdependent and reciprocal. In the 1600s Descartes separated mind from body (Brown, Barrett, & Padilla, 1998), a philosophy embedded in Western medicine and culture (Mackelprang & Mackelprang, 2005). We believe this is a false dichotomy. As Damasio (1994) states, the physiological operations of the mind are structural and functional and can be fully understood only in the context of our interactions with the environment. As Sapolsky (1998) states, "We have come to recognize the vastly complex intertwining of our biology and emotions, the endless ways in which our personalities, feelings, and thoughts both reflect and influence events in our bodies . . . and a critical shift in medicine has been the recognition that many of the damaging diseases of slow accumulation can be either caused or made far worse by stress" (p. 3).

We argue that physical and psychological characteristics are not distinct and separate; they are really the same. On an individual level, one of the authors has a disability that is associated with the structural differences in the area of his brain controlling motor function. The other author has atypical brain function that can also be shown by diagnostic tests showing atypical electrical-chemical activity in the brain. Professionals may "diagnose" his atypical brain activity and function as pathological, yet the author embraces the experiences and perspectives gained from these characteristics. As Sapolsky (1998) suggests, disease and illness associated with disabilities are stress related, often because of environmental influences that make life with a disability more difficult.

On the social or what Bronfenbrenner (2005) calls the micro-system level external influences on biosocial functioning are reciprocal; that is, relationships are dependent on the commitment and actions of interacting parties. It is critical to determine the nature and the levels of support (Crewe & Zola, 1983), including both physical and emotional supports. For example, some people may provide much physical support, such as personal attendant care or assistance with shopping. Others may provide no physical care but may provide emotional support. In addition to the strength of the support, conflict should also be assessed. Sometimes strong support comes at a high price when conflict is present; therefore, people should be encouraged to assess the biosocial benefits and costs of their social supports. The type of relationship is also important. For example, the connection people have with professionals who provide services is usually temporary and is much different from that of family and friends.

Psychosocial Domain

The psychosocial domain involves people's emotional and cognitive functioning in their social environments. For professionals to justify their involvement and receive reimbursement for services, *DSM-IV TR* diagnoses may be required. If so, assessment is, by necessity, pathology based. In playing the reimbursement game, human service professionals may learn to engage in labeling an individual with an innocuous diagnosis, such as an anxiety or adjustment disorder (Saleebey, 1996). In contrast, the social model recognizes that individuals have problems, but assessments focus on strengths. Human service professionals work as consultants in conjunction with individuals to identify strengths, potentials, and capabilities. They emphasize supporting people's capacities rather than fixing their problems. Workers rely on those with whom they work to identify their own needs. The individual's perceptions, rather than the professional's expectations, are paramount. The difference between the traditional and social approaches was repeatedly illustrated to one of the authors in his work with persons with neurological disabilities. The following example was typical.

> Late one afternoon I received a call from a nurse and a resident physician to consult on the case of thirty-year-old Bill, who had paraplegia resulting from a fall. Bill was well known to me and had been doing very well during inpatient rehabilitation for his spinal cord injury. I had met with Bill, his wife, and their young children on a number of occasions in the month he had been hospitalized. However, the nurse and physician were very upset because Bill was nearing discharge and he had "not dealt emotionally with his paraplegia." When I asked them what they saw as the problem, they told me Bill was in denial. I asked how they reached that conclusion. They replied, "He has never been depressed and is too pleasant all the time." "Sounds good to me," I responded. "Yes, but he needs to begin to deal with his disability," they stressed. I replied that in repeated conversations with Bill and his family, they said that they felt they were coping with things well. I saw nothing to indicate anything different.
>
> I expressed concern that their expectations of Bill placed him in a no-win situation. If Bill didn't become depressed, he was in denial. Bill could become psychologically healthy only by experiencing emotional states they considered pathological (e.g., depression, anger, anxiety). They assumed the lack of pathology meant pathology, and they would be satisfied that he was healthy only if he became depressed. Their latent expectations could even produce unnecessary difficulties.

In the months following this incident, Bill and his wife sought the author out on a number of occasions. In one instance, they asked for help finding social support from others with spinal cord injuries. On another occasion, they sought sexual education and counseling. Assessment and counseling were provided in the context of enhancing strengths rather than fixing dysfunction.

Although an acute disability such as paraplegia can be traumatic and produce a range of emotional responses, we reject the idea that disabilities automatically cause psychosocial problems. A social model recognizes the tremendous resources people possess in dealing with life's experiences. It acknowledges the importance and reciprocal nature of social supports people use. Individual coping problems are often a result of others' reactions to and expectations of disability.

Human service workers are cautioned to listen to individuals' personal perceptions of the emotional impact of their disabilities as well as the nature of their social supports, rather than assuming people will react in a certain way. This concept is illustrated in a study of persons with long-term spinal cord injuries by Mackelprang and Hepworth (1987). Two of their findings ran counter to extant beliefs of professionals, and a third illustrated the impact of support systems (Mackelprang, 1986). First, it was widely assumed that the higher a person's spinal cord injury, the lower the level of adjustment he or she would experience. Instead, the study found that those with lower injuries (lumbar and sacral) had lower levels of adjustment than people with thoracic and low cervical injuries. Second, people with spinal cord injuries reported less emotional distress overall than was expected. Third, the study revealed that people with strong religious beliefs reported better levels of social and emotional adjustment than nonreligious respondents; however, they also reported that expectations and relationships with others in their faith communities were a source of significant stress. For example, some felt that others judged them because they had not had the faith to be healed of their "affliction." This study supports the notion that people's perceptions of their disabilities are the most critical factor in psychological assessment. The assumption that persons with disabilities are in greater need for professionals to determine their emotional status is an ableist notion.

Cowger (1994) offers twelve principles of assessment, all of which underlie the need for the human service practitioner to seek the perceptions of the person with whom he or she is working. First of all, the individual's understanding of the facts and issues is of foremost importance. Second, believe in the credibility and ability of the person. Third, look for what the person wants. Do not bring into the assessment process preconceived notions and biases. Fourth, move the assessment toward an emphasis on personal and environmental strengths. Fifth, look for strengths on a multidimensional level—address individual, family, and community strengths. Sixth, use language that the person understands and relates to. The use of professional jargon should be avoided. Seventh, make the assessment process a combined effort; this should be easy if you believe in the person. Eighth, and much related to the preceding principle, reach a mutual agreement on the assessment. Ninth, do not blame the victim. In working with persons with disabilities, it is easy to make their "laziness" or their "dependency" the cause of the problem that needs to be addressed. Tenth, avoid cause-and-effect analysis in assessment. Humans are far too complex for the human service practitioner to figure out the cause. Eleventh, "assess, do not diagnose" (Cowger, 1994, p. 267). Diagnosis assumes pathology and dysfunction. Last, see difference and uniqueness as strengths. This is easy to do when the cultural domain is addressed as it intersects with disability.

The psychosocial domain includes intersections between what Bronfenbrenner (2005) describes as micro systems and meso systems. Effective assessment is concerned with the impact of social systems on people's lives and the impact people can have on those systems. Psychosocial assessment should encompass neighborhoods, health care organizations, churches, schools, social agencies, and businesses in which people are employed. It is critical that the influences of these systems be addressed in assessment. For example, Brown (1996) chronicles the low income and employment levels of persons with disabilities, which traditionally have been attributed to people with disabilities being less capable than persons without disabilities. However, it is clear that people with disabilities are denied opportunities and subjected to much discrimination in employment. Assessment of the psychosocial domain must include the opportunities and obstacles people face in their social and community contexts rather than focusing primarily on the individual. It is also important to assess the individual's ability to affect meso systems. For example, people now have recourse against organizations such as schools and businesses that practice discrimination. When institutional discrimination occurs, assessment can identify the sources of and factors contributing to discrimination and the resources to combat it. Initially, the individual with a disability may be the primary beneficiary; however, assessments that include meso-level influences have farther-reaching consequences when institutional ableism and societal barriers that affect others as well are identified. This is illustrated in the following example of a student seeking a degree in education.

> Javier, a thirty-five-year-old Latino with a visual disability seeking a bachelor of science in education, filed an action with the ADA compliance committee of his university concerning discrimination he experienced in student teaching. He had been removed from his internship without warning. Reasons given for his termination were lateness in showing up for work, poorly prepared lesson plans, non-attendance of school functions, and failure to control students in class. Initially, Javier sought support to deal with his personal failure through a local organization for persons with visual disabilities. As the independent living specialist discussed Javier's situation, they jointly assessed a number of institutional procedural problems that hindered Javier's success. First, Javier had requested that the school accommodate his disability by finding a site near his home. Instead, he was placed in a school several miles from his home that had no public transportation access. As a result, he was dependent on others for transportation, which was inconsistent, and it was impossible for him to attend extracurricular activities. Second, his mentor teacher's style of mentoring was hands off; little attempt was made to orient Javier geographically. Finally, when students took advantage of Javier's visual disability, which limited his ability to teach effectively, the teacher did not consult with Javier to develop strategies to better control the class. Instead, the teacher stated that these problems were caused by Javier's disability, which limited his ability to teach effectively.
>
> In spite of these practices, Javier initially internalized his mentor teacher's view of his failure and regarded his dismissal as being caused by his inadequacies. By exploring micro-level as well as meso-level factors of psychosocial functioning, Javier began to recognize the environmental conditions that contributed to his problems. He was also able to identify areas in which he needed to grow to become an effective teacher. However, he began to reject the notions that the problem resided exclusively in himself. As a result, he filed a complaint

against the educational department of his university because it failed to reasonably accommodate his disability. Had his counselor focused only on emotional adjustment, his problems would have been assessed as coming from a lack of personal adjustment rather than the school environment. Javier's complaint was successful.

Social Structural Domain

Effective assessment must include an analysis of societal values and the laws, policies, and structures that support and are supported by those values, or what Bronfenbrenner (2005) labels the exo-system and macro-system levels. Rounds, Weil, and Bishop (1994) address the need for a multicultural perspective in dealing with families of children with disabilities. Within assessment and practice, several elements must be applied in maintaining the cultural domain. Cultural diversity must be not only recognized but valued. Different ethnic cultures deal with disability in different ways. In most cases, these differences need to be accounted for and regarded as strengths. Culture affects when and how certain individuals or families seek assistance; it affects how individuals participate in the human service framework. Practitioners must also be aware of their own cultural perspectives and how that affects the assessment process. Human service practitioners must recognize and understand the different levels of culture and how they interact. Fee (1994) points out the myriad of cultural levels within human service delivery systems for persons with disabilities. There is the ethnic culture of the individual and his or her family, the culture of the human service practitioner, the culture of the human service system, and the culture of Disability. All these cultures play into the process of assessment.

An important tool at the social structural level of social model assessments is the ethnographic interviewing technique. Originally utilized by anthropologists to obtain objective information about various ethnic cultures, this technique has been expanded into an interviewing process that can help human service practitioners understand the worldview from any cultural perspective. Green (1982) defines an ethnographic interview as one that is used to provide a description of the problem of the person the practitioner is working with from that person's worldview. The person with whom the practitioner is working becomes the teacher, guiding the practitioner into an understanding of his or her world. The ethnographic interviewing process assumes that language is the bridge to understanding the various cultures that are a part of the service provision. Words may have meanings that are understood only within a certain cultural context, even though the word may be used outside that culture. The human service practitioner must explore these words to get an understanding of the person's worldview. An example from disability culture is the term *crip*. *Cripple* has a certain meaning to mainstream culture. If a person without a disability refers to someone with a disability as crip, it is construed as pejorative. Within disability culture, however, when the term is used between persons with disabilities, it is one of kinship and belonging. Persons with disabilities may use the term in referring to themselves or to each other. But the term *supercrip* is one of disdain for a person with a disability. It means someone who is trying to prove that he or she is not disabled. To be called a supercrip by another person with a disability is not a good thing. Without this inside knowledge, the human service practitioner is at a loss to really understand the world of disability. But in order to find these pieces of information, the practitioner must ask within an ethnographic perspective (Green, 1982).

In the social component of assessment, it is important to recognize the many societal elements affecting persons with disabilities (Bilbao, Kennedy, Chatterji, Ustun, Barquero, & Barth, 2003) in terms of their biosocial, psychosocial, and social structural functioning. The flow of energy in support systems is also important—the social model recognizes that not only are people affected by their environments, but they affect their environments as well. The independent living movement is built around the concept of people affecting their environments. On the social structural level, Herling (1996) states that "only the systematic and intentional building of local organizations owned by, and dedicated to the empowerment of people with disabilities will change the societal structures that perpetuate injustice. [The] primary goal is to organize [people] with disabilities and empower them to take an active role in shaping their lives and circumstances" (p. 26).

Therefore, a systematic evaluation of the impact that people have—and have the potential to have—on their environments is crucial. This can be facilitated through a personal-professional collaboration in assessing all systems—biosocial through social structural.

Social-ecological assessment evaluates the impact of social structures and institutions on people's lives. For disabled persons it starts with an acknowledgment of the power differences and social conditions that disempower them and make them vulnerable to abuse and devaluation (Sobsey, 1994). For example, in assessing the employment of a person with a health-related disability, it may be essential to evaluate the impact of health policies and practices, vocational agencies, and business. This is illustrated in the following case.

> Erica was a twenty-seven-year-old woman diagnosed with schizophrenia who approached a vocational rehabilitation agency for help finding work. Since age twenty, Erica had been in and out of psychiatric institutions. She had a high school diploma, but few skills to make her employable. She had begun taking Clozaril six months earlier with very positive results. Hallucinations and delusions had subsided, and her isolation decreased dramatically. She became more social and desired to seek employment. Unfortunately, the social barriers were formidable. Erica was supported by SSI and received Medicaid, which paid for her Clozaril. Since she was unskilled and had a psychiatric history, she could

only find employment in low-paying jobs that had no benefits. If she took a job at this level, she would lose her SSI and Medicaid coverage. The costs of medication and ongoing mental health treatment made the price of employment prohibitive. When Erica sought vocational rehabilitation, she was informed that they could find her a lower-paying job but could not afford to provide her with the education she desired to obtain adequate employment.

An evaluation of the biosocial and psychosocial domains of Erica's life would focus on her mental health disability as the cause of her unemployment. A social structural evaluation, however, uncovers the institutional barriers to self-sufficiency. This assessment clarifies the lack of resources to reach goals. The federal/state Medicaid system makes it nearly impossible for some persons to work and live because working renders them ineligible for needed health and mental health coverage. The SSI system allows people to work for a short time, but ineligibility can be a significant deterrent. State and federal funding of vocational rehabilitation agencies makes people unable to procure essential services. Whereas individuals and small groups can have a relatively strong impact at the biosocial and psychosocial levels, it generally takes a collective effort to change societal systems, policies, and practices. Assessments of the environment by groups of people can lead to collective action and social change that is impossible for individuals alone to achieve. Passage of laws such as the Americans with Disabilities Act is an example of collective action. The movement of persons with intellectual disabilities out of institutions and into the community is another example of institutional change brought about by grassroots efforts and the collective voices of advocates.

UNIVERSAL DESIGN AND UNIVERSAL ACCESS

To fully assess people in their environments, a comprehensive assessment of the environment is critical. A fair question to use to guide assessment is, To what extent are communities and society designed to be inclusive of people and groups with diverse characteristics, both typical and atypical? Social policies upon which affirmative action and reasonable accommodation practices are based have been critical to the advancement of devalued groups, including persons with disabilities. Implicit in affirmative action and reasonable accommodation is the need to redress or provide relief to people who have been disadvantaged by society. When special laws and policies are needed to provide equal opportunities, it is assumed that laws and policies disadvantage them in the first place. We argue for the promotion of a society that uses universal design and promotes universal access for all. Rather than creating a society for those who are considered normal, then making special accommodations for those who differ from the norm, we should embrace people of all diverse characteristics, which could lead to a society universally accessible to all. For example, curb cuts and power doors were originally designed to accommodate people with mobility disabilities. However, these accommodations make society more accessible for parents pushing strollers and people whose arms are full. One of the authors has excellent hearing but routinely uses captions to watch television when working out at his fitness club. The first functional typewriters were developed to help blind persons communicate; however, keyboards are essential in the lives of most people who are reading these words. Recently, when traveling through Europe using the Eurorail, one of the authors, who is monolingual in English, was relieved to find universally accessible signage that guided him to trains—thus negating his need to read German, Italian, French, Swiss, Flemish, Danish, and Dutch.

The principle of universal access grew out of the concept of universal design, which was developed in professions such as architecture and engineering and applied to the physical world. Ron Mace, a physically disabled wheelchair-using architect, is credited with coining the term *universal design* to describe environments and communities that are designed to be accessible to the greatest extent possible to everyone, regardless of their age, characteristics, capabilities, or status in life (North Carolina State University, College of Design, 2006).

Mace, an advocate for disabled persons and a proponent of universal design, saw the benefits of universal design extending far beyond the disability community. He became internationally recognized as an architect, product designer, and educator whose philosophy challenged convention and provided a design foundation for a more usable world. Shortly before his death, Mace (1998) spoke of his belief that universal design benefits everyone. Universal design's "focus is not specifically on people with disabilities, but all *people.* . . . We tend to discount people who are less than what we popularly consider to be 'normal.' To be 'normal' is to be perfect, capable, competent, and independent. Unfortunately, designers in our society also mistakenly assume that everyone fits this definition of 'normal.' This just is not the case."

Mace joined forces with a working group of architects, product designers, engineers, and environmental design researchers at the Center for Universal Design at North Carolina State University who define universal design as "The design of products and environments to be useable by all people, to the greatest extent possible, without the need for adaptation or special design" (Connell, Jones, Mace, Mueller, Mullick, Ostroff, et al., 1997). Their seven principles of universal design, listed below, were initially developed for the physical environment but have wide applicability. In the two examples of each principle, note how the principles of universal design benefit not only disabled users, but a wide range of people.

1. Equitable use. The design is useful and marketable to people with diverse abilities. Designs provide identical or equivalent use for all,

with privacy and safety in mind, and without segregating or stigmatizing diverse users.

- ○ Bathrooms with stalls that are large enough for wheelchairs
- ○ Men's and women's bathrooms

2. Flexibility in use. The design accommodates a wide range of individual preferences and abilities.
   - ○ Ramp and power doors in a public library
   - ○ Power doors in a grocery store for shoppers with large bags of groceries

3. Simple and intuitive. The design is easy to understand and use regardless of the user's experience, knowledge, language skills, or current concentration level.
   - ○ Web site with alt tabs to guide visually impaired users
   - ○ Web site with prominently marked graphics to guide users

4. Perceptible information. The design communicates necessary information effectively to the user, regardless of ambient conditions or the user's sensory abilities.
   - ○ Captioned television for deaf persons
   - ○ Television marketing ad in which a phone number is simultaneously spoken and shown on the screen

5. Tolerance for error. The design minimizes hazards and the adverse consequences of accidental or unintended actions.
   - ○ Spell checks for people with cognitive disabilities, who tend to confuse the letters *d* and *b* and *p* and *q*
   - ○ Keyboard that corrects spelling errors before documents are printed

6. Low physical effort. The design can be used efficiently and comfortably with a minimum of fatigue.
   - ○ Bathrooms with under-sink access for wheelchair users
   - ○ Baby diaper changing table in men's and women's bathrooms

7. Size and space for approach and use. Appropriate size and space is provided for approach, reach, manipulation, and use regardless of the user's body size, posture, or mobility.
   - ○ Drinking fountains of multiple heights accessible to people of short stature
   - ○ Drinking fountains of multiple heights accessible to children

We believe an accurate social-ecological assessment based on the social model must include a critical analysis of the extent to which communities and societies are constructed and organized to welcome the broadest range of diversity, including, but not limited to, all types of disabilities. Principles of universal access are a way of measuring this goal against the current reality.

SUMMARY

Human service professionals working with disabled persons invariably engage in assessments. Traditional assessment models have focused on the presence or absence of pathology, and an assessment of problems is essential in many contexts. However, the exclusive focus on pathology has had negative consequences in long-term involvement. This is especially true in human services. By attending primarily to problems, assessments can fail to account for individual strengths. A deficiency focus can lead to the devaluing and, in some cases, dehumanizing of people. The individual pathology focus also fails to recognize the complexity of experiences and relationships.

The approach that best meets the needs of persons with disabilities takes a social model rather than individual pathology approach to disability. Effective assessments are contextual; that is, the context in which the assessment occurs determines the nature and extent of the assessment. There are several elements in approaching assessment from a social perspective. A critical component of the independent living approach is that individuals identify their own needs. In the social model, a critical element of assessment is the environment. The social model emphasizes people's strengths and potential. It acknowledges that disabled persons have impairments but contends that they are not defined by their disabilities. The social model of disability emphasizes the importance of institutionalized oppression and devaluation to which people with disabilities have been subjected. It also acknowledges that disabled people have the right to control their resources and to determine how resources are expended.

We have introduced you to social-ecological assessment, which is based on the social model. Social-ecological assessments attend to the multiple and interrelated influences on people's lives: biosocial, psychosocial, and social structural. Finally, we introduced you to the concept of universal access. Ultimately, to fully embrace diversity, we cannot settle for a society that is designed for the majority and makes allowances for those who do not fit the mold. Instead, we must strive for a society that is set up for all: minority and majority, disabled and nondisabled.

DISCUSSION QUESTIONS

1. What are some of the issues around a medical model of assessment? What are the advantages and disadvantages of using it in work with persons with disabilities?
2. Explain the individual components of a social model of assessment. How could you use it if you are working in a health facility that requires a pathologically based assessment model?
3. Relate the micro, meso, and macro components of the social model of assessment to Cowger's (1994) statement "Assessment that focuses

on deficits provides obstacles to clients exercising personal and social power and reinforces those social structures that generate and regulate the unequal power relationships that victimize clients" (p. 264).

4. Compare the following two assessments in terms of descriptions of disability, impairment, and function:

Mr. Anderson is an African American male, age nineteen, with an average IQ, who was severely injured in a motorcycle accident. Mr. Anderson never completed high school. His injury resulted in partial paralysis of both his arms and legs. He has limited hand movement. Mr. Anderson suffers chronic depression, for which he takes medication.

Mr. Anderson is severely limited in his mobility. He is confined to a wheelchair and totally dependent on attendants or family members to prepare his food, bathe him, attend to his bowel program, and so on. His family was uncooperative in his rehabilitation. They missed appointments. They did not follow through on suggestions to make the apartment more accessible. Mr. Anderson appears to have limited ambition toward education or employment. He rarely gets out in the community, other than in his immediate neighborhood. He does not take advantage of community resources made available to him.

Mr. Anderson is a nineteen-year-old African American male with partial paralysis from a motorcycle accident who lives with his mother and his younger brother in a housing project. Several of his relatives live in the same project, and they stop in frequently to visit. His family is very close. They agreed that that he will stay with them rather than be institutionalized or live on his own. Mr. Anderson has trained his family to provide his attendant care under his supervision. Attendants from a local agency also provide personal care. With assistive devices, he is able to feed himself and transfer between bed and wheelchair. His emotional status has improved significantly since he began using antidepressants.

Mr. Anderson gets along well in the neighborhood, using a wheelchair for community mobility. The apartment building is wheelchair accessible; however, he lacks financial resources to make his bathroom completely accessible. He uses a portable commode chair to make do. He visits other family members frequently. He gets out into the neighborhood quite often, and various store owners watch out for him.

Mr. Anderson visits the local Radio Shack, where Ralph Henderson, the owner, takes time to show him how to use a computer on display. Mr. Anderson is giving Ralph $10 a week toward the purchase of a computer. Mr. Anderson has talked about obtaining a GED and is thinking about going to school to learn computer programming.

What assumptions are being made in the first assessment? What are the assumptions in the second assessment? What things are left out of the first assessment? What components are missing in the second assessment? Which assessment more accurately reflects the perceptions of the person in question?

5. Martin and Julie Torgesson are proudly awaiting the confirmation of eight-year-old Martin Jr. Martin, a deacon in the congregation, and Julie, who is active in the women's auxiliary, anticipate that much of their community will attend the Sunday picnic following the confirmation. Martin's parents are active in preparations and fondly recall the confirmations of their three older children, of whom Martin is the second son. Though the confirmation will be attended by their families and a few other members of their congregation, the Torgessons have worked with Pastor James and the church board to invite lapsed members and non-church members to the subsequent festivities in the hopes of engaging them in church and community fellowship. Martin Jr.'s sister Bryn was confirmed only eighteen months earlier, when she turned eight, and his younger siblings, twins Marj and Damon, look forward to their confirmation in three years. Of course Esther, at age two, is too young to understand what was happening but could still feel the excitement in the air.

Like the other children, Esther was born at home, but soon after her birth, Martin and Julie were informed that she had trisomy 21, otherwise known as Down syndrome. The Torgesson's consider Esther their "little gift from God" and once a week take Esther to a program for children with intellectual disabilities in the city, an hour's drive from their home. Costs for this program are covered under the Individuals with Disabilities Education Act. A major concern for the Torgessons, however, is that they just learned Esther needs heart surgery to correct a defect associated with her Down syndrome.

To understand the Torgessons, let's take a look at their family and community history. Of proud northern European Protestant heritage, Martin Sr. is the fourth-generation son to take over operation of the five-hundred-acre grain farm from his father in their northwestern community of 1,200—if you include the outlying farms. Julie is a third-generation community member whose parents ran a farm just ten miles from Martin's. While Martin manages the farm's commercial operations, Julie is responsible for the household and also the large garden, chickens for eggs, the steer butchered annually for beef, and the milk cow.

Martin and Julie moved into the family home when Martin took over operation of the farm, and his parents, who are in their sixties and both in good health, still reside there, though they travel frequently. Julie is the oldest of four siblings, and her parents, who are in their fifties, still operate their farm. Martin and Julie knew each other from their childhoods and within a year of Julie's graduation from high school, two years after Martin's, they married. Both had looked forward to continuing the farming family tradition since their youth.

Though excited about the upcoming event, there are several stresses the Torgessons are facing. Though they are moderately self-sufficient in raising their own food, their farm's survival lasts year to year. First, small farms have become increasingly rare as large conglomerates buy land and operate on smaller profit margins per acre. Second, crop prices fluctuate from year to year, and the weather is always an uncertainty. Thus, the Torgessons are frequently forced to borrow money every spring in the hopes that their harvests will cover expenses each fall. And now, they are faced with Esther's impending heart surgery.

In addition to stresses with the farm, recent family events are affecting their lives. Martin's mother was just diagnosed with breast cancer. Though it is stage 1 cancer and highly treatable, the costs will exceed Medicare coverage, and the diagnosis has rocked their world. In addition, Julie just received news that her younger sister Ruth has just separated from her husband and moved back to their parents' home with her two daughters, ages seven and five. Circumstances of the marriage and separation were especially distressing. Ruth met her husband in high school when their respective schools, located twenty-five miles apart, played each other in basketball. Ruth was a cheerleader, and her future husband, Troy, was a player for the other team. Both were seniors when they met, and by April, Ruth was pregnant. They married shortly after graduating, and Ruth moved in with Troy and his parents, where they lived until they had their first baby. Subsequently, Troy obtained work at the town's paper mill, working there until the present time. Ruth's marriage has been rocky for years; Troy has repeatedly abused alcohol, and there have been domestic violence incidents. However, recently problems worsened when their oldest daughter told a teacher that her daddy had touched her in a bad place. Ruth has always been considered rebellious by the family (who had never been fond of Troy), but although her return home has increased family stress greatly, she was welcomed home with open arms. A final stressor is related to Martin's older brother Reuben, who is in the military. As the oldest Torgesson son, Reuben had the option of taking over the family farm; however, from a young age he expressed his desire to "get out of Hicksville," and he joined the Marines immediately after his eighteenth birthday. Reuben's grandfather had served in the army in World War II, and an uncle in the Marines in Vietnam, and Reuben was proud to follow in a family tradition—as well as to see the world. Reuben has been deployed to the Middle East in the "war on terror," but his exact whereabouts are classified. The family does, however, assume Reuben is in harm's way.

Your task is to engage in an evaluation of the Torgesson family. Assume a role as a human service worker in one of three contexts: (1) you are a counselor seeing Martin and Julie for marriage counseling; (2) you are a health care worker involved in Esther's case relative to surgery; (3) you are a financial aid worker for the state.

   a. Assess the biosocial, psychosocial, and social structural domains relative to this family.
   b. Outline the three elements of an evaluation: history (what), evaluation (so what), and plan (now what).
   c. How would the application of the principle of universal access to health care affect your evaluation?
   d. Now, assume that you are a loan officer at the local credit union, and Martin and Julie are approaching you for a loan to purchase a new tractor to replace their current dilapidated tractor. How would the current social structural policies and practices influence your decisions relative to loaning them money?

SUGGESTED READINGS

Blotzer, M. A., & Ruth, R. (1995). On sitting with uncertainty: Treatment considerations for persons with disabilities. In M. A. Blotzer & R. Ruth (Eds.), *Sometimes you just want to feel like a human being: Case studies of empowering psychotherapy with people with disabilities* (pp. 15–24). Baltimore: Paul H. Brookes.

Brown, W. V. (1996). *In search of freedom: How people with disabilities have been disenfranchised from the mainstream of American society.* Springfield, IL: Charles C. Thomas.

Cowger, C. D. (1994). Assessing client strengths: Clinical assessment for client empowerment. *Social Work, 39*(3), 262–268.

Szymanski, E. M., & Trueba, H. T. (1994). Castification of people with disabilities: Potential disempowering aspects of classification in disability services. *Journal of Rehabilitation, 60*(3), 12–20.

REFERENCES

Bilbao, A., Kennedy, C., Chatterji, S., Ustun, B., Barquero, J. L. & Barth, T. (2003). The ICF: Applications of the WHO model of functioning, disability and health to brain injury rehabilitation. *NeuroRehabilitation, 18*(3), 239–250.

Blotzer, M. A., & Ruth, R. (1995). On sitting with uncertainty: Treatment considerations for persons with disabilities. In M. A. Blotzer & R. Ruth (Eds.), *Sometimes you just want to feel like a human being: Case studies of empowering psychotherapy with people with disabilities* (pp. 15–24). Baltimore: Paul H. Brookes.

Bronfenbrenner, U. (Ed.). (2005). *Making human beings human: Bioecological perspectives on human development*. Thousand Oaks, CA: Sage.

Brown, P. J., Barrett, R. L., & Padilla, M. B. (1998). Medical anthropology: An introduction to the fields. In P. J. Brown (Ed.), *Understanding and applying medical anthropology* (pp. 10–19). Mountain View, CA: Mayfield.

Brown, W. V. (1996). *In search of freedom: How people with disabilities have been disenfranchised from the mainstream of American society*. Springfield, IL: Charles C. Thomas.

Condeluci, A. (1995). *Interdependence: The route to community* (2nd ed.). Winter Park, FL: GR Press.

Connell, B., Jones, M., Mace, R., Mueller, J., Mullick, A., Ostroff, E., et al. (1997). *The Center for Universal Design, version 2.0*. Retrieved April 10, 2006, from http://www.design.ncsu.edu/cud/about_ud/udprinciplestext.htm

Cowger, C. D. (1994). Assessing client strengths: Clinical assessment for client empowerment. *Social Work, 39*(3), 262–268.

Crewe, N. M., & Zola I. K. (1983). *Independent living and physically disabled people: Developing, implementing and evaluating self help rehabilitation programs*. San Francisco: Jossey-Bass.

Damasso, A. R. (1994). *Descartes' error: Emotion, reason, and the human brain*. New York: Avon.

DeJong, G. (1979). *The movement for independent living: Origins, ideology, and implications for disability research*. East Lansing: Michigan State University, Center for International Rehabilitation.

Fee, F. A. (1994). An introduction to multicultural issues in spinal cord injury rehabilitation. *SCI Psychosocial Process, 7*(3), 104–107.

Fine, M., & Asch, A. (1993). Disability beyond stigma: Social interaction, discrimination, and activism. In M. Nagler (Ed.), *Perspectives on disability: Text and readings on disability* (2nd ed., pp. 61–74). Palo Alto, CA: Health Markets Research.

Green, J. W. (1982). *Cultural awareness in the human services*. Englewood Cliffs, NJ: Prentice Hall.

Hahn, H. (1991). Alternate views of empowerment: Social services and civil rights. *Journal of Rehabilitation, 57*(4), 17–19.

Hepworth, D. H., Rooney, R. H., Larsen, J., Rooney, G. D., & Strom-Gottfried, K. (2005). *Direct social work practice: Theory and skills* (7th ed.). Pacific Grove, CA: Brooks/Cole.

Herling, D. (1996). Keeping promises: Coalition of Montanans concerned with disabilities. *Rural Exchange, 9*(2), 26–28.

Mace, R. (1998). *A perspective on universal design*. Retrieved April 10, 2006, from http://www.design.ncsu.edu/cud/newweb/about_center/ronmacespeech.htm

North Carolina State University, College of Design. (2006). *Center for universal design*. Retrieved April 10, 2006, from http://ncsudesign.org/content/index.cfm/fuseaction/alum_profile/departmentID/1/startRow/3

Mackelprang, R. W. (1986). *Social and emotional adjustment following spinal cord injury*. Unpublished doctoral dissertation. University of Utah. Salt Lake City.

Mackelprang, R. W., & Hepworth, D. H. (1987). Ecological factors in the rehabilitation of people with severe spinal cord injuries. *Social Work in Health Care, 13*, 23–38.

Mackelprang, R. W., & Mackelprang, R. D. (2005). Historical and contemporary issues in end-of-life decisions: Implications for social work. *Social Work: Journal of the National Association of Social Workers, 50*(4), 315–324.

Mackelprang, R. W., & Salsgiver, R. O. (1996). People with disabilities and social work: Historical and contemporary issues. *Social Work, 41*(1), 7–14.

Miley, K. K., O'Melia, M., & DuBois, B. L. (1995). *Generalist social work practice: An empowering approach.* Boston: Allyn & Bacon.

Rosenthal, M. (1989). Psychosocial evaluation of physically disabled persons. In B. W. Heller, L. M. Flohr, & L. S. Zegans (Eds.), *Psychosocial interventions with physically disabled persons* (pp. 43–57). New Brunswick, NJ: Rutgers University Press.

Rounds, K. A., Weil, M., & Bishop, K. K. (1994). Practice with culturally diverse families of young children with disabilities. *Families in Society: Journal of Contemporary Human Services, 38*, 3–13.

Saleebey, D. (1996). The strengths perspective in social work practice: Extensions and cautions. *Social Work, 41*(3), 296–305.

Salsgiver, R. O. (1996). Perspectives on families with children with disabilities. *SCI Psychosocial Process, 9*(1), 18–23.

Sapolsky, R. M. (1998). *Why zebras don't get ulcers.* New York: Freeman.

Schuler, A. L., & Perez, L. (1991). Assessment: Current concerns and future directions. In L. H. Myer, C. A. Peck, & L. Brown (Eds.), *Critical issues in the lives of people with severe disabilities* (pp. 101–106). Baltimore: Paul H. Brookes.

Sobsey, D. (1994). *Violence and abuse in the lives of people with disabilities: The end of silent acceptance?* Baltimore: Paul H. Brooks.

Strom, K. (1992). Reimbursement demands and treatment decisions: A growing dilemma for social workers. *Social Work, 37*(5), 398–403.

Szymanski, E. M., & Trueba, H. T. (1994). Castification of people with disabilities: Potential disempowering aspects of classification in disability services. *Journal of Rehabilitation, 60*(3), 12–20.

Trieschmann, R. B. (1980). *Spinal cord injuries: Psychosocial, social, and vocational adjustment.* New York: Pergamon.

14

Models of Practice

I had a real role model here at the center for independent living—my supervisor, a licensed clinical social worker. Since that
time, there has never been a doubt in my mind that I am a person
with a disability. It is so much a part of who I am today. It feels
liberating. I swore to myself I would never hide anything about
my disability.

—Abby Kovalsky, Jewish Family and Children's Services,
San Francisco, California

STUDENT LEARNING OBJECTIVES

1. To be able to identify how traditional models of practice stem from an
   individual pathological perspective
2. To be able to analyze the functional use and limitations of the individual
   pathological perspective in human service provision
3. To be able to identify the strengths and limitations of the strengths-based,
   empowerment, case management, and independent approaches to
   human service provision
4. To be able to compare and contrast the provision of case management
   and independent living models of practice on the individual level, the
   community level, and the societal level
5. To understand the mechanisms by which effective practice models view
   the disability community as a source of change and power

MODELS OF PRACTICE IN HUMAN SERVICE PROVISION

There are numerous models of practice in the human service field. Among
the more noted and fundamental models of practice with individuals and
families are psychoanalysis; Gestalt psychology; cognitive, behavioral, existential, problem-solving, and client-centered therapy; the task-centered
model of social work; crisis counseling; ego psychology; transactional analysis; psychosocial theory; and the life model and casework approaches
(Turner, 1986). Some of the more recent models are case management, generalist and advanced generalist, empowerment, strengths-based, and brief
intervention approaches (Johnson, 1995). Some contemporary professional

practice models approach intervention not just with individuals and families but at the systems level as well. This includes intervention to solve problems in agencies and organizations, neighborhoods, and communities (Neugeboren, 1991).

Most traditional models of practice stem from an individual pathological perspective. These models see individuals and families in need as dysfunctional or impaired. Traditional approaches have proved valuable for large numbers of people. They have helped people overcome problems, develop strengths, and enhance their lives. We acknowledge the importance of these models in individual and family practice. However, traditional models do not account for the devaluation and oppression experienced by disabled people as a group. As a rule, society views disability as a problem, and people with disabilities as innately deficient. Therefore, the individual repair focus of traditional therapies can reinforce ableism and classism by failing to recognize the environment as a primary locus of problems for persons with disabilities. Traditional models focus on helping individuals cope with or overcome problems associated with their disabilities rather than emphasizing the social devaluation and institutional ableism associated with having a disability.

The professional emphasis on making the individual as "perfect" as possible originally stemmed from the Enlightenment period (Mackelprang & Salsgiver, 1996; Rhodes, 1993). Later versions of this perspective have taken into account the environment as a factor in people's problems; however, they have stressed helping individuals cope with the environment rather than changing the environment to meet people's needs. Traditional models view people with disabilities in the role of patient or client. Physicians, counselors, social workers, therapists, rehabilitation workers, and other professionals apply their expertise and knowledge to the patient or client in order to "cure" the affliction or abnormality. The patient or client, in turn, is expected to play a passive role in responding to the expertise and knowledge of the professional (Tower, 1994). Environmental intervention is contemplated only as a means of helping the individual cope, and it is rarely attempted as a way of changing a dysfunctional system (Mackelprang, 1986).

More recent models of practice offer alternative approaches and are particularly applicable to persons with disabilities. Here we discuss four current approaches. The first two, the strengths and empowerment approaches, provide conceptual frameworks that focus on potential and capabilities. The third, case management, is a widely used professional modality that acknowledges the need for community and personal involvement. In each of the first three models, professionals assume leadership responsibilities for clients. The fourth, the independent living model, which was developed and nurtured within the disability community, is built on a foundation of self-determination and civil rights for persons with disabilities in which people in need are seen as participants or consumers of services.

THE STRENGTHS APPROACH AND POSITIVE PSYCHOLOGY

It is critical that human service professionals see people with disabilities as people, not as disabilities housing people. It has been far too common and easy for human service practitioners to view people from a deficit-focused, pathology-based perspective (Cowger, 1994; Hepworth, Rooney, Larsen, Rooney, & Strom-Gottfried, 2005), especially persons with disabilities. In contrast, when approaching people from a strengths perspective (Saleebey, 1992), human service practitioners focus on capabilities, capacities, and opportunities rather than limitations. Just as importantly, as Cowger (1994) suggests, practitioners begin to "nourish, encourage, assist, enable, support, stimulate, and unleash the strengths within people, to illuminate the strengths available to people in their own environment, and to promote equity and justice at all levels of society" (p. 246).

The strengths view of practice also "comes from an awareness that US culture and helping professionals are saturated with psychosocial approaches based on individual, family, and community pathology, deficits, problems, abnormality, victimization, and disorder. A conglomeration of businesses, professions, institutions, and individuals—from medicine to the pharmaceutical industry, from the insurance industry to the media—assure the nation that everyone has a storehouse of vulnerabilities" (Saleebey, 1996, p. 296).

Similar to the strengths perspective is positive psychology. The Positive Psychology Center (2007) emphasizes strengths and virtues that enable individuals and communities to thrive. Positive psychology has three central concerns: positive emotions, positive individual traits, and positive institutions. Understanding positive emotions entails the study of contentment with the past, happiness in the present, and hope for the future.

Seligman (2002) suggests that positive psychology can be divided into three life goals. A person who is living a *pleasant life* or life of enjoyment is able to experience the positive emotions and feelings that come from healthy living. A person who is living a *good life* has achieved a match between his or her strengths and interests and life activities. A person who is living a *meaningful life* has a sense of purpose and satisfaction with his or her contributions to society and culture, and a sense of belonging in social groups and in the community.

Practitioners who use approaches such as the strengths perspective and positive psychology focus on the capabilities and potential of the individuals with whom they work. In addition, rather than concentrating exclusively on the individual, they attend to the environment. They acknowledge the influence of communities, social structures, and institutions. Practice transcends efforts to help individuals improve their lives and becomes political, as "its thrust is the development of client power and the equitable distribution of societal resources" (Cowger, 1994, p. 264). For example, in dealing with the lack of housing, practitioners using a strengths or positive psychology approach could consider several areas. They might assist with personal problems that individuals who cannot obtain housing might experience, such as isolation and depression. They could also work to help them obtain accessible and affordable housing. In addition, they could work within the community to increase the availability of such housing and to influence social policy. Finally, they might work with persons with disabilities individually and collectively to facilitate their involvement to affect their communities and to influence public policies.

Human service practitioners employing strengths or positive psychology approaches work to help clients nurture and generate their individual strengths and control their own lives. In conjunction with individual with disabilities, they work to make communities respond equitably to all people. They acknowledge societal structures and economic forces and work to promote social policies and structures that are based on principles of social justice. Practice then becomes a consumer-driven partnership that encompasses micro, meso, and macro levels of intervention.

EMPOWERMENT

The empowerment approach gained popularity in the last decades of the twentieth century. Empowerment seeks to help people take control over their lives. It shares many components of the strengths perspective. Gutierrez (1990) defines this practice model as "a process of increasing personal, interpersonal, or political power so that individuals can take action to improve their life situations. Empowerment theory and practice have roots in community organization methods, adult education techniques, feminist theory, and political psychology" (p. 142).

Miley, O'Melia, and DuBois (1995) view the empowerment intervention model as focusing on three areas: the client's strengths, the resources that exist in the client's neighborhood and community, and a vision that solutions are possible. The outcome of empowerment is the client's increased control over the social and organizational environment (Cohen, 1994; Emener, 1991).

Solomon (1976) outlines the roles of a human service provider in the empowerment process. A key role is that of *resource consultant*. Practitioners link clients with resources in their neighborhoods or communities. At times, these resources may be national in scope. Of course, for the practitioner, this means having knowledge of the array of available resources in the community. The resource consultant fosters independence, not dependency, by actively involving the client in the process of finding and utilizing resources: "It involves linking clients to resources in a manner that enhances their self-esteem as well as their problem-solving capacities. The consultant's knowledge of the resource systems and expertise in using these systems are placed at the disposal of the client and his participation in the process from identification to location to utilization is intensive" (Solomon, 1976, p. 347).

The human service provider also acts as a *sensitizer* by helping the client discover past or present life situations that may hinder self-fulfillment and empowerment. It is within this role that the practitioner helps the client perceive stereotypes and societal barriers that, on a personal level, reinforce self-doubt and in some cases self-hatred. Solomon sees the practitioner's role of *teacher/trainer* as crucial in the empowering process. This role focuses specifically on helping the client master tasks related to solving problems of social living. Last, Solomon (1976) describes one of the most important roles of the practitioner: *placing the client in the role of service provider*. This results in two things: "It provides an opportunity for the client to step out of the supplicant role of one who seeks advice into the more favored position of helper or one who provides service" (p. 354). It also allows the individual receiving the help from the client to gain wisdom and insight from someone who has been through it, someone who has experienced the problem and situation firsthand. In the independent living model, this is known as peer counseling. The knowledge gained from the experience of living with the disability often surpasses the knowledge of the practitioner who only has theoretical insight and practice wisdom.

Gutierrez (1990) outlines additional empowerment techniques. First, the practitioner accepts the client's perceptions of problems and needs. In doing this, the practitioner is acknowledging the client's competence and the individual's right to self-determination and personal control. In addition, the practitioner helps the individual assess existing strengths and build new ones. The practitioner should also facilitate a power assessment with the client on both the personal and neighborhood/community levels: What are the conditions resulting in powerlessness? What sources of power exist for the client? Furthermore, the practitioner advocates for the client to help him or her get needed services and resources. Practitioners do not empower clients; people empower themselves. Professionals can be tools to help people identify, nurture, and develop internal competencies and external resources for self-empowerment.

CASE MANAGEMENT

In the last decade of the twentieth century, case management emerged as a preeminent method of providing human services. Case management is similar to the old casework model of practice in social work (Moore, 1990); however, ideally case management emphasizes professional involvement with systems that affect clients rather than focusing primarily on micro-system interventions. Rothman (1991) presents this succinct definition of case management: "Case management incorporates two broad junctions: (1) providing individualized advice, counseling, and therapy to clients in the community and (2) linking clients to needed services and supports in community agencies and informal helping networks. Case management, in professional terms, is both micro and macro in nature. It entails both individual practice and community practice in integrated form" (pp. 520–521). In addition, case management assumes long-term care management with a coordination of a wide range of services from the community.

In utilizing case management techniques with persons with severe disabilities, the case manager does an assessment and seeks the required services for the individual, which may include housing, health and mental health care, socialization, day activities/recreation, and education. As the necessary services are obtained and utilized, the case manager continually monitors each case to ensure that the services are maintained. Case managers must be extremely knowledgeable about the groups they serve. They work in numerous settings, including group homes, long-term care facilities, acute care settings, and foster care environments (Netting, 1992). They utilize various roles such as counselor, advocate, educator, and mediator on behalf of their clients (Mackelprang & Salsgiver, 1996). A strength of the case management approach is the attention given to multiple system levels. In addition, professionals assume a variety of roles and functions in response to client needs.

Case management, however, has significant limitations. In this approach, professionals are the experts on whom clients or "cases" rely for services. Case managers, not clients, maintain control over decisions. In addition, current case management has evolved in an era of cutbacks and cost containment. Quality and access to care have been limited to reduce costs. Therefore, case managers have been forced to reduce services and limit client eligibility. The limitations of case management are due, in part, to the fact that case management is practiced primarily under the auspices of agencies and institutions that adopt mainstream perceptions of people with disabilities. Therefore, case managers are often in roles that perpetuate professional control and "case" dependence.

On a social structural level, case management developed and evolved in the late 1980s and 1990s, a time of increasing demand for and diminishing resources in health, mental health, and social services. Frankel and Gelman (2004) state that the goals of case management are to ensure access, facilitate coordination, and reduce fragmentation of services. They differentiate between case management and managed care, and its goals of coordinating care, reducing unnecessary services, and reducing costs. While the objectives of case management as described by Frankel and Gelman are laudable, in an era of managed care, case managers are often compelled to act as gatekeepers and forced to limit access to care (Johnson & Mackelprang, 1995). Consider the example of case management in a nonprofit publicly funded mental health program. The agency charges a monthly fee per client regardless of the level of services provided each client. In addition, the agency is penalized if the proportion of clients referred for inpatient services exceeds a predetermined formula. Consequently, case managers are faced with competing demands to provide adequate services and to hold costs down by limiting services and seeking the least expensive treatments. In medicine, primary health care providers experience similar constraints, as they are discouraged from providing tests and referring patients to specialists. In fact, some managed care contracts provide monetary incentives for limiting costs and access to care.

THE INDEPENDENT LIVING MODEL

Though case management is an extant model of professional practice, a more progressive model of involvement is the independent living model of practice, where, in effect, consumers manage their own cases—their own lives. Whereas case management's roots are deeply embedded in professional practice, the independent living (IL) model is derived from the minority perspective and the social model of viewing disability. The minority perspective assumes that people with disabilities are minorities and have been denied opportunities that nondisabled persons take for granted. The social model assumes that the greatest obstacles facing persons with disabilities are devaluation, lack of opportunity, and oppression (DeJong, 1979).

Civil rights laws such as the ADA and other national laws, the 2007 UN convention on disability rights, and policies such as affirmative action and reasonable accommodation have been implemented to address and to redress the obstacles disabled persons face. These laws and policies are re-shaping the discussion of disability as pathology to discussion of disability as a form of diversity and as a civil rights issue.

The IL perspective differs from traditional approaches to disability, which begin with the assumption that individual deficiencies are the primary reasons that people seek services (DeLoach, Wilkins, & Walker, 1983). In defining problems, the IL model first looks to the social and environmental deficiencies with which a person with a disability lives (Zola, 1983). This contrasts sharply with professional models that assume problems arise primarily from within individuals. The IL perspective suggests that problems reside primarily within nonadaptive and hostile environments. Pity, lack of physical access, and limited opportunities are the primary problems facing people with mobility disabilities, not their need to use wheelchairs for mobility. The primary problems for people with intellectual disabilities have been institutions that segregate and limit their opportunities, not their personal limitations. Fear, segregation, and stereotyping have been the primary constraints for persons with mental health disabilities. Lack of opportunity, not lack of capability, has been the primary problem for persons with disabilities as a group.

Traditional models view people with disabilities as patients and clients. The independent living model views persons with disabilities as individuals, citizens, consumers, and/or participants in service. The roles of professionals under the IL model are also different. They may be considered experts in their fields; however, that expertise does not translate into control over people's lives (White, Gutierrez, & Seekins, 1996). Instead, they act as consultants and assistants. Their roles are akin to those of financial investment consultants, who educate and sell investment packages to consumers. However, decisions rest with consumers, who decide whether they act on the advice of their consultants (Zola, 1983). In the IL model, consumers or participants may rely on physicians, social workers, and others for advice in a similar manner.

In the IL model, consumers are responsible for their own decisions about their lives. They may utilize the services of professionals such as physicians, social workers, nurses, and vocational counselors. However, professionals rely on the individual's direction rather than ordering or prescribing *for* the client.

A new role is also critical to the IL model. Peer or independent living counselors are key participants in this model. IL counselors work with consumers, as do other professionals. However, IL counselors are likely to have disabilities themselves and are committed to individual self-determination and control. Mackelprang and Salsgiver (1996) provide the following example of the contrasting approaches:

> Sharon is a 32-year-old woman who received social work case management services after an automobile accident in which she experienced a spinal cord injury resulting in quadriplegia. During Sharon's hospitalization, her social worker provided case management services, facilitating the procurement of Medicaid, ordering medical equipment such as a wheelchair, procuring the services of a home health agency for home nursing visits, arranging for vocational rehabilitation services, and working with Sharon's family to prepare for her discharge from the hospital. Similar case management services were provided for six months following discharge; the social worker generally informed Sharon of the services she would be providing, and Sharon also made requests for services.
>
> Six months after discharge from the hospital, Sharon became involved with a local independent living center for peer counseling and independent living training. When she had trouble with Medicaid, she asked the IL counselor to intervene on her behalf. Similarly, she asked the IL counselor to procure a commode chair. Rather than meet her requests as the social worker had done, the IL counselor taught Sharon to self-advocate with Medicaid and guided her through the process of ordering medical equipment so she could do so in the future. In addition, the counselor informed Sharon how she could gain access to a program in which she could hire and direct her attendants rather than having nurses and aides assigned to her. Sharon developed the knowledge and skills to direct her own personal care, including hiring, firing, and money management, essentially reclaiming control over her life. (p. 12)

In the preceding example, Sharon's social worker, acting in the role of case manager, thought the best way to help was to provide services. In contrast, the IL counselor sought to help Sharon develop the skills and recognize her ability to control the systems affecting her. The IL counselor assumed Sharon was capable of independence. Sharon needed physical attendant care; however, she learned to independently direct her care, to access systems, and to self-advocate. Though Sharon needed the social worker's help initially following her injury, she was capable of taking control of her life once the crisis of her spinal cord injury was over.

In the IL model, all helping professionals, including IL counselors, are expected to function within the parameters set by the individual consumer, who retains ultimate control (Tower, 1994). Just as financial consultants must leave decisions to individuals, IL proposes that individuals retain control over interventions and treatments, physical and psychosocial therapies, and other decisions. In multidisciplinary/interdisciplinary teamwork, the head of the team is the consumer. Professionals may consult, recommend, and suggest, but self-determination is paramount. Human service workers are often needed to help people make decisions by educating and counseling them and helping them obtain resources; however, this is done under the control and direction of the consumers.

In the IL model, the expectations for persons with disabilities differ greatly from other practice models. First, people with disabilities are perceived as competent. Traditional models of practice assume they need others, usually professionals, to take control and make decisions, essentially assuming people with disabilities are incompetent. The IL model presupposes that people with disabilities are fully functioning human beings (Zola, 1983). Traditional models treat people with disabilities as the "worthy poor," who receive services and financial sustenance from a sympathetic society. The IL model expects society to remove barriers that deny full participation to persons with disabilities; at the same time, it places higher expectations on people with disabilities by assuming they are capable of functioning in and contributing to society. The IL perspective sees persons with disabilities as part of the larger society, not as in debt to society for its generosity. Their disabilities make them different from persons without disabilities; however, the commonality of their humanity is far more important. Thus, persons with intellectual disabilities are able to live in society, and to participate and function with persons with and without disabilities. Blind individuals, given an accessible environment, are able to function in the same roles as persons who are sighted. Conversely, there is a societal expectation that barriers will be removed and opportunities for full participation will be provided. Traditional professional intervention rests upon the underlying assumptions of perfection and normalcy. A person with a disability takes a passive role in the process and patiently waits for the professional to use his or her expertise to "fix" the problem and make him or her "normal."

Persons with disabilities may need to rely on professionals to make decisions at times. A person with a spinal cord injury who has a urinary tract infection may need to rely on a physician to direct care and prescribe an appropriate antibiotic. However, the physician is still responsible for fully informing the person and obtaining his or her consent for treatment. Likewise, a family seeking counseling needs to rely on the counselor or therapist to employ an approach that meets the needs of the family. Yet the provider is responsible for reaching mutually acceptable agreements about the expectations of therapy.

The IL model also recognizes that people with disabilities, like all persons, are sometimes unable to make decisions in specific situations. For example, some people with intellectual disabilities may be unable to understand how to manage complex financial affairs and may need help managing their personal finances. Some people with depression may have times when depression immobilizes them and they need help from others to manage their affairs. The IL model of intervention recognizes these circumstances. However, it begins with the assumption that people with disabilities are capable (Tower, 1994). The burden of proof lies in determining when people need help rather than in proving people do not need others to direct their lives.

To achieve the overall goal of independence for persons with disabilities, IL intervention focuses on five objectives:

1. Providing consumers with information about local, regional, and national resources and establishing ways the consumer can access these resources and services
2. Facilitating attendant care for persons who need it
3. Offering peer counseling
4. Working with individuals to obtain affordable and accessible housing
5. Teaching personal and political advocacy (McAweeney, Farchheimer, & Tate, 1996)

The IL model requires that the practitioner be knowledgeable about local, regional, and national resources. The practitioner must teach the consumer about resources that are available and about how to access them (Saxton, 1983). For example, the IL model requires practitioners to be knowledgeable about local attendant care services and to teach consumers how to access these services and how to hire, fire, and manage attendants (DeJong & Wenker, 1983). The IL model assumes that counseling for persons with disabilities is provided by persons with disabilities if the service participant so chooses. Nondisabled counselors need to be aware of peer counselors in the local community and any peer support groups that may exist (Saxton, 1983). The IL model also requires practitioners to be knowledgeable about local accessible housing and services that can make existing housing accessible (Wiggins, 1983). In addition, it requires practitioners to be advocates on three levels. First, a key role is to teach persons with disabilities to be self-advocates in getting the services and resources they need. Second, practitioners teach persons with disabilities how to be politically active and can engage them in political processes. Third, the IL model expects human service practitioners themselves to become involved in advocating increased services and accessibility (Tower, 1994).

In conclusion, the IL model recognizes that the strength of the disability community, like any minority group, must ultimately come from within. Human service practitioners and other nondisabled professionals can provide services and be valued allies; however, disabled people and the disability community must have the right, responsibility, and opportunity to control their own collective destiny. In recent decades, disabled people have been effective self-advocates in promoting laws and policies that are removing barriers to participation. Ultimately, social justice commands that societies must be universally accessible for all persons, regardless of race, ethnicity, sex and gender, sexual orientation, disability, or other characteristics. Policies like reasonable accommodation have been great stepping stones for inclusion, but ultimately independent living will be achieved as universally accessible communities and societies evolve.

SUMMARY

Recent models offer alternative approaches that are particularly applicable to persons with disabilities. These include the strengths-based and empowerment approaches as well as case management and independent living models.

Practitioners using the strengths perspective focus on the capabilities and potential of individuals with whom they work. In addition, rather than concentrating exclusively on the individual, they attend to the environment. They acknowledge the influence of communities, social structures, and institutions.

The empowerment intervention model focuses on three areas: the client's strengths, the resources that exist in the client's neighborhood and community, and a belief that solutions are possible, as well as a vision of the multidimensional form of these solutions. The outcome of empowerment is client control over the social and organizational environment. The practitioner in this model has four roles: resource consultant, sensitizer, teacher/trainer, and service provider. Additional empowerment techniques include accepting the client's perception of the problem, assessing and increasing client strengths, assessing the limits and potential sources of power related to the client, and advocating for the client.

Case management emphasizes professional involvement with systems that affect clients rather than focusing primarily on micro-system interventions. The case manager, after assessment, seeks the required services for the individual. These may include housing, health and mental health care, socialization, day activities/recreation, and education. After the necessary services have been obtained, the case manager continually monitors each case to ensure that the services are maintained. Case managers must be extremely knowledgeable about the various target groups being serviced. Case managers must also balance competing goals of coordination and access with cost containment and fiscal restraint.

Within the framework of the independent living model of practice, consumers manage their own cases—their own lives. The IL model suggests that problems reside primarily within nonadaptive and hostile environments. Lack of opportunity, not lack of capability, is the primary problem for persons with disabilities as a group. The IL model is consumer driven, with individual and political advocacy at its core. It recognizes that persons with disabilities are involved in a human rights struggle.

We encourage human service practitioners to adopt a strengths-based perspective. Professionals will find competence and potential only when they actively seek them in people. We applaud the political component in empowerment-based practice. Only by looking at individuals in their larger contexts will we see the institutional and societal barriers that devalue people and limit their opportunities and be able to determine how to overcome those barriers. Case management has evolved as a mainstream human service practice method but has limitations, particularly given current social political contexts. We find that as a current practice model, the consumer-driven IL approach utilizes many of the best concepts of the three professional approaches to practice with persons with disabilities. Unlike traditional models and approaches to professional practice, the IL approach gives persons with disabilities the tools they need to live independent lives, to self-advocate, and to lead the way to the development of a just society that provides universal access for all.

DISCUSSION QUESTIONS

1. Compare and contrast the four models of practice presented in this chapter.
2. What elements of the strengths-based model particularly apply to the social model of practice with disabled persons?
3. What are the strengths of the case management approach to social service practice? What are the limitations? Given the context in which you currently practice or hope to practice in the future, what roles would be important for a case manager?
4. How do managed care and case management complement and clash with each other?
5. Using the four models presented in this chapter, formulate a model of intervention that you could use with persons with disabilities.

6. Apply the principles of universal access to a professional setting. How would the environment change if these principles were used?

SUGGESTED READINGS

DeJong, G. (1979). *The movement for independent living: Origins, ideology, and implications for disability research*. East Lansing: Michigan State University, Center for International Rehabilitation.

Mackelprang, R. W., & Salsgiver, R. O. (1996). People with disabilities and social work: Historical and contemporary issues. *Social Work, 41*(1), 7–14.

Saleebey, D. (Ed). (1992). *The strengths perspective in social work practice*. New York: Longman.

Solomon, B. B. (1976). *Black empowerment: Social work in oppressed communities*. New York: Columbia University Press.

Tower, K. D. (1994). Consumer-centered social work practice: Restoring client self-determination. *Social Work, 41*(l), 191–196.

REFERENCES

Cohen, M. B. (1994). Overcoming obstacles to forming empowerment groups: A consumer advisory board of homeless clients. *Social Work, 39*(6), 742–749.

Cowger, C. D. (1994). Assessing client strengths: Clinical assessment for client empowerment. *Social Work, 39*(3), 262–269.

DeJong, G. (1979). *The movement for independent living: Origins, ideology, and implications for disability research*. East Lansing: Michigan State University, Center for International Rehabilitation.

DeJong, G., & Wenker, T. (1983). Attendant care. In N. M. Crewe & I. K. Zola (Eds.), *Independent living for physically disabled people* (pp. 157–170). San Francisco: Jossey-Bass.

DeLoach, C. P., Wilkins, R. D., & Walker, G. W. (1983). *Independent living: Philosophy, process, and services*. Baltimore: University Park Press.

Emener, W. G. (1991). An empowerment philosophy for rehabilitation in the 20th century. *Journal of Rehabilitation, 57*(4), 7–13.

Frankel, A. J., & Gelman, S. R. (2004). *Case management*. Chicago: Lyceum Books.

Gutierrez, L. M. (1990). Working with women of color: An empowerment perspective. *Social Work, 35*(2), 149–153.

Hepworth, D. H., Rooney, R. H., Larsen, J., Rooney, G. D., & Strom-Gottfried, K. (2005). *Direct social work practice: Theory and skills* (7th ed.). Pacific Grove, CA: Brooks/Cole.

Johnson, H. W. (1995). *The social services: An introduction*. Itasca, IL: F. E. Peacock.

Johnson, P., & Mackelprang, R. W. (1995). Managed care: Balancing costs, quality and access. *SCI Psychosocial Process, 8*(4), 175–178.

Mackelprang, R. W. (1986). *Social and emotional adjustment following spinal cord injury*. Unpublished doctoral dissertation. University of Utah, Salt Lake City.

Mackelprang, R. W., & Salsgiver, R. O. (1996). People with disabilities and social work: Historical and contemporary issues. *Social Work, 41*(1), 7–14.

McAweeney, M. J., Farchheimer, M., & Tate, D. B. (1996). Identifying the unmet independent living needs of persons with spinal cord injury. *Journal of Rehabilitation, 62*(3), 29–35.

Miley, K. K., O'Melia, M., & DuBois, B. L. (1995). *Generalist social work practice: An empowering approach*. Boston: Allyn & Bacon.

Moore, S. T. (1990). A social work practice model of case management: The case management grid. *Social Work, 35*(5), 444–448.

Netting, F. E. (1992). Case management: Service or symptom. *Social Work, 37*(2), 160–164.

Neugeboren, B. (1991). *Organization, policy, and practice in the human services*. Binghamton, NY: Haworth Press.

Positive Psychology Center. (2007). *Positive psychology*. Retrieved December 10, 2007, from http://www.ppc.sas.upenn.edu/

Rhodes, R. (1993). Mental retardation and sexual expression: An historical perspective. In R. W. Mackelprang & D. Valentine (Eds.), *Sexuality and disabilities: A guide for human service practitioners* (pp. 1–27). Binghamton, NY: Haworth Press.

Rothman, J. (1991). A model of case management: Toward empirically based practice. *Social Work, 36*(4), 520–522.

Saleebey, D. (Ed.). (1992). *The strengths perspective in social work practice*. New York: Longman.

Saleebey, D. (1996). The strengths perspective in social work practice: Extensions and cautions. *Social Work, 41*(3), 296–305.

Saxton, M. (1983). Peer counseling. In N. M. Crewe & I. K. Zola (Eds.), *Independent living for physically disabled people* (pp. 171–186). San Francisco: Jossey-Bass.

Seligman, M. E. P. (2002). *Authentic happiness: Using the new positive psychology to realize your potential for lasting fulfillment*. New York: Free Press.

Solomon, B. B. (1976). *Black empowerment: Social work in oppressed communities*. New York: Columbia University Press.

Tower, K. D. (1994). Consumer-centered social work practice: Restoring client self-determination. *Social Work, 41*(1), 191–196.

Turner, F. S. (Ed.). (1986). *Social work treatment: Interlocking theoretical approaches*. New York: Free Press.

White, G. W., Gutierrez, R. T., & Seekins, T. (1996). Preventing and managing secondary conditions: A proposed role for independent living centers. *Journal of Rehabilitation, 62*(3), 14–22.

Wiggins, S. E. (1983). Specialized housing. In N. M. Crewe & I. K. Zola (Eds.), *Independent living for physically disabled people* (pp. 219–244). San Francisco: Jossey-Bass.

Zola, I. K. (1983). Developing new self-images and interdependence. In N. M. Crewe & I. K. Zola (Eds.), *Independent living for physically disabled people* (pp. 49–50). San Francisco: Jossey-Bass.

15

Practice Guidelines

If you [professionals] don't believe that disabled people can
achieve, get out of the way. [The professionals] need to learn as
much as they can to help ensure that disabled people are given
the tools we need in order to move ahead in our lives. Professionals who work with kids need to give their parents positive images
of their children's abilities and possibilities. They should not limit
people's thinking; they should help expand people's horizons.
They need to understand the implications of discrimination and
bias in order to allow people to remedy those problems. They
need to be part of the solution, not part of the problem.

—Judy Heumann, assistant secretary, Office of
Special Education and Rehabilitation Services

STUDENT LEARNING OBJECTIVE

To develop intervention skills with persons with disabilities based upon
strengths, self-management, independent living, and empowerment
approaches.

Six principles guide our approach to working with persons with disabilities.
First, we assume that people are capable or *potentially* capable (Cowger,
1994; DeJong, 1979; Gutierrez, 1990; Saleebey, 1992; Solomon, 1976; Tower,
1994; Zola, 1983). When people lack insight, knowledge, and skills, professionals are responsible for helping them become insightful, knowledgeable,
and skillful. For example, professionals may need to help people with intellectual disabilities develop knowledge and skills to manage financial matters
to the greatest extent of their ability. It is the human service professional's
responsibility to facilitate the mobilization of resources to help people
achieve their greatest potential. When people lack the ability for the whole,
we assume they are capable of parts of the whole. For example, persons
with intellectual disabilities may not be able to handle all their financial matters but should manage the elements they are capable of handling. Similarly,
people with quadriplegia may be physically unable to dress themselves;

however, they are capable of directing who provides attendant care and how and when it is provided.

We should constantly evaluate people's capacities and potential. As people develop, their capabilities grow. New capabilities should continually be assessed, nurtured, and maximized. When determining capacities, we adopt the minority view and work to reject the imposition of the dominant society's views of the capabilities of disabled persons individually and as a group (Zola, 1983). As an illustration of the minority view, one of the authors spent several years of his childhood and adolescence in an institution because the dominant culture determined he needed to be made as physically "normal" as possible. The majority decided that institutionalization, multiple surgeries, and removal from his family and community were necessary for him to function adequately and fit into society. Dominant cultural and professional values led professionals to make decisions that were inhumane and dehumanizing to a child. Like others with disabilities, the author needed adequate resources, advocates who valued persons with disabilities, and role models with disabilities. Instead, he was institutionalized, isolated, and ostracized by society. (His story is told in the case examples at the end of the chapter.)

Second, we reject traditional methods of practice that assume that the problem with disability lies with the person and that individuals with disabilities must change or be "fixed" before they can function adequately in society (Blotzer & Ruth, 1995; DeJong, 1979; Emener, 1991; Hahn, 1991; Zola, 1983). We reject the pathological interpretation of disability, along with its belief that disability requires grief and mourning, "equating disability to death" (Salsgiver, 1996, p. 18).

Third, we believe that any model of practice for working with disabled persons must assume that disability is a social construct and that a primary emphasis on intervention must be political in nature (DeJong, 1979; Fine & Asch, 1993; Tower, 1994; Zola, 1983). As a whole, persons with disabilities constitute a unique group that brings contributions and experiences that enhance society. As a minority group, they have suffered oppression just as people of color, women, gays and lesbians, and older persons have suffered oppression (Mackelprang & Salsgiver, 1996). The solutions to problems faced by persons with disabilities rest primarily in access to society's resources and rewards. Environmental, attitudinal, and policy barriers to participation in society must be eliminated.

Fourth, we believe there is a Disability history and culture. Even though different people may have different disabilities, they have more in common than they have differences. Because of the shared experience of oppression, containment, and isolation, it is imperative that anyone working with persons with disabilities be knowledgeable of the history of oppression that this group has experienced. In addition, they need to be aware of political figures, advocates, and conveyors of Disability culture and how they have contributed to the fight for respect and disability rights. Furthermore, practitioners need to be highly knowledgeable about political advocacy. They must be willing to help consumers become politically involved (Tower, 1994).

Fifth, although disabled individuals and disabled people as a group have experienced oppression, we strongly believe that there is joy to be found in disability and richness in the experience of living with disability. Models of practice for working with persons with disabilities must view "disability as different and not necessarily dysfunctional." They should "view a child with a disability as one more panel of color, which makes up the glorious tapestry of human existence" (Salsgiver, 1996, p. 23). Indeed, we believe that disability is beautiful and that most people with disabilities are actually happy with themselves and their lives (Hahn, 1993; Mackelprang & Altshuler, 2004).

Sixth, we believe that persons with disabilities have, *without question,* the right to control their lives (DeJong, 1979). This means that the consumer controls the professional's involvement. This means that the professional brings expertise to the consumer, which he or she can reject or accept, or reject in part or accept in part (DeJong, 1979; Hahn, 1991; Zola, 1983). Consumers have the right to walk or roll away from services and interventions they believe are not in their best interests. The natural place for persons with disabilities, even if professionals disagree with their choices, is in control of their own lives, living independently of custodial environments, with the same rights and opportunities as nondisabled persons.

INTEGRATING A POSITIVE DISABILITY IDENTITY

In addition to the preceding principles of practice, we believe human service practitioners must also be aware of the need for persons with disabilities to develop healthy self-identities. This changes the focus of human service practice from repairing individuals to helping people develop a healthy self-identity in a society that accepts and values them, disability and all. This process has many similarities to the process of positive identity development for sexual orientation/sexual identity minorities (Chan, 1989; Coleman, 1982; Troiden, 1993). Like sexual minorities, persons with disabilities may experience a coming out process as they integrate disability into their self-images. In our experience, positive disability identity develops differently in different people; there are no stages people must experience to reach an ultimate positive disability identity. However, human service practitioners may identify processes that are commonly experienced. The processes listed here are based on the work of Onken (Onken & Mackelprang, 1997), who applied them to persons with disabilities and to sexual orientation/sexual identity minorities. They can aid professionals in identifying consumers' experiences.

Preawareness conformity is characterized by an unquestioning acceptance of societal stereotypes and oppression. The person is unaware of alternate positive views of disability and attributes problems to personal deficits. *Contact* occurs when an individual is exposed to challenges to ableist views of disability. The individual may be oblivious to the personal implications of ableist oppression but may begin to feel different from others because of his or her disability. In the *denial or avoidance* stage, the person rejects the implications of ableism and oppression. Some may acknowledge the implications for others but deny being personally affected, some attempt to pass as nondisabled, and some distance themselves from others with disabilities and reject membership in this marginalized population. *Comparison* is a process in which the person begins to develop an awareness of the reasons for which he or she feels different. The individual develops a heightened sense of not fully belonging in ableist society and begins to recognize the disadvantages of having a disability in ableist society and the sense of disempowerment that it brings. As a result of this increased awareness, the person may begin to feel *confusion and dissonance*. There can be a growing sense of personal isolation and lack of group identity. The person may acknowledge that he or she is a member of the disability community but may be reluctant or refuse to claim membership. There may be a feeling of "I'm not like them" or "I don't want to be around them." Feelings of isolation can lead to *tolerance,* as the person begins to acknowledge membership in the disability community. The individual may seek out others with disabilities to increase socialization and avoid isolation and may experience a heightened sense of alienation in an ableist society. *Connection* occurs as an individual experiences feelings of kinship and begins to develop an identity with the community of persons with disabilities. Disability is seen in a positive light. Respect for others with disabilities grows, and a positive disability identity is enhanced. *Immersion and resistance* occur for some people, who may react in the extreme by rejecting and retreating from ableist society and maintaining nearly exclusive contact with the disability community. Persons involved in the Deaf separatist movement (as well as the lesbian separatist movement) provide examples of this process. Some find permanent happiness in this state. *Acceptance and pride* are related to immersion and resistance, but reactions are less extreme. An individual may begin to actively challenge ableist practices and beliefs, and a sense of disability pride develops. An example of this is the adoption and proud use of labels (e.g., "cripple," "gimp," "crazy") that have commonly been used to demean. *Introspection and synthesis* occur when an individual balances personal and community disability identity with other identities, memberships, and relationships. There is a renewed appreciation for diversity, a sense of the value of universally accessible multicultural societies. An individual feels comfortable with disability as a form of diversity, continues to acknowledge the societal impli-cations of living with a disability, and may feel less anger and stridence. "The person seeks to be competent in disabled-nondisabled (and/or sexual minority-sexual majority) interactions, including ongoing self-assessment, attention to the dynamics of difference, and expansion of knowledge, resources, and adaptations in order to better connect with people regardless of difference. The person is comfortable in challenging and in developing allies in challenging ableist (and/or heterosexist) practices and beliefs and corresponding oppression" (Onken & Mackelprang, 1997, pp. 25–26).

HUMAN SERVICE PRACTICE FUNCTIONS

The six pillars outlined above, combined with a disability-affirming approach, guide our practice with disabled persons and communities. They provide a foundation of empowerment with a strengths orientation that takes into account the biosocial, psychosocial, and social structural systems in which persons live. Given these pillars, effective human service practitioners must function at multiple societal system levels. We believe that effective clinical or direct practice must involve intervening at the institutional and societal levels. Similarly, administrators and community practitioners must make decisions in the interests and with the input of individuals with disabil-ities and the disability community.

In this section, we outline the four major functions of human service practitioners working with persons with disabilities: counselor, teacher, bro-ker, and political/policy activist. Within each of these practice domains, practitioners may engage in a variety of roles such as mediation, advocacy, facilitation, enabling, education, referral, and therapy.

The functions of counselor and teacher are manifested primarily at the micro- and meso-systems levels with interventions directed toward biosocial and psychosocial well-being. The function of broker spans micro, meso, and macro levels, and interventions occur in all three social-ecological domains. The function of political activist/policy activist plays out primarily in the meso and macro arenas, with interventions occurring in the social structural domain. Functions may overlap with each other; however, to be comprehen-sive, we discuss them as discrete entities. All these functions are based on a consumer-driven independent living approach. All are based on the belief that actions at one level influence other levels. In other words, personal actions and interventions are political and affect the community, and politi-cal interventions are done with individuals in mind.

The human service practitioner as counselor

The function of counselor is multifaceted and goes well beyond the tradi-tional role of clinical psychotherapist. We see Solomon's role of sensitizer

(1976), in which practitioners sensitize consumers to the oppression that persons with disabilities experience and how oppression can affect sense of self, self-esteem, and the ability to gain personal and political power, as a critical component of the counseling function for human service practitioners working with persons with disabilities. Sometimes awareness of oppression lies buried, which prevents people from developing the self-concept necessary for success defined in their terms. Sometimes the denial that allows persons with disabilities to survive and mature (Wright, 1983) also can become a hindrance when attitudinal, social, and environmental factors begin to destroy the "reality" found in the denial. In the role of counselor, the human service practitioner helps disabled persons develop an understanding of that process and understand themselves and their disability identity in a positive light (Blotzer & Ruth, 1995; Sullivan & Scanlan, 1990). Therefore, an understanding of the impact of oppression on persons with disabilities is crucial to the counseling role of human service practitioners.

Wright (1983) makes the following statement concerning people with physical disabilities, which can be applied to all persons with disabilities: "Physical limitations per se may produce suffering and frustrations, but the limitations imposed by the evaluative attitudes toward physique cut far deeper and spread far wider; they affect the person's feelings about himself as a whole. One of man's basic strivings is for acceptance by the group for being important in the lives of others, and for having others count positively in his life. As long as physical disability is linked with shame and inferiority, realistic acceptance of one's position and one's self is precluded" (p. 14).

The function of counselor requires the exploration of this domain. Sometimes counselors and consumers/participants must explore the personal effects of this negativity and stereotyping. It may be especially difficult when people explore the effects of these perceptions on how their family members, loved ones, and others perceive and treat them. For example, persons with physical disabilities whose parents subjected them to futile surgeries and other painful procedures as advised by health care providers may harbor a multitude of feelings. They may acknowledge their parents' love but harbor resentment toward them for the unnecessary pain they suffered. They may struggle to form a positive disability identity. They may also need help reestablishing and redefining relationships with family and friends. In these instances, practitioners may utilize multiple roles, such as that of the therapist to help individuals adjust to events and traumas associated with their disability, mediator of communication between disabled individuals and others, and facilitator of referrals to resources.

When disabilities are acquired later in life, counselors can help consumers in a number of ways. They can provide therapy to help individuals and loved ones cope with the adjustment and personal loss many experience. Just as importantly, they can help them understand ableist societal attitudes and help them develop new perspectives on disabilities. Peer counselors can often fill this valuable role by exposing individuals to competent, adjusted persons with disabilities who can guide them in dealing with devaluation and stereotyping.

There are a variety of other counseling roles that human service practitioners can fill. Group counselors can facilitate groups of persons with disabilities in coming together to share personal experiences and life stories. Interaction and sharing help people develop Disability identity and culture. Resource counseling is a role in which practitioners counsel consumers and teach them about community resources and how to utilize them. Family counselors can help consumers and their loved ones understand and cope with the vicissitudes of life. Educational counseling is a role in which practitioners teach participants about a variety of concerns, such as biosocial and sexual functioning.

The primary function of disability counseling is to help individuals cope with life and function within their social environments and society. Counselors can facilitate the coming out process discussed earlier in the chapter. It is critical that counseling be participant driven and that it focus on people's strengths and potential. Counseling is provided in the context of helping people understand the ableist society in which they live and how to use their strengths to chart a positive life course and to overcome oppression and reject devaluation.

The human service practitioner as teacher/consultant

A second major function in human service practice is that of teacher/consultant. The human service practitioner teaches the participant only about those areas about which the consumer seeks to learn. In other words, the teacher is a consultant rather than an educational director. Teaching by the human service practitioner covers three basic areas: (1) personal techniques for identifying capabilities and for dealing with the results of oppression, (2) self-management and self-advocacy, and (3) political advocacy. Consulting in the first two areas is similar to the counseling function. However, we place them separately because of the strong social and community emphasis involved in teaching about these areas.

Learning about strengths and capabilities and about the pernicious effects of oppression helps people eschew dependency, which creates non-assertiveness and passivity (Sussman, 1977). Passive, conforming behavior results in social isolation (Orr, Thein, & Aronson, 1995) and the inability to function successfully in employment and in the political process. The first step in helping overcome dependency and passivity is to teach the person about the societal forces imposing negative stereotypes, about incorporating disability into the definition of self, and about developing assertiveness

(Joiner, Lovett, & Goodwin, 1989). Smith's (1975) classic model of assertiveness training is still relevant for practice today. It involves teaching about the dynamics of guilt and shame and how to develop assertive verbal and behavioral skills. Assertiveness also involves self-disclosure and individual persistence in getting needs met.

The next step in teaching and consulting involves helping people modify their expectations and acknowledge and demand their rights. For example, individuals can be helped to develop personal assertiveness in a job interview by recognizing their strengths and asserting their needs. In addition, employees can convey the expectation that employers make workplaces accessible. Expectations of access expand to the community as individuals begin to expect accessible communities as a basic human right and as a societal responsibility.

The second area of teaching lies with self-management and self-advocacy. Rather than acting as a case manager, we see the role of the human service practitioner as teaching personal management skills to persons with disabilities so that they can manage their lives themselves. Based upon the IL model of practice, areas of teaching in self-management and advocacy include peer education and support, transportation, attendant care, accessible housing, and personal advocacy.

As discussed previously, the sharing of the disabled experience is crucial in the lives of persons with disabilities. There are some experiences that can only be understood within the disability community. Consumers can derive great benefit from contact with peer counselors, role models, and others with disabilities. Human service practitioners must first have knowledge of neighborhood and community resources offering peer support and of disability advocacy groups. They may need to show disabled individuals how to link with services in person, by phone, and/or electronically. Practitioners may need to make referrals and pave the way so that persons with disabilities can begin to involve themselves in the disability community.

Self-advocacy may also entail teaching a person with a disability to use public transportation. If public transportation is not available, the human service practitioner may have to help arrange alternative transportation, but the consumer must be fully involved in this process (Cole, 1983). When accessible transportation is problematic, the human service professional may need to teach the consumer how to begin the political process and facilitate pressuring local government and government transit agencies to develop accessible transportation (Bowe, 1983).

Self-advocacy is also critical in other areas. Some consumers with disabilities need attendant care. They may need to be taught how to access attendants through independent living centers, local government agencies, or private means (DeJong & Wenker, 1983). In addition, consumers may request training in how to manage personal attendants. Attendant management training includes interviewing, hiring, training, and firing attendants.

Human service practitioners must be knowledgeable about management issues and techniques in order to teach them to consumers. Consumers may need education to avoid problems such as physical abuse and the development of romantic relationships with attendants. Strategies for boundary maintenance between employee and employer can help prevent these problems.

Another important area in which many persons with disabilities request training is the acquisition of accessible housing. This means that persons with disabilities may need to modify existing housing or seek out accessible housing. The human service professional may need to be aware of or have access to existing accessible housing options. In addition, the human service practitioner may be able to help the consumer access private contractors who provide modification services (Wiggins, 1983). Just as with the issue of transportation, it may be necessary for the human service professional to help the consumer advocate the addition of accessible housing and the enforcement of existing codes and laws requiring both public housing entities and private buildings to be wheelchair accessible.

Another component of self-management is personal advocacy, which involves teaching consumers techniques for asserting their rights and acquiring the things they need or desire. Becoming a self-advocate begins with an understanding of the impact of oppression and lack of opportunity. Then consumers need to develop assertiveness skills, as discussed earlier, and to work within the agency or organization providing the services to achieve their goals. At times, self-advocacy involves going outside existing social agencies and institutions. For example, consumers may seek legal solutions or redress to force institutions to meet their needs.

In our model, the final educational role for the human service professional centers on political advocacy. The passage and implementation of disability policies discussed in chapter 5 were accomplished in large measure due to the political efforts and social activism of disabled persons and advocacy groups. Shapiro (1993) chronicles the movements controlled and directed by persons with a variety of disabilities, which resulted in a range of historic U.S. legislation, including the Rehabilitation Act of 1973 and the Americans with Disabilities Act of 1990. Subsequent efforts by disabled people and disability rights groups have produced laws and policies to enhance the lives of disabled people worldwide.

Social activism and education begins with the practitioner being knowledgeable of these various political undertakings and communicating the importance of political activity to the consumer (Tower, 1994). The next step involves helping the consumer access the local groups involved with political advocacy around disabilities. National and international disability advocacy groups have proliferated in recent decades and can be easily found on the Internet. The independent living movement has spread to multiple continents and continues to gain momentum. Practitioners can teach consumers about the political decision-making process and how to connect with local, regional, national, and international political and policy representatives. They can provide disabled persons with lists of the politicians who represent them and can help mobilize consumers to access them. Strategies ranging from cooperation to co-optation to confrontation can also be taught. Consumers can be taught skills such as how to testify before legislative bodies, interview with the media, and participate in political demonstrations. Tower (1994) states: "Consumers need good role models if they are to become more autonomous. In direct practice social workers can demonstrate good advocacy skills, teach strategies for effective communication, and coach clients through the maze of policies and procedures. They can commiserate about the inequities and absurdities that are ubiquitous to the human services. Meanwhile, they can encourage their clients to take purposeful action to improve their condition through self-advocacy and organization with peers" (p. 195).

In teaching self-advocacy, human service professionals should not be directive. However, by developing political knowledge and skills and passing them along to consumers, human service practitioners can facilitate consumer empowerment.

The human service practitioner as broker

Human service practitioners may be called upon to act as social brokers. Brokers identify and help consumers gain access to resources. It is important for human service practitioners to involve consumers in the brokering process as much as possible and to help consumers develop brokering and self-advocacy skills. Effective brokering requires human service practitioners to know which agencies within the community provide the services that disabled individuals need. Next, brokering may require practitioners to know how to utilize agency personnel and policies effectively. For example, there may be a certain administrator or supervisor in an agency or a particularly conscientious worker with whom the human service practitioner can broker to access services. Brokering requires practitioners to pass on their knowledge of how to access resources to consumers and to help them develop personal brokering skills. They can teach consumers how to make phone calls, write letters, and participate in meetings with bureaucrats. Consumers may also need to learn how to connect the services of various agencies and how to organize others with disabilities. Practitioners can strategize, advise, and support consumers as they begin to broker for themselves (Tower, 1994). Finally, practitioners can organize groups of disabled people and their allies to influence policy and practice.

Brokering and facilitating self-advocacy requires work on the micro-, meso-, and macro-systems levels as practitioners assess situations and intervene with individuals as they come in contact with larger systems and communities. Interventions at these levels require helpers to assess community strengths and limitations. Direct service practitioners must consider the impact that meso and macro systems have on people and, reciprocally, how people and groups can affect these systems. In conjunction with participants, they can plan and implement strategies to enhance the responsiveness of larger systems.

Meso- and macro-level practitioners also act as social brokers in working to help communities become more responsive to people's needs. They may act as consultants to help individuals and groups of people with disabilities learn how to affect communities. Because professionals often hold status and power, they may fill the role of advocates in working to create positive community environments. Community developers and social planners can broker disability-friendly environments as well as call policy developers within agencies and organizations. The role of mediator can also be valuable in connecting people and organizations as well as in interceding between organizations.

Human service professionals who work at all systems levels on behalf of persons with disabilities should remember that their ultimate goal is to help people self-advocate by realizing their own personal potential and by using their skills. The various roles used should be directed at helping persons take control. We can use our expertise to help people examine their problems and needs. We can advocate adequate resources and accessible communities. Ultimately, however, it is persons with disabilities who offer the strongest voice and direct the struggle for self-determination.

The human service professional as political/policy activist

Our model stresses that human service professionals work at the meso and macro levels for political change around issues relating to persons with disabilities. Political/policy activism requires practitioners to advocate for individuals and social causes. Traditionally, however, there have been conflicts of interest between professions and communities of disability. For example, large institutions that rely on the medical model of treatment have been used for centuries to warehouse persons with intellectual and mental health disabilities. As these facilities close down, human service jobs, including nursing, social work, and medical jobs, are lost, and human service professionals are forced to find different roles. Practitioners may need to acknowledge that political advocacy on behalf of disabled persons and groups can have negative effects on their traditional professional roles. We believe, however, that there is a place for the human service professions if we are proactive in working with persons with disabilities to carve out niches that focus on their strengths and their empowerment. Human service professions can join forces with consumer-directed organizations and movements. Collaboration between professional organizations and these groups increases trust and understanding and fosters consumer-professional interdependence (Condeluci, 1996). The convergence of diverse groups of persons with and without disabilities has led to the passage of civil rights laws and the implementation of disability policies worldwide. Public support for entities such as centers for independent living has grown as disabled people and the disability community have advocated for themselves in conjunction with professionals and other allies. Policy makers have listened and acted in response to the increased power shown by activists and other advocates. As the human service professions begin to welcome increasing numbers of persons with disabilities as colleagues and peers, we will be increasingly equipped to act in the roles of advocates, brokers, community planners, and policy developers.

This means that human service professionals must be taught political skills by human service educators (Tower, 1994). It means that human service professionals must become involved with local, state, and national elections by volunteering time and money. And it means that human service professionals must access politicians and policy makers to support laws, policies, and programs that empower and promote the independence of persons with disabilities.

CASE EXAMPLES

We include several case examples here to illustrate and identify major points made throughout this chapter and to help readers apply the principles used in the text.

The Author

An understanding of the impact of oppression on persons with disabilities is crucial to the counseling role of human service practitioners. The life experience of one of the authors, Richard Salsgiver, reflects the impact of devaluation and oppression, the importance of role models and the disability community, and the resilience of human beings. The author was born with cerebral palsy, was institutionalized between the ages of six and twelve, and received a master's degree in social work and a doctorate in history as an adult. He moved to California in 1984 at the age of thirty-eight. As you read his story, identify the impact that the dominant view of disability has had on his life. Take into account the decisions made concerning him during his childhood, his self-perceptions, and the process of coming out with a disability to himself and others. In addition, identify the role a counselor played in this process.

I came to California in 1984 after being a successful mental health worker in a private psychiatric/school facility in western Pennsylvania. My first job in California was as a social worker working with people with intellectual disabilities at the Golden Gate Regional Center in San Francisco. The first day on the job I met a person, herself a person with a disability, who would become a lifelong friend. When I referred to myself over lunch as "handicapped," she jumped down my throat. She informed me that the correct term was "person with a disability." I replied that it didn't really matter what I called myself. She replied that it did. She proceeded to tell me about the independent living movement, a story (which I didn't realize at the time) that would change my whole life.

In Pennsylvania, my friends and professional colleagues rarely acknowledged my disability. I never perceived myself as a person with a disability. I remember catching a glimpse in a store window of myself walking with my crutches, and being taken aback and feeling that this was not really me. I negated my need for accommodation. I bought a three-story house that sat on a bank with stairs leading up to the entrance. It had no garage. Even though it was hell getting to it in the winter, I never let my disability enter into my decision to purchase the house.

At my work, issues of accessibility were not even an afterthought. I remember going to a social work conference where I slipped and fell on the ice. The injury to my hip was so severe that I could get into my car only with great difficulty. I pulled myself in and drove home; however, I could hardly get into the house. The next day, when I took two students to the local community college to meet with the admissions counselor, I refused to acknowledge the pain in my hip or the fact that I could hardly walk with my crutches. I had to prove that I was not like the rest of them. This incident is representative of my attitude at the time, supported by my friends and colleagues, that I was not really handicapped.

In California, things began to change. I quickly became immersed in the independent living movement. I took a management position at the Center for Independent Living in Belmont, California. There I became involved not only in the practice of independent living but in politics and political advocacy on all levels. In 1986, I moved into the executive directorship of the California Association of the Physically Handicapped (now the Center for Independent Living) in Fresno, California. Here I was truly engulfed in disability. The majority of my staff were persons with disabilities. The members of my board of directors were persons with disabilities. The professionals at the state and national levels with whom I worked were mostly persons with disabilities. I began to feel resentment and anger, and I didn't know why. I began to hate to come to work and to hate dealing with my staff and board. My hatred and anger turned into depression, and I sought help. One of my staff members told me about a local social worker in private practice she had met at a party, and who seemed really good. I called him. Fortunately, the therapist understood disability and the oppression around disability. He opened up points of understanding that had been hidden in me for years. We explored my years of institutionalization and society's stereotypes of persons with disabilities. We explored the impact of the stereotypes on my family and how that influenced their treatment of me. This knowledge helped me understand my anger and resentment toward my colleagues and other persons with disabilities. That knowledge allowed me to embrace myself as a person with a disability as a positive self-loved being. It allowed me to embrace other people with disabilities as truly beautiful and whole.

In the years since I started integrating my disability into my concept of self, I have witnessed others as they have struggled with the shame and internalized ableism and sought to embrace themselves, disability and all. I have seen persons with disabilities acting as mentors, helping others integrate disability into their definition of who they are. One tremendous source of personal strength is my tie to an international disability community that is just beginning the long journey of changing how society perceives us. This community has fostered a collective disability pride and identity.

Robert and Lisa

The following is the case example of Robert and Lisa (pseudonyms), two young nursing facility residents with quadriplegia from neuromuscular disabilities who were able to leave the nursing facility in which they lived and begin living in the community. Their case, which was mentioned briefly in chapter 13, provides readers an opportunity to assess human service practices. Contrast the impacts of the social model and the medical model approaches used to identify their problems and apply intervention strategies. Had a traditional model of intervention been employed, what strategies would likely have been used to help Robert and Lisa? What was the impact of self-determination and community resources in their lives? What systems and system levels were targets for professional intervention? Identify professional functions and roles utilized. In what areas of personal advocacy and self-management did Robert and Lisa participate? Identify community resources employed to enhance their lives. Describe the relationship and power balances between professionals and consumers.

> Robert and Lisa were in their mid-twenties. Both resided in a large nursing facility with a unit devoted to young residents (under sixty years of age). Robert had come to the nursing facility to leave his small community and live in an urban area. Lisa left her parents' home because she wanted to "break away" and live "on my own." When they met in the nursing facility, they fell in love. They wanted to room together, but the nursing facility staff, with the strong concurrence of Robert and Lisa's families, refused.
>
> A social work consultant was brought in by the nursing facility with the consent of Robert and Lisa. Nursing facility staff members were concerned that Robert and Lisa were not ready for a sexual relationship, emphasizing their physical limitations. They also identified Robert as borderline mentally retarded and depressed. Lisa was diagnosed with depression and as lacking social skills. Robert and Lisa were upset that the nursing facility did not allow them freedom and self-determination.

The social worker was initially sought to provide counseling for the couple. Individual and couples counseling were provided; however, it was clear that meso-level interventions were needed. Robert and Lisa both expressed a strong desire to live in the community and become more autonomous.

At the meso level, the social worker began acting as a mediator between the couple and the nursing facility so that Robert and Lisa could spend more time together in their courtship. The social worker helped the couple articulate their needs. They were able to reach an agreement about dating outside the facility and were allowed to alter their schedules and activities inside the facility. The facility had to expend more resources to meet their demands. Robert's borderline diagnosis had been used to withhold decision-making authority from him. He now wanted to challenge this pattern. The nursing facility's corporate office used this diagnosis to stop the couple from rooming together because of concerns about liability if they became sexually active. The social worker acted as a broker by helping Robert contact a legal center that provided services to persons with disabilities. They helped Robert assert his right to self-determination by having him judged competent to handle his own affairs. The nursing facility was then forced to deal with Robert exclusively rather than relying on the wishes of Robert's parents, which sometimes conflicted with Robert's desires. This opened the door for Robert and Lisa to room together.

Robert's and Lisa's case forced the nursing facility to reassess its practices relative to unmarried persons rooming together. The social worker was instrumental as a policy developer in helping the facility develop policies that would allow for greater self-determination of its residents.

The role of community developer was critical for the social worker. Robert, Lisa, and others in similar situations were catalysts for creating non-institutional community living situations for persons with disabilities. With the involvement of several consumers, professionals, and agencies, community living resources were developed to allow people with physical disabilities to live outside institutions. Robert, Lisa, and others were anxious to let people know they were in nursing facilities not by choice or need, but because there were no resources for them to live outside nursing facilities. The social worker acted as an educator to help them make their stories known and to self-advocate. At the same time, Mona, a woman with a spinal cord injury, went public with a news story chronicling her plight of being forced to live in a nursing facility. She demonstrated that she could live in an apartment with attendant care, at much less cost to the state than living in an institution. Robert and Lisa attended a city council meeting to ask them to set aside public housing for people with needs similar to theirs. The social worker who worked with Robert and Lisa, along with other human service workers, acted as a consultant to help them determine effective strategies, but Robert and Lisa were responsible. At the request of consumers, human service workers acted as advocates to help increase access to housing, transportation, and community independent living services.

Eventually, Robert and Lisa located housing outside the nursing facility. The community housing authority provided subsidized accessible housing, and the state social services agency provided funding for personal care attendants. Lisa (and Mona) moved into individual apartments. Robert moved to a residence with three roommates with disabilities. He continued to consult a human service professional for financial planning help but controlled his personal affairs. By the time they moved out of the nursing facility, Robert and Lisa's relationship had developed platonically, and they remained friends.

Theron Sloan

The case of Theron Sloan (pseudonym) is an additional example of the use of multiple professional roles in direct service provision. Identify the roles of the direct practitioner. What was the power balance between Theron and the practitioner? What are the strengths and weaknesses of the approach used by the clinician on a systems level? What are the advantages and disadvantages of this approach for nondisabled family members of persons with disabilities? What were the circumstances that allowed Theron to use other professionals as resources? How were Theron's relationships with other professionals influenced?

Theron Sloan was a twenty-seven-year-old male with a disability from a closed head injury sustained in a motorcycle accident that occurred six months prior to his seeking help from a social worker. As a result of his head injury, Theron had left-sided weakness and was on medication for seizures. He also had short-term memory problems and would lose control emotionally under stress. He had worked, prior to his disability, as an accountant. His primary reason for seeking counseling was for help with depression. The social worker began individual counseling and worked with Theron on issues of self-esteem and reclaiming control over his life. He also began to educate Theron on strategies to help him compensate for his memory difficulties, such as keeping a log of activities and writing down his plans and activities at the beginning of each day.

Early in the relationship, the social worker realized Theron was having marital difficulties and suggested that Theron consider marriage counseling. When Theron declined, the social worker respected his wishes and did not push for marriage counseling, even though he knew marital problems were an ongoing stress. Although the social worker was not employed in an independent living center, he used an IL approach, reasoning that Theron was capable of deciding on interventions that were in his best interests.

During counseling, Theron revealed that he had been having difficulty with his physician, whom he felt was unresponsive to his needs. He was frustrated because he wanted to work again but was unable to return to his previous employer. In addition, he felt socially isolated from others. The social worker could have acted as a case manager by arranging for various services. Using an independent living counselor approach, however, he began planning with Theron to address his problems. Theron wrote out a list of his frustrations with his physician; he and the social worker then role-played a conversation with his physician about the concerns on the list. The social worker identified a vocational rehabilitation counselor with whom Theron could work. Theron called the counselor from the social worker's office, using the social worker as support. The social worker also gave Theron the names of key people in the head injury community who could act as resources. In these activities, the social worker used the roles of consultant and broker.

Theron maintained his relationship with the social worker for a period of several months. At one point, Theron disclosed that he and his wife were having sexual problems and requested help. The social worker, acting as a marital therapist, provided help for the couple's sexual problems. The social worker also referred Theron to a physician to evaluate the effects of his physical problems and medications on his sexual functioning.

A. Bruce Benet

In reviewing the case of A. Bruce Benet (pseudonym), identify elements of self-advocacy and personal empowerment. Discuss the impact of defining Bruce's personal problems in their social context. What was the value of a peer counselor in this scenario?

A. Bruce Benet had developed a malignant tumor at the base of his spine, which, when removed, left him paralyzed from the waist down. He was released from a local rehabilitation hospital and referred to a peer counselor at the local independent living center. Bruce exhibited long periods of depression with occasional outbursts of anger. At his first session, he was an hour late for his appointment. The lift on the local transit bus broke halfway into the process of loading Bruce and his wheelchair. The driver told him that all the lifts on the buses were in poor repair but the county refused to allocate money to fix them. Upon arriving at the independent living center, he was furious. He told the peer counselor (after he waited for another hour because of the counselor's next appointment) what had happened. The peer counselor suggested that he attend the local transit advisory meeting, where citizens can give input on transit issues. The peer counselor informed Bruce of the place and time of the next meeting. When Bruce expressed his intent to attend, the peer counselor told Bruce to let him know at the next session what had happened.

At the next session, Bruce was like a different person. He was neither angry nor depressed, but intense. Attending the meeting was a singular event for Bruce. He told the counselor that at the meeting there were two other wheelchair users angry about the same thing—lifts on public buses that didn't work. The county representative blew off their statements, saying that there was simply no money to fix the buses. After the meeting, Bruce got together with the other two concerned citizens at the local watering hole. They decided to form a political action group to force the county to put more resources into making public transit accessible.

The peer counselor, a wheelchair user himself, listened intently. He offered to come to the next meeting of the group to discuss different political strategies that might work. He also referred Bruce to a friend of his who worked for one of the county supervisors interested in public transit. This gave Bruce access to the formal decision-making system. As Bruce began to self-advocate, not only did he start to feel better about himself, but he was making a contribution to the larger disability community. He began to apply his understanding that his problems extended beyond himself to the social system and societal institutions.

SUMMARY

Six principles guide our approach to working with persons with disabilities. First, we assume that people are capable or potentially capable. Second, we reject traditional methods of practice that assume that the problem with disability lies with the person and that individuals with disabilities must change or be "fixed" before they can function adequately in society. Third, we believe that any model of practice applied to work with persons with disabilities must assume that disability is a social construct and that the primary emphasis on intervention must be political in nature. Fourth, we believe in an identity and culture of Disability. Fifth, although persons with disabilities experience oppression, we strongly believe that there is joy to be found in disability. Sixth, we believe that persons with disabilities must be the ones in control of their lives. This means that the consumer controls the professional.

These six principles are the pillars of our practice model. This model rests upon these pillars and upon principles of strengths-based practice and empowerment. Furthermore, we adopt a social model of disability with a consumer-driven model of practice. Our practice model proposes four fundamental functions for the human service practitioner working with persons with disabilities: counselor, teacher, broker, and political activist or advocate. Several roles are involved in these functions. The functions of counselor and teacher are used basically on the micro and meso levels. Brokers function at all three levels, whereas the role of political activist or advocate plays out in the meso and macro arenas.

DISCUSSION QUESTION

Apply the model of practice presented in this chapter to the following scenario. You are a rehabilitation social worker at a major rehabilitation hospital in the Midwest. You have been presented with the following case:

> Anthony Mares is a forty-three-year-old male with blindness as a result of a progressive degenerative eye condition. Married, with three children (ages fifteen, thirteen, and six), Anthony worked for twenty years, until recently, as an auto mechanic. His wife, Patty, forty-one, has worked as a homemaker. She has also worked part-time as a billing clerk. The Mares are buying a home in a small community that is twenty-five miles from the city in which your hospital is located. Anthony is depressed over his recent loss of sight. He exhibits a depressed affect and displays anger toward hospital staff, and his wife states he is "rejecting" her. You have been referred to the case because he is causing trouble for staff and because he needs help with discharge from the hospital, which is due to occur in three days.

How would you assess Anthony and his family using a strengths perspective? Compare how you would view working with Anthony from a traditional and a social model of intervention. What are the functions and roles you might use in working with Anthony? Discuss strategies you might use to help Anthony in empowerment.

SUGGESTED READINGS

Blotzer, M. A., & Ruth, R. (1995). *Sometimes you just want to feel like a human being: Case studies of empowering psychotherapy with people with disabilities.* Baltimore: Paul H. Brookes.

Hahn, H. (1993). Can disability be beautiful? In M. Nagler (Ed.), *Perspectives on disability: Text and readings on disability* (2nd ed., pp. 213–216). Palo Alto, CA: Health Markets Research.

Tower, K. D. (1994). Consumer-centered social work practice: Restoring client self-determination. *Social Work, 41*(1), 191–196.

Wright, B. (1983). *Physical disability—a psychological approach* (2nd ed.). New York: Harper & Row.

REFERENCES

Blotzer, M. A., & Ruth, R. (1995). *Sometimes you just want to feel like a human being: Case studies of empowering psychotherapy with people with disabilities.* Baltimore: Paul H. Brookes.

Bowe, F. (1983). Accessible transportation. In N. M. Crewe & I. K. Zola (Eds.), *Independent living for physically disabled people* (pp. 205–218). San Francisco: Jossey-Bass.

Chan, V. C. (1989). Issues of identity development among Asian American lesbians and gay men. *Journal of Counseling & Development, 68,* 16–20.

Cole, J. A. (1983). Skills training. In N. M. Crewe & I. K. Zola (Eds.), *Independent living for physically disabled people* (pp. 187–204). San Francisco: Jossey-Bass.

Coleman, E. (1982). Developmental stages of the coming out process. *Journal of Homosexuality, 7*(2/3), 31–43.

Condeluci, A. (1996). *Interdependence: The route to community* (2nd ed.). Winter Park, FL: GR Press.

Cowger, C. D. (1994). Assessing client strengths: Clinical assessment for client empowerment. *Social Work, 39*(3), 262–269.

DeJong, G. (1979). *The movement for independent living: Origins, ideology and implications for disability research.* East Lansing: Michigan State University, University Center for International Rehabilitation.

DeJong, G., & Wenker, T. (1983). Attendant care. In N. M. Crewe & I. K. Zola (Eds.), *Independent living for physically disabled people* (pp. 157–170). San Francisco: Jossey-Bass.

Emener, W. G. (1991). An empowerment philosophy for rehabilitation in the 20th century. *Journal of Rehabilitation, 57*(4), 7–13.

Fine, M., & Asch, A. (1993). Disability beyond stigma: Social interaction, discrimination, and activism. In M. Nagler (Ed.), *Perspectives on disability: Text and readings on disability* (2nd ed., pp. 61–74). Palo Alto, CA: Health Markets Research.

Gutierrez, L. M. (1990). Working with women of color: An empowerment perspective. *Social Work, 35*(2), 149–153.

Hahn, H. (1991). Alternative views on empowerment: Social services and civil rights. *Journal of Rehabilitation, 57*(4), 17–20.

Hahn, H. (1993). Can disability be beautiful? In M. Nagler (Ed.), *Perspectives on disability: Text and readings on disability* (2nd ed., pp. 213–216). Palo Alto, CA: Health Markets Research.

Hepworth, D. H., Rooney, R. H., & Larsen, J. (1997). *Direct social work practice: Theory and skills* (5th ed.). Pacific Grove, CA: Brooks/Cole.

Joiner, J. G., Lovett, P. S., & Goodwin, L. K. (1989). Positive assertion and acceptance among persons with disabilities. *Journal of Rehabilitation, 55*(3), 22–30.

Mackelprang, R. W., & Altshuler, S. (2004). A youth perspective on life with a disability. *Journal of Social Work in Disability and Rehabilitation, 3*(3), 39–52.

Mackelprang, R. W., & Salsgiver, R. O. (1996). People with disabilities and social work: Historical and contemporary issues. *Social Work, 41*(1), 7–14.

Onken, S. J., & Mackelprang, R. W. (1997). *Building on shared experiences: Teaching disability and sexual minority content and practice.* Presented at the Annual Program Meeting, Council on Social Work Education, Chicago.

Orr, E., Thein, R. D., & Aronson, E. (1995). Orthopedic disability, conformity and social support. *Journal of Psychology, 129*(2), 203–220.

Saleebey, D. (Ed.). (1992). *The strengths perspective in social work practice.* New York: Longman.

Salsgiver, R. O. (1996). Perspectives on families with children with disabilities. *SCI Psychosocial Process, 9*(1), 18–23.

Shapiro, J. P. (1993). *No pity: People with disabilities forging a new civil rights movement.* New York: Times Books.

Smith, M. J. (1975). *When I say no I feel guilty: How to cope using skills of systemic therapy.* New York: Dial Press.

Solomon, B. B. (1976). *Black empowerment: Social work in oppressed communities.* New York: Columbia University Press.

Sullivan, P. M., & Scanlan, J. M. (1990). Psychotherapy with handicapped sexually abused children. *Developmental Disabilities, 18*(2), 21–24.

Sussman, M. B. (1977). Dependent disabled and dependent poor: Similarity of conceptual issues and research needs. In S. Tubbins (Ed.), *Social and psychological aspects of disability* (pp. 247–249). Baltimore: University Park Press.

Tower, K. D. (1994). Consumer-centered social work practice: Restoring client self-determination. *Social Work, 41*(1), 191–196.

Troiden, R. R. (1993). The formation of homosexual identities. In L. D. Garnets & D. C. Kimmel (Eds.), *Psychosocial perspectives on lesbian & gay male experiences* (pp. 191–217). New York: Columbia University Press.

Wiggins, S. F. (1983). Specialized housing. In N. M. Crewe & I. K. Zola (Eds.), *Independent living for physically disabled people* (pp. 219–244). San Francisco: Jossey-Bass.

Wright, B. (1983). *Physical disability—a psychological approach* (2nd ed.). New York: Harper & Row.

Zola, I. K. (1983). Developing new self-images and interdependence. In N. M. Crewe & I. K. Zola (Eds.), *Independent living for physically disabled people* (pp. 49–59). San Francisco: Jossey-Bass.

Index

Page numbers followed by *f* refer to figures